Data Science Advancements in Pandemic and Outbreak Management

Eleana Asimakopoulou
Hellenic National Defence College, Greece

Nik Bessis
Independent Researcher, UK

A volume in the Advances in Data
Mining and Database Management
(ADMDM) Book Series

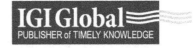

Published in the United States of America by
    IGI Global
    Engineering Science Reference (an imprint of IGI Global)
    701 E. Chocolate Avenue
    Hershey PA, USA 17033
    Tel: 717-533-8845
    Fax: 717-533-8661
    E-mail: cust@igi-global.com
    Web site: http://www.igi-global.com

Library of Congress Cataloging-in-Publication Data

Names: Asimakopoulou, Eleana, 1976- editor. | Bessis, Nik, 1967- editor.
Title: Data science advancements in pandemic and outbreak management /
  Eleana Asimakopoulou and Nik Bessis, editors.
Description: Hershey, PA : Engineering Science Reference, [2021] | Includes
  bibliographical references and index. | Summary: "This book demonstrates
  how strategies and state-of-the-art information technologies have and/or
  could be applied to serve as the vehicle to advance pandemic and
  outbreak management including revisiting and critically reviewing past
  and current approaches, identifying good and bad practices and further
  developing adaptation for future pandemics and outbreaks"-- Provided by
  publisher.
Identifiers: LCCN 2020052951 (print) | LCCN 2020052952 (ebook) | ISBN
  9781799867364 (hardcover) | ISBN 9781799867371 (paperback) | ISBN
  9781799867388 (ebook)
Subjects: LCSH: Epidemiology. | Emergency management--Information
  technology.
Classification: LCC RA648.5 .D38 2021 (print) | LCC RA648.5 (ebook) | DDC
  614.40285--dc23
LC record available at https://lccn.loc.gov/2020052951
LC ebook record available at https://lccn.loc.gov/2020052952

This book is published in the IGI Global book series Advances in Data Mining and Database Management (ADMDM) (ISSN: 2327-1981; eISSN: 2327-199X)

British Cataloguing in Publication Data
A Cataloguing in Publication record for this book is available from the British Library.

All work contributed to this book is new, previously-unpublished material.
The views expressed in this book are those of the authors, but not necessarily of the publisher.

For electronic access to this publication, please contact: eresources@igi-global.com.

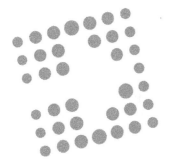

Advances in Data Mining and Database Management (ADMDM) Book Series

ISSN:2327-1981
EISSN:2327-199X

Editor-in-Chief: David Taniar, Monash University, Australia

MISSION

With the large amounts of information available to organizations in today's digital world, there is a need for continual research surrounding emerging methods and tools for collecting, analyzing, and storing data.

The **Advances in Data Mining & Database Management (ADMDM)** series aims to bring together research in information retrieval, data analysis, data warehousing, and related areas in order to become an ideal resource for those working and studying in these fields. IT professionals, software engineers, academicians and upper-level students will find titles within the ADMDM book series particularly useful for staying up-to-date on emerging research, theories, and applications in the fields of data mining and database management.

COVERAGE

- Web-based information systems
- Web Mining
- Database Testing
- Sequence analysis
- Cluster Analysis
- Enterprise Systems
- Heterogeneous and Distributed Databases
- Data Mining
- Profiling Practices
- Data Quality

IGI Global is currently accepting manuscripts for publication within this series. To submit a proposal for a volume in this series, please contact our Acquisition Editors at Acquisitions@igi-global.com or visit: http://www.igi-global.com/publish/.

Titles in this Series

For a list of additional titles in this series, please visit: *http://www.igi-global.com/book-series*

Analyzing Data Through Probabilistic Modeling in Statistics
Dariusz Jacek Jakóbczak (Koszalin University of Technology, Poland)
Engineering Science Reference • © 2021 • 331pp • H/C (ISBN: 9781799847069) • US
$225.00

Applications of Big Data in Large- and Small-Scale Systems
Sam Goundar (British University Vietnam, Vietnam) and Praveen Kumar Rayani (National
Institute of Technology, Durgapur, India)
Engineering Science Reference • © 2021 • 377pp • H/C (ISBN: 9781799866732) • US
$245.00

*Developing a Keyword Extractor and Document Classifier Emerging Research and
Opportunities*
Dimple Valayil Paul (Department of Computer Science, Dnyanprassarak Mandal's College
and Research Centre, Goa University, Goa, India)
Engineering Science Reference • © 2021 • 229pp • H/C (ISBN: 9781799837725) • US
$195.00

Intelligent Analytics With Advanced Multi-Industry Applications
Zhaohao Sun (Papua New Guinea University of Technology, Papua New Guinea)
Engineering Science Reference • © 2021 • 392pp • H/C (ISBN: 9781799849636) • US
$225.00

*Handbook of Research on Automated Feature Engineering and Advanced Applications
in Data Science*
Mrutyunjaya Panda (Utkal University, India) and Harekrishna Misra (Institute of Rural
Management, Anand, India)
Engineering Science Reference • © 2021 • 392pp • H/C (ISBN: 9781799866596) • US
$285.00

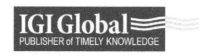

701 East Chocolate Avenue, Hershey, PA 17033, USA
Tel: 717-533-8845 x100 • Fax: 717-533-8661
E-Mail: cust@igi-global.com • www.igi-global.com

Table of Contents

Section 1
Overview of Technologies for Pandemic Management

Chapter 1
A Review of Technologies in Emergency Medicine and Sophisticated
Collective Decision-Making in the Era of the Fight Against the Pandemic 1
 Georgios Kolostoumpis, Stelar Security Technology Law Research UG,
  Germany

Chapter 2
Overview of IoT and Machine Learning for E-Healthcare in Pandemics and
Health Crises.. 16
 Mohsin Raza, Edge Hill University, UK
 Muhammad Awais, Edge Hill University, UK
 Imran Haider, Capital University of Science and Technology, Pakistan
 Muhammad Usman Hadi, University of Aalborg, Denmark
 Ehtasham Javed, University of Helsinki, Finland

Chapter 3
Data Analytics Epidemic Modelling and Human Dynamics Approaches for
Pandemic Outbreak 44
 Marcello Trovati, Edge Hill University, UK

Section 2
Data Science Practices in Pandemic Management

Section 3
Technology-Driven Challenges and Implications in Pandemic Management

Detailed Table of Contents

Section 1
Overview of Technologies for Pandemic Management

*Georgios Kolostoumpis, Stelar Security Technology Law Research UG,
Germany*

For last decade, one of the most popular ideas in healthcare services increased computational power. In this global health crisis, several new diseases have emerged in different geographical areas with pathogens including Ebola, zika, and coronavirus. The authors promise emergency technologies to prevent the concerningly rapid spread of coronavirus disease in the era on fight against pandemic. However, a digital revolution and sophisticated clinical decision tools play a key role in the support of system in public health globally. Emphasis is on an innovation introduction by various advance technologies to achieve with a various issue linked to this viral pandemic. Regardless, future research could continue to explore how different innovative technologies and support systems are helping in the fight against pandemics such as coronavirus.

Mohsin Raza, Edge Hill University, UK
Muhammad Awais, Edge Hill University, UK
Imran Haider, Capital University of Science and Technology, Pakistan
Muhammad Usman Hadi, University of Aalborg, Denmark
Ehtasham Javed, University of Helsinki, Finland

The outbreak of COVID-19 has severely affected the healthcare infrastructure. The limitations of conventional healthcare urge the use of the digital technologies to lessen the overall load on the healthcare infrastructure and assist healthcare workers/staff. This chapter focuses on digital technologies to enable smart healthcare solutions to sustain and improve health services. The chapter focuses on two main driving technologies (internet of things [IoT] and artificial intelligence [AI]), pioneering automation and digitalization of healthcare. The enabling technologies possess the potential to transform the healthcare with emergence of new and novel research directions to realize and address healthcare needs. Therefore, it is essential to focus on key driving and complementing technologies to establish multidisciplinary research solutions with cross-platform design coupled with translational learning to unlock the potentials of next generation healthcare.

Chapter 3

A pandemic is a disease that spreads across countries or continents. It affects more people and takes more lives than an epidemic. Examples are Influenza A, HIV-1, Ebola, SARS, pneumonic plague. Currently, the ongoing COVID-19 pandemic is one of the major health emergencies in decades that has affected almost every country in the world. As of 23 October 2020, it has caused an outbreak with more than 40 million confirmed cases, and more than 1 million reported deaths globally. Also, as of 23 October 2020, the reproduction number (R) and growth rate of coronavirus (COVID-19) in the UK range is 1.2-1.4. Due to the unavailability of an effective treatment (or vaccine) and insufficient evidence regarding the transmission mechanism of the epidemic, the world population is currently in a vulnerable position. This chapter explores data analytics epidemic modelling and human dynamics approaches for pandemic outbreaks.

Section 2
Data Science Practices in Pandemic Management

Chapter 4

Big data have the potential to change the way responders make sense of crisis situations, respond, and make decisions concerning the crises. At the same time, however, the explosion to the amount of crisis-related data can create an information overload to the crisis responders, and a challenge for their efficient management and utilisation. Crisis big data streams for epidemics may lack, for instance, key demographic identifiers such as age and sex, or may underrepresent certain age groups as well as residents of developing countries. Relevant metadata information needs therefore to be obtained and validated in order to trust make predictions and decisions based on the big data set. Crisis-related big data must be meaningful to the responders in order to form the basis of sound decisions. The aim of the chapter is to review all issues pertaining to the use of metadata for big data in emergency/ crisis management situations.

 Ibrahim Sabuncu, Yalova University, Turkey
 Mehmet Emin Aydin, University of the West of England, UK

Social media analytics appears as one of recently developing disciplines that helps understand public perception, reaction, and emerging developments. Particularly, pandemics are one of overwhelming phenomena that push public concerns and necessitate serious management. It turned to be a useful tool to understand the thoughts, concerns, needs, expectations of public and individuals, and supports public authorities to take measures for handling pandemics. It can also be used to predict the spread of the virus, spread parameters, and to estimate the number of cases in the future. In this chapter, recent literature on use of social media analytics in pandemic management is overviewed covering all relevant studies on various aspects of pandemic management. It also introduces social media data sources, software, and tools used in the studies, methodologies, and AI techniques including how the results of the analysis are used in pandemic management. Consequently, the chapter drives conclusions out of findings and results of relevant analysis.

 Marcello Trovati, Edge Hill University, UK
 Eleana Asimakopoulou, Hellenic National Defence College, Greece
 Nik Bessis, Independent Researcher, UK

A quick decision-making process in response and management of epidemics has been the most common approach, as accurate and relevant decisions have been demonstrated to have beneficial impacts on life preservation as well as on global and local economies. However, any disaster or epidemic is rarely represented by a set of single and linear parameters, as they often exhibit highly complex and chaotic behaviours, where interconnected unknowns rapidly evolve. As a consequence, any such decision-making approach must be computationally robust and able to process large amounts of data, whilst evaluating the potential outcomes based on specific decisions in real time.

Chapter 7

Tariq Soussan, Edge Hill University, UK

Marcello Trovati, Edge Hill University, UK

Social media platforms are widely used to share opinions, facts, and real-time general information on specific events. This chapter will focus on discussing and presenting data analytics approaches which combine a variety of techniques based on text mining, machine learning, network analysis, and mathematical modelling to assess real-time data extracted from social media and other suitable data related to pandemic outbreaks. The use of real-time insights regarding pandemic outbreaks provides a valuable tool to inform and validate existing modelling techniques and methods. Furthermore, this would also support the discovering process of actionable information to facilitate the decision-making process by enhancing the most informed and appropriate decision, based on the available data. The chapter will also focus on the visualisation and usability of the insight identified during the process to address a non-technical audience.

Chapter 8

Isa Inuwa-Dutse, University of St Andrews, UK

Conventional preventive measures during pandemics include social distancing and lockdown. Such measures in the time of social media brought about a new set of challenges – vulnerability to the toxic impact of online misinformation is high. A case in point is COVID-19. As the virus propagates, so does the associated misinformation and fake news about it leading to an infodemic. Since the outbreak, there has been a surge of studies investigating various aspects of the pandemic. Of interest to this chapter are studies centering on datasets from online social media platforms where the bulk of the public discourse happens. The main goal is to support the fight against negative infodemic by (1) contributing a diverse set of curated relevant datasets; (2) offering relevant areas to study using the datasets; and (3) demonstrating how relevant datasets, strategies, and state-of-the-art IT tools can be leveraged in managing the pandemic.

Section 3
Technology-Driven Challenges and Implications in Pandemic Management

Chapter 9

    Iman Hussain, University of Wolverhampton, UK
    Chloë Allen-Ede, University of Wolverhampton, UK
    Lukas Jaks, University of Wolverhampton, UK
    Herbert Daly, University of Wolverhampton, UK

A pandemic crisis inevitably puts great pressure on different aspects of societal and commercial infrastructure. Paths for information and goods designed and optimised for stable conditions may fail to meet the needs of emergency situations, whether suddenly imposed or planned. This chapter discusses the effects of the 2020 pandemic on food supply chains. These issues are considered as problems of information sharing and systemic behaviour with implications for both people and technology. Based on work in Wolverhampton, UK, the effect of the 2020 lockdown period on local businesses and charities is considered. In response to these observations, the design and development of Lupe, a prototype application to support the distribution and trading of food during periods of lockdown, is described. The aim of the system is to integrate the needs of consumers, businesses, and third sector organisations. The use of blockchain technology in the Lupe system to provide appropriate functionality and security for data is explored. Initial evaluations of the prototype by stakeholders are also included.

Chapter 10

    Thu Yein Win, University of Gloucestershire, UK
    Hugo Tianfield, Glasgow Caledonian University, UK

The recent COVID-19 pandemic has presented a significant challenge for health organisations around the world in providing treatment and ensuring public health safety. While this has highlighted the importance of data sharing amongst them, it has also highlighted the importance of ensuring patient data privacy in doing so. This chapter explores the different techniques which facilitate this, along with their overall implementations. It first provides an overview of pandemic monitoring and the privacy implications associated with it. It then explores the different privacy-preserving approaches that have been used in existing research. It also explores the strengths as well as their limitations, along with possible areas for future research.

Chapter 11

Guru K., SRM Valliammai Engineering College, India
Umadevi A., SRM Valliammai Engineering College, India

The World Health Organization (WHO) declared COVID-19, an infectious disease caused by the virus SARS-CoV-2, as a pandemic in March 2020. More than 2.8 million people tested positive at the time of publication. Infections are exponentially increasing, and immense attempts are being made to tackle the epidemic. In this chapter, the authors aim to systematize data science works and evaluate the fast-growing community of recent studies. They also analyze public datasets and repositories that can be used to map COVID-19 dissemination and mitigation strategies. As part of that, they suggest a library review of the papers produced in this short period of time. Finally, they emphasize typical issues and pitfalls found in the surveyed works on the basis of these observations. Data science, narrowly established, will play a critical role in the global COVID-19 pandemic response. This chapter addresses the implications of data science for policymakers and strategists and allows them to resolve the threats, possibilities, and pitfalls inherent in using data science for tackling the COVID-19 pandemic.

Preface

Pandemics are disruptive, they cause crisis yet they occur every now and then. According to the UN the coronavirus COVID-19 pandemic is the defining global health crisis of our time and the greatest challenge we have faced since World War Two. Within the first three months, the spread of the virus around the world and in particular, in more than 196 countries, challenged public and private health systems and governments worldwide, leading the World Health Organization (WHO) to declare a global pandemic. The director-general of WHO when referring to COVID-19 referred to that this is not just a public health crisis alone but it is a crisis that will touch every sector. During the last two decades society had suffered by epidemic outbreaks, including the SARS in 2003 and the H1N1 in 2009. Pandemic is not a term to use lightly or carelessly and, if misused, can cause unreasonable fear, or unjustified acceptance that the challenge is over, potentially leading to unnecessary suffering and loss. However, humans are not always capable of avoiding the risks and consequences of such situations. Thus, there is a need to prepare and plan in advance actions in identifying, assessing and responding to such events in order to manage uncertainty and support sustainable livelihood and wellbeing. A detailed assessment of a continuously evolving situation needs to take place and several aspects have to be brought together and examined before the declaration of a pandemic.

Various health organisations, crisis management bodies and authorities at local, national and international levels are involved in the management of pandemics. There is no better time to revisit current approaches in order to advance the disciplines and cope with these new and unforeseen threats. As countries must strike a fine balance between protecting health, minimizing economic and social disruption and respecting human rights, there has been an emerging interest in lessons learnt and specifically in revisiting past and current pandemic approaches. Such approaches involve the strategies and practices from several disciplines and fields, to name a few, healthcare, management, IT, mathematical modelling and data science. Reviewing these approaches as a means to advance in-situ practices and prompt future directions could alleviate or even prevent human, financial and environmental compromise, loss and social interruption via state-of-the-art technologies and frameworks. According to the UN, humanity needs leadership and solidarity to defeat pandemics. Leadership without science cannot support such issues in their full potential and therefore the scope of this book is to bring these aspects together.

THE PURPOSE OF THE BOOK

The primary goal of the book is to demonstrate how strategies and state-of-the-art IT have and/or could be applied to serve as the vehicle to advance pandemic and outbreak management. The achievement of such a goal implies the contribution of various practitioners, scholars in the area and researchers from many disciplines who are willing to offer their expertise and skills in advancing their discipline both as a theory and practice. The book also aims to provide conceptual and practical guidance to relevant stakeholders including managers of relevant organizations. It helps assist in identifying and developing effective and efficient approaches, mechanisms, and systems using emerging technologies to support their effective operation.

The overall mission of the book is to introduce both technical and non-technical details of management strategies and advanced IT, data science and mathematical modelling and demonstrate their application and their potential utilization within the identification and management of pandemics and outbreaks. It also prompts revisiting and critically reviewing past and current approaches, identifying good and bad practices and further developing the area for future adaptation. The book has collected vast experience of many leaders and as such, is a definitive state-of-the-art collection suggesting future directions for healthcare stakeholders, decision makers and crisis management officials in identifying applicable theories and practices in order to mitigate, prepare for, respond to and recover from future pandemics and outbreaks.

WHO SHOULD READ THE BOOK

The projected audience is broad, ranging from those currently working in or those who are interested in joining interdisciplinary, multidisciplinary and transdisciplinary collaborative management of pandemics and outbreaks. Specifically, audiences who are: (1) researchers and practitioners in the areas of pandemic and outbreak detection and management; pandemic assessment; contingency planning and business continuity; emerging technologies and advanced IT; artificial intelligence, data science and mathematical modelling; big data and data management; smart systems, cyber-physical systems and industry 4.0; (2) managers and decision makers in the central and local authorities, research institutes and scientific centers and the industry; (3) academics, instructors, researchers and students in colleges and universities

ORGANIZATION OF THE BOOK

Eleven self-contained chapters, each authored by experts in the field, are included in this book. The book is organized into three sections according to the thematic topic of each chapter. Thus, it is quite possible that a paper in one section may also address issues covered in other sections. However, the following three sections reflect most of the topics sought in the initial call for chapters. These are:

Section 1: Overview of Technologies for Pandemic Management includes three chapters.
Section 2: Data Science Practices in Pandemic Management includes five chapters.
Section 3: Technology-Driven Challenges and Implications in Pandemic Management includes three chapters.

A brief introduction to each of the chapters follows.

In Chapter 1, "A Review of a Technologies in Emergency Medicine: Sophisticated Collective Decision-Making in Era on Fight Against Pandemic," G. Kolostoumpis presents how digital revolution and sophisticated clinical decision tools play a key role in the support of system in public health globally. It also discusses how different types of innovative technologies and support systems are helping in era on fight against pandemic such as corona virus.

In Chapter 2, "Overview of IoT and Machine Learning for E-Healthcare in Pandemics and Health Crises," Raza et al, presents the limitations of conventional healthcare urging the use of the digital technologies to lessen the overall load on the healthcare infrastructure and assist healthcare workers/staff. It focuses on digital technologies to enable smart healthcare solutions to sustain and improve health services. Two main driving technologies (Internet of Things (IoT) and Artificial Intelligence (AI)), pioneering automation and digitalization of healthcare are discussed.

In Chapter 3, "Data Analytics Epidemic Modelling and Human Dynamics Approaches for Pandemic Outbreak," M. Trovati describes the key features of epidemic spread. This chapter presents a review of data analytics epidemic modelling and human dynamics approaches for pandemic outbreaks.

In Chapter 4, "The Importance of Big Data Metadata in Crisis Management," B. Karakostas highlights that the explosion to the amount of crisis related data can create an information overload to the crisis responders and a challenge for their efficient management and utilisation. To this end the aim of the chapter is to review all issues pertaining to the use of metadata for Big Data in emergency/crisis management situations.

In Chapter 5, "Pandemic Management With Social Media Analytics," I. Sabuncu and M. E. Aydin focus on the social media analytics that appears to be a useful tool to understand the thoughts, concerns, needs, expectations of public and individuals, and supports public authorities to take measures for handling pandemics. It also introduces social media data sources, software and tools used in the studies, methodologies and AI techniques including how the results of the analysis are used in pandemic management.

In Chapter 6, "Deep Learning Approaches in Pandemic and Disaster Management," M. Trovati, E. Asimakopoulou, and N. Bessis present that a computationally decision-making approach must be able to process large amounts of data - which is rarely represented by a set of single and linear parameters- in order to manage the dynamic nature of a disaster or epidemic.

In Chapter 7, "Information Extraction From Social Media for Epidemic Models," T. Soussan and M. Trovati focus on discussing and presenting data analytics approaches which combine a variety of techniques based on text mining, machine learning, network analysis, and mathematical modelling to assess real-time data extracted from social media and other suitable data related to pandemic outbreaks. The chapter also focusses on the visualisation and usability of the insight identified during the process to address a non-technical audience.

In Chapter 8, "Towards Combating Pandemic-Related Misinformation in Social Media," I. Inuwa-Dutse presents studies centering on datasets from online social media platforms where the bulk of the public discourse happen. Its main goal is to support the fight against negative infodemic by contributing a diverse set of curated relevant datasets; offering relevant areas to study using the datasets; and by demonstrating how relevant datasets, strategies and state-of-the-art IT tools can be leveraged in managing the pandemic.

In Chapter 9, "Ensuring Food Supply and Security During Localised Lockdowns: An Information and Technology-Based Approach," I. Hussain, C. Allen-Ede, L. Jaks, and H. Daly discuss the effects of the 2020 pandemic on food supply chains and highlights the challenges and implications for both people and technology. A prototype application to support the distribution and trading of foods during periods of lockdown is described. The aim of the system is to integrate the needs of consumers, businesses and third sector organisations. The use of blockchain technology has been explored.

In Chapter 10, "Privacy-Preserving Pandemic Monitoring: A Survey," T. Y. Win and H. Tianfield highlight the importance of ensuring patient data privacy in pandemic management. This chapter provides an overview of pandemic monitoring and the privacy implications associated with it. It then explores the different privacy-preserving approaches that have been used in existing research. It also explores the strengths as well as their limitations, along with possible areas for future research.

In Chapter 11, "Strategies for Upskilling in Data Science After COVID-19 Pandemic," G. K. and A. Umadevi analyse public datasets and repositories that can be used to map COVID-19 dissemination and mitigation strategies. As part of that, we suggest a library review of the papers produced in this short period of time. This chapter addresses the implications of data science for policymakers and strategists and allows them to resolve the threats, possibilities, and pitfalls inherent in using data science for tackling the COVID-19 pandemic.

Acknowledgment

It is our great pleasure to comment on the hard work and support of many people who have been involved in the development of this book. It is always a major undertaking but most importantly, a great encouragement and somehow a reward and an honor when seeing the enthusiasm and eagerness of people willing to advance their discipline by taking the commitment to share their experiences, ideas and visions towards the evolvement of a collaboration like the achievement of this book. Without their support the book could not have been satisfactory completed.

We wish to thank all the authors who, as distinguished scientists despite busy schedules, devoted so much of their time preparing and writing their chapters.

We are deeply indebted to our family for their love, patience and support throughout this rewarding experience.

Eleana Asimakopoulou
Hellenic National Defence College, Greece

Nik Bessis
Independent Researcher, UK

Section 1
Overview of Technologies for Pandemic Management

Chapter 1

A Review of Technologies in Emergency Medicine and Sophisticated Collective Decision-Making in the Era of the Fight Against the Pandemic

Georgios Kolostoumpis
https://orcid.org/0000-0001-9768-9526
Stelar Security Technology Law Research UG, Germany

ABSTRACT

For last decade, one of the most popular ideas in healthcare services increased computational power. In this global health crisis, several new diseases have emerged in different geographical areas with pathogens including Ebola, zika, and coronavirus. The authors promise emergency technologies to prevent the concerningly rapid spread of coronavirus disease in the era on fight against pandemic. However, a digital revolution and sophisticated clinical decision tools play a key role in the support of system in public health globally. Emphasis is on an innovation introduction by various advance technologies to achieve with a various issue linked to this viral pandemic. Regardless, future research could continue to explore how different innovative technologies and support systems are helping in the fight against pandemics such as coronavirus.

DOI: 10.4018/978-1-7998-6736-4.ch001

INTRODUCTION

Recently, a new type of viral infection emerged in China suggesting a novel coronavirus disease 2019 (COVID-19) and it has widely spread worldwide in the early months of 2020. The relating to the observation and treatment of actual patients rather than theoretical or laboratory studies severity, rapid transmission, and human losses due to coronavirus disease have led the World Health Organization to declare it a pandemic. During pandemic outbreaks, short - quick data sharing is critical as it allows for a better understanding of the origins and spread of the infection and can deliver as a basis for effective prevention, treatment, and care. A high volume of patients demanding care, treatment to balance it healthcare systems globally. There are increasing appeals on March 11, 2020, as the WHO announced the explosion of beginning of a current situation during pandemic. Looking forward, to our attempts could prove quite beneficial to the literature is the idea that requires modern technologies like Artificial Intelligence, Internet of Things, Big Data, Internet of Medical Things, Machine learning methods and sophisticated clinical decision – making tools in the support of system in public health globally, as a highlighting significant results and achievements by authors (Schurink, C. A. M., Lucas, P. J. F., Hoepelman, I. M., & Bonten, M. J. M., 2005). Thus, navigating a path out of the pandemic crisis through appropriate decisions requires careful consideration of the information, technology available.

Reviewing subsequent and more recent literature by authors (Davenport, T., & Kalakota, R., 2019), to address this global novel pandemic, World Health Organization, scientists, and physicians in medical industry are searching for new innovative technology to screen infected patients in a various stages, find the best clinical trials, by manage of the virus, trace contract of the infected citizen. Latest, scientifically international finding identified that artificial intelligence techniques could be the key in every aspect of the COVID-19 crisis response to finding high-quality predictive models that are promising engaged by various public health stakeholders as they result in a better scale-up, reliable and reach human in specific daily clinical tasks.

A DIGITAL COMMUNICATION DURING THE CRISIS OF PANDEMIC

In walking on an exciting decade in Health and Science with the development and maturation of several digital technologies it could be applied to tackle major health issues and diseases. Moreover, other solutions like next generation technologies such as Big Data, Artificial Intelligence, Blockchain Technology, Internet of Things, and next generation of telecommunication like 5G, may be used for fight against coronavirus as we explore the huge potential to augmenting strategies for tackling pandemic:

1. Prevention, detection, surveillance, monitoring of a pandemic situation
2. Mitigation of impact to pandemic

Mentioning positive aspects of others' authors work as (Alsafi, Z., Abbas, A. R., Hassan, A., & Ali, M. A., 2020), summarize, the importance of communication, during the pandemic it is a critical step with a potential role is our communication between healthcare systems (i.e., health workers, physicians, scientists, etc), government bodies, public and local authorities must be clear, collaborative, and real – time according with above technology we have on our hands. Due to the fact a multiple - social media platforms, are on the way to protect an appropriate risk communication for an ongoing flexibility media presence could be provide a real-time update on the actual number of citizen to receive accurate information about coronavirus and government initiatives. As defined by the *World Health Organization[1]*, is "the exchange of real-time information, advise and opinion between physicians, scientists, citizens threats to their social-economic well-being".

Digital technologies and decision – making tools during the ongoing COVID-19 response is crucial for a coordinated response to public health systems globally. It is critical to note that public health systems globally focuses on increasing the efficiency and effectiveness of a high-level response measurements and activities before, during, and after a public health event to ensure optimal response decision-making and strategy. Hence, the focus of tackling the direct impact of current situation with COVID-19, in many healthcare settings, it is crucial to maintain core and critical healthcare service. The initial re-action in many countries should be planning to communicate via "*virtual technology*", that could be set up through the use of tele-monitoring, clinical consultations via peripheral sites which can be interpreted remotely by physicians. Although, the citizens continue to receive standard health care and communication while reducing physical crowding of patients into clinics, hospitals premises. Outlining, as the key medical activities such as research, education, experiments can be performed via virtual e-learning platforms which are increasingly being exploitation to eliminate physical face – to – face meetings.

In the first wave of pandemic crisis, several authors have attempted (Singh, R. P., Javaid, M., Haleem, A., & Suman, R., 2020), to explain us how a complex medical centre contribute with a different way during the period of pandemic using Internet of Things methodologies that allows in medical staff offering a daily clinical function, for the patients. Most of these services interconnected with various devices such as smart patient bed, scanning instruments, biosensors, wearable devices, etc. which are able to detect, and attack with easy rapid measurement of molecules in body fluids such as heart rate, blood pressure, etc. for diagnosis, treatment, and monitoring purposes. In the meantime, the daily administrative tasks are possible achieved through its use of various electronic tools in hospital management, by way of:

1.   Managing the inventory;
2.   Management the assets such as capital value instruments and implants;
3.   Identifying daily issues in hospital via improving the administrative of patient's flow using cloud computing, access to applications and resources services to provide easy, productivity and efficiency to a healthcare worker, scientists.

In fact, the use of a global research database by WHO, we are gathering the update international multilingual scientific findings and knowledge on COVID-19. Therefore, big data gradually provides an innovative progress of our current technology which can take the opportunity for performing computationally analysis to reveal trends, clinical studies on a large amount of data about the virus, pandemic, and measures to fight against COVID-19 and its after – effects. It remains, a big challenging for tractable models that yield fast answers given at the large uncertainty facts, figures, data, during an emergency, and because efficiently models are more easily explained, communicated, and use the evidence to have outbreaks as effectively possible.

BLOCKCHAIN TECHNOLOGY TO ADDRESS THE CRISIS DURING THE COVID-19 PANDEMIC

As a foundational technology that promises to provide new solutions to old problems, blockchain technology is increasingly being applied in innovative ways that are significant to the challenges created by the latest updates for COVID-19. As a further matter, author (Mettler, M., 2016), mentions that a Blockchain has shown the quality of being able to adjust to a new condition, in a latest year leading to its in-corporation focus on a range of applications including also on a healthcare system. The current pandemic crisis has highlighted the potential of blockchain technology, as a unique opportunity to test and adopt more open transparent, patient-focused, and robust system of information management that may significantly contribute more effectively to the fight against the pandemic and emergency technology in near future.

As demonstrated, a few researchers like (Li, J., & Guo, X. 2020), have addressed the issue, from the beginning of current pandemic, it should be noted that every day, a new set of baffled data are reported concerning the number of positive and negative covid-19 tests, patients hospitalized, hospital beds in covid-19 clinics are occupied, ventilator shortfalls, deaths, etc. These numbers allow the officials and public to track the progress of disease to avoid infection in a real time and as they become available, making it a data-driven pandemic.

Showing cause and effect authors, (Fusco, A., Dicuonzo, G., Dell'Atti, V., & Tatullo, M., 2020), presents evidence that blockchain technology, could assist combat the pandemic as scientists, engineers, researchers from different fields has been increasingly applied to healthcare management, as a strategic tool to strengthen operative protocols and to create, manage, the proper basis for an efficient and effective evidence-based decisional process.

Several studies globally have presented according with authors surveys (Bodas, M., & Peleg, K., 2020), blockchain applications, provide the assistance to promptly trace persons who have been exposed to an infected person as an advantage to promote and protect public health that can be limit the continuing spread of the infection. Therefore, blockchain technologies are enable privacy preserving for each person to share only personal data, information without sharing other medical data in a secure environment with governmental health organizations without revealing their identity or contributing that information to centralized corporate database may assist to identify other citizen who come into contact with a people who has tested positive for coronavirus.

Scientists globally are dealing with a difficult situation for the development of vaccines, preventing the spread of infection and quick identification of viral carries since coronavirus is extremely contagious. Indeed, one of the most prominent fact blockchain potential use cases on a digital health and remote patient monitoring according with a satisfy different requirements, such as data sharing, security, and data access.

Meanwhile, authors (Marbouh, D., Abbasi, T., Maasmi, F., Omar, I. A., Debe, M. S., Salah, K., & Ellahham, S., 2020), presented consequently with other critical examples should also include the healthcare Internet of Things concept where patient has the digital health monitored by a smart devices like trace the patients as holds a full access authorization of their data in terms of, they can choose whom they would like that block to be shared with in the healthcare network. Patient can choose even to share the information for a time limit also for validation purposes.

For example, lots of new insurance policies may just need to do some verifications and the access to patient data can be provided to the insurance company for that time. With the smart devices if the patient has established an emergency alerting to the hospital or general practice, the doctor or the practice can get alerted with the situation. This can be lifesaving and less time-consuming process with legacy. A significant, a key role in a near future how digital healthcare specifically, it may to use and improve blockchain technology for Coronavirus disease 2019, safe in a clinical practice. Moreover, adopting blockchain technology and public ledgers maximizes cost savings by take-away intermediaries that handle manual transactions.

In the same way a blockchain tracking system for validating the pandemic data from diverse sources to mitigate the spread of falsified or modified data. solution promotes trust, transparency, traceability and streamlines the communication between physicians and engineers in the global pandemic network. According with latest updates of current pandemic crisis we believe Blockchain technology have the potential as an innovative ways that fight against of current and each pandemic crisis in the near future.

APPROACHES BASED ON ARTIFICIAL INTELLIGENCE FOR CONTROL AND PREVENT THE SPREAD OF CORONAVIRUS

In the era of Big Data, Artificial Intelligence and medicine offer a cutting-edge algorithms, application of information science to define disease, medicine, therapeutics and identifying targets with the minimum error. Public Health Organisations requiring immediate action for decision-making technologies to control this virus and assist them in getting proper suggestions in a real – time to avoid its spread. To address the Coronavirus disease 2019, resource allocation problem, it is necessary to understand complex data, un-structured clinical information related to the prioritization criteria and resources in question.

Artificial Intelligence will play an important role in understanding, suggesting, screening, analysing, spreading, predicting, and tracking of current patients where this virus will affect in future by collecting and analysing all previous data. Indicating that AI can also be present as an important assistant to detect, diagnose and prevent the spread of the virus. By introducing AI algorithms that identify patterns and irregularities are already working to predict and detect the spread of virus, while image recognition systems are to go faster for a medical diagnosis. In the meantime, authors, (Bullock, J., Luccioni, A., Pham, K. H., Lam, C. S. N., & Luengo-Oroz, M., 2020) investigated further evidence as they identified similarities and differences in the evolution of the pandemic across countries and regions using AI tools investigate the scale and spread of the "infodemic" with the purpose of the action of widely spreading of misinformation and disinformation, as well as the emergence of hate speech. Moreover, scientists from different fields are examine the spread of misinformation *"which they identify using external fact-checking organizations"* and find that information from both reliable and less-reliable sources propagates in similar patterns, but that user engagement with posts from the latter is lower across major social media streams. In a nutshell, AI can contribute to the fight against pandemic by maximized safety during the period of pandemic. Expressing opinions and probabilities authors (Hollander, J. E., & Carr, B. G., 2020), provide us a lot of studies regarding the current pandemic creates a vital challenges.

There is still considerable point for AI can assist a limited healthcare workers, to delivery fast and reliable healthcare services using latest machinery and equipment developed from the application of scientific knowledge. We have now seen how heavy loaded the daily processes in health sector using the smartphone app which can collects in a real-time from patients' symptoms, signs, travel locations, history data, using a variety of algorithms only for suspected cases are examined by medical staff. In the current case of corona virus, lots of algorithms by AI can be process large amounts of an un-structured various text data and can predict the arithmetic values for more than one cases by area and which types of populations will be most at high – risk, as well as to evaluate strategies for preventing and controlling the spread of the epidemic. The involvement of AI application can quickly analyse of any symptoms and thus alarm the patients and the healthcare authorities has led authors such as (Xie, X., Zhong, Z., Zhao, W., Zheng, C., Wang, F., & Liu, J., 2020), analysed case studies and the contribution in the literature review. In the sufficiently great steps of covid-19 treatment by the state of being precise and reduces complexity and time taken, as the medical staff specialized with corona virus disease not only focused on the medical care of the patient, but also identifies the high-risk patients, and control this infection in a real-time.

During the first waves of pandemic authors (Mahrouf, M., Lotfi, E. M., Maziane, M., Hattaf, K., & Yousfi, N., 2017), remarkably, have been extending the usage of traditional mathematical modeling for infections and viruses may assist simplify the process of understanding virus dynamics. Simulate and model different scenarios using differential equations in virology and epidemiology to may impair or prevent with the action of widely spreading the virus.

This confirms substantiates previous findings in the literature, having been reported a traditional mathematical modelling of the dynamics and containment of COVID-19 with various ways in use by authors (Car, Z., Baressi Šegota, S., Anđelić, N., Lorencin, I., & Mrzljak, V., 2020), wishing to test the possibility of modeling using comparatively methods, for the extremely important in the prediction of their impact with standard modeling that can be provide satisfactory models with comprehend the intricacies contained within the data. We will appreciate an Artificial Neural Network training models how relevant and fast can be achieved a model which including a maximal number of recovered and infected patients across all countries in each time unit. There is a considerable a vast amount of literature on with this in mind AI and computational methods have emerged as very vital tools that can complement experimental techniques with the use of traditional mathematical modeling as mentioned above. In numerous areas in biomedical field AI can help bridge information gaps among experiments through reporting in different temporal and spatial domains in addition to their considerable predictive models and powers.

Scientists and physicians are working so close with AI applications and machine learning techniques to provide faster decision-making, which at this stage is cost-effective tools with a valuable assistance of imaging technologies like CT scan, MRI, and X-ray with efficiency active role in the enemy of coronavirus disease. As AI methods and X-ray collaborate can be used in parallel for accurate detection of virus and can likewise be find a quick answer and explanation providing precise treatment in a small medical teams. Based on AI an intelligent platform can extract the visual features of this disease, and this would assist in regarded to be monitoring and treatment of the influence for a particular person as mentioned by authors (Haleem, A., Vaishya, R., Javaid, M., & Khan, I. H., 2020). It has the ability of make adequate preparation for patients updated day-to-day and provide solutions by physicians to be followed during the treatment. Artificial Intelligence is a forthcoming and powerful tool to indicate who or what is at early infections due to coronavirus and also make it easier in monitoring the situation in life of a particular group of the infected patients.

In particular, artificial neural networks are a crucial importance role at this stage provide us assistance for a drug studies by analysing the current data and each case for disease. Outlining the possible future, AI-based approaches could mitigate the Covid-19 pandemic and similar upcoming infectious disease threats by practical purpose for delivery, design, and development providing a faithful representation of a drug for disease.

Understanding the moving parts of Artificial intelligence, we like to think of clinical process, as the overarching concept that encompasses AI to assist scientists for development drug and therapies for fight the current pandemic disease. At the first step to identify and clearly understand the needs of coronavirus disease and then analysing the available data that will be useful for drug delivery design and development. Mentioning positive aspects of others' work (Chan, H. S., Shan, H., Dahoun, T., Vogel, H., & Yuan, S., 2019), formulating, innovative techniques based on the recommendations of a long clinical process for drug discovery are:

1. Target selection and validation;
2. Compound screening and lead optimization;
3. Preclinical studies; and
4. Clinical trials.

At latest years, many impressive Artificial Intelligence methods and tools have been developed that can make the above processes more cost-efficient in a real-time image based on standards to automated and optimized to substantially speed up the drug discovery process. The bottom line is that we are faced the workload of healthcare workers due to a sudden and massive increased in the numbers of patients during pandemic. As we mentioned earlier, the role of Artificial Intelligence is used to reduce the workload of physicians, engineers, scientists, in the early stages of diagnosis providing treatment, monitoring using all the digital technologies bring nearer decision-making efforts, offers the best training to healthcare workers.

We have repeatedly seen examples, as mentioned authors (Vaishya, R., Javaid, M., Khan, I. H., & Haleem, A., 2020), that real – time data analysis of Artificial Intelligence can impact in the near future patient care and think, for showing the capacity to develop new guidelines, instructions, in the future. Actually, we will obtain the skills needed which can reduce the workload daily in hospitals, medical centers and healthcare works.

INTERNET OF THINGS (IoT) USED IN REFERENCE TO A DAILY TASK FOR FIGHT PANDEMIC

Honestly, as we discussed in the beginning of our chapter, the Internet of Things (IoT) is an indispensable component of the system, including all the network elements like as: software and hardware components, connectivity of the network and any additional electronic or computer devices, by supporting in data interaction and collection. Thus, if we divide corona virus on the medical and diagnostic devices in health centres or hospitals into things and modulate these things to be sufficiently intelligent to operate on their own, we can establish a behaviour for every subsystem. The challenge is to understand each thing separately. We thus, to understand the behaviour of things used to help control coronavirus, it is necessary to understand the main subcomponents of each thing; then, we must understand the behaviour of each subsystem to understand the behaviour of the thing as a whole and how to enable it to connect and communicate with other things via the internet.

A crucial challenge for the advancement of digital health is efficient and effective integration of incomplete or heterogeneous information about coronavirus disease from different sources and different types, such as interoperability solutions, insufficient availability, and existence of current information silos. All this contradicting information is hindering the development of effective applications. Different information types must be integrated, such as clinical information (including EHRs), information extracted from the biomedical literature by text mining, and high-throughput information on how drugs or chemicals interact in different circumstances.

In the same way authors (Haleem, A., Javaid, M., & Khan, I. H.., 2020), mentioned that Internet of things are still looking for a cost-effective and practical solutions in a typical daily functioning without having any human involvement at any level. It handles all cases smartly to provide ultimately strengthened service to the patient and healthcare. IoT seems to be an excellent way to screen the infected patient. In healthcare, this technology is ready to give assistance to maintain quality supervision with real-time information. With an appropriate implementation of this technology, scientists, physicians, government, healthcare workers can create a better healthcare environment to fight with coronavirus disease.

An alternative approach to be grateful for remote sessions, such as telecare, telemonitoring, as has also become feasible with various tools, techniques, and concepts via Internet approach assist health sector and crucial domains in medicine to fight against for global pandemic. The major essential roles of proposed Internet of Medical Things make the appropriate services to the available healthcare data.

INTELLIGENCE SYSTEMS PROVIDE DECISION-MAKING AND THINKING DURING THE PANDEMIC DISEASE

Intelligent computing systems can support decision-making even when the problems are complex. A great deal of success has been achieved in integrating expert systems into intelligent systems. Suggested, expert systems may face difficulties in acquiring and processing Coronavirus disease 2019 knowledge. Thus, to recognize the involved patterns and the skills acquired through experience gained from different fields, it is vital to combine data mining with intelligent computing systems to determine the information gathered and the patterns involved, which may include clustering algorithms, neural network algorithms, regression algorithms, and Bayesian algorithms

Numerous other challenges may also emerge, including privacy breaches, ethical concerns, and lack of information security. Thus, the ability to share, analyse, and gather information about Coronavirus disease 2019 in the actual time during which a process with different devices may add to the difficulty of maintaining patient privacy.

The mining of a relatively great size COVID-19 data sets may present difficulties in terms of computation and storage. For instance, authors (Riche, N. H., Hurter, C., Diakopoulos, N., & Carpendale, S., 2018), provide us an example, combining various types of information in heterogeneous Coronavirus disease 2019, data sets with global information systems can be complicated. Additionally, numerous experts are needed to formulate the data mining process. Finally, the quality of data mining results depends on the level of diversity of the gathered COVID-19 data set.

This can be seen as data mining play of great importance and many benefits from large sets of data, helps scientists, physicians, to discover patterns in improving the quality of treatment as author highlighting (Ranjan, J., 2009), to findings. In particular, powerful high-speed processes can be established to examine the enormous amounts of information related to Coronavirus disease 2019 and can provide a knowledge base for a specific area of disease information. Additionally, the diagnosis and prediction of pandemic can be automated, and data mining can enhance decision-making processes.

Given the fact, our expert systems we attempting to calculate a conservative estimates of the resources that will be needed to fight for Coronavirus disease 2019, we find that the resources needed are beyond the available capacities of health care facilities. To achieve an accurate estimation of these resources, estimations should include human resources (such as health workers, including physicians, therapists, and nurses) and other facilities (including numbers of medical centers, emergency departments, intensive care units, ventilators, oxygen concentrators, oxygen cylinders, oxygen plants, liquid oxygen, medications, critical medical supplies, and pulse oximeters). It is very important to assess all these resources before establishing any action plan for resource allocation.

An Expert System for fight against pandemic, in the therapeutic area is very complex but it is still requires coordination, expertise of many variables and estimations that must be guided by comprehensive and accurate information based on IoT technology. On the other hand, at this stage we can provide information about numbers, sizes, capacities, and risks related to both resources and the affected populations worldwide. The realization of such expert systems will mainly depend on sharing and collecting data; this can be greatly facilitated by the IoT.

CONCLUSION

Furthermore, the ideas of aggregation of repositories and information technology platforms, it can be concluded that capabilities can be valuable to analyse, predict, and clarify (treat) COVID-19 contaminations. All of the above technologies was chosen because it is one of the most feasible and rapid ways to assist oversee profitable, effects for healthcare services . Coronavirus disease, as the first major epidemic of the 21st century with collaboration with emerging technology can improve and assist citizens to fight in this infection. Nowadays, modern technologies like Blockchain, AI, and other available resources for a various clinical services can be interconnected via applications, tools, devices as result to completely changed the operations and services in health sector. The majority of digital revolution and sophisticated decision - making tools who responded to current pandemic felt that to recognize early stages symptoms of infection and furthermore assists in checking the particular condition of the exposure patients until the treatment of disease. Highlighting limitations of previous studies - authors (Pedrycz, W., Ichalkaranje, N., Phillips-Wren, G., & Jain, L. C., 2008), mentioned, *"Artificial Intelligence is not only applied to replace Human Interactions, but to provide decision – making for clinicians on what they are modelled for*". Current pandemic has reminded us of the importance of data for decision-making. However, there is still a need for while the quality merits of a determined by data-driven response are well-evidenced, it is a great value for governments to recognise that benefits of having more data do not always outweigh costs of collecting it – particularly in resource appearing forced environments. Consequence of this governments need to set clear priorities that align to their human capacity. Any data collection ensure that the enabling high quality of infrastructure of technologies are in place to turn this information into actionable, targeted solutions.

In the current global pandemic situation, we are fighting with enemy of coronavirus and we are focus on a cost-effective solutions to contribute to our society with multiple intelligence resources and the power of technology. Scientists in health and medical science are attempting to take such challenges, to grow new theories, approaches to describe new study problems, to generate user-centred explanations, and to edify ourselves and the overall civilian.

REFERENCES

Alsafi, Z., Abbas, A. R., Hassan, A., & Ali, M. A. (2020). The coronavirus pandemic: adaptations in medical education. International Journal of Surgery.

Bodas, M., & Peleg, K. (2020). Self-Isolation Compliance In The COVID-19 Era Influenced By Compensation: Findings from a recent survey in Israel: public attitudes toward the COVID-19 outbreak and self-isolation: a cross sectional study of the adult population of Israel. *Health Affairs*, *39*(6), 936–941. doi:10.1377/hlthaff.2020.00382 PMID:32271627

Bullock, J., Luccioni, A., Pham, K. H., Lam, C. S. N., & Luengo-Oroz, M. (2020). Mapping the landscape of artificial intelligence applications against COVID-19. *Journal of Artificial Intelligence Research*, *69*, 807–845. doi:10.1613/jair.1.12162

Car, Z., Baressi Šegota, S., Anđelić, N., Lorencin, I., & Mrzljak, V. (2020). Modeling the spread of COVID-19 infection using a multilayer perceptron. *Computational and Mathematical Methods in Medicine*, *2020*, 2020. doi:10.1155/2020/5714714 PMID:32565882

Chan, H. S., Shan, H., Dahoun, T., Vogel, H., & Yuan, S. (2019). Advancing drug discovery via artificial intelligence. *Trends in Pharmacological Sciences*, *40*(8), 592–604. doi:10.1016/j.tips.2019.06.004 PMID:31320117

Davenport, T., & Kalakota, R. (2019). The potential for artificial intelligence in healthcare. *Future Healthcare Journal*, *6*(2), 94–98. doi:10.7861/futurehosp.6-2-94 PMID:31363513

Fusco, A., Dicuonzo, G., Dell'Atti, V., & Tatullo, M. (2020). Blockchain in healthcare: Insights on COVID-19. *International Journal of Environmental Research and Public Health*, *17*(19), 7167. doi:10.3390/ijerph17197167 PMID:33007951

Haleem, A., Javaid, M., & Khan, I. H. (2020). Internet of things (IoT) applications in orthopaedics. *Journal of Clinical Orthopaedics and Trauma*, *11*, S105–S106. doi:10.1016/j.jcot.2019.07.003 PMID:31992928

Haleem, A., Vaishya, R., Javaid, M., & Khan, I. H. (2020). Artificial Intelligence (AI) applications in orthopaedics: An innovative technology to embrace. *Journal of Clinical Orthopaedics and Trauma*, *11*, S80–S81. doi:10.1016/j.jcot.2019.06.012 PMID:31992923

Hollander, J. E., & Carr, B. G. (2020). Virtually perfect? Telemedicine for COVID-19. *The New England Journal of Medicine*, *382*(18), 1679–1681. doi:10.1056/NEJMp2003539 PMID:32160451

Li, J., & Guo, X. (2020). *Covid-19 contact-tracing apps: A survey on the global deployment and challenges*. arXiv preprint arXiv:2005.03599.

Mahrouf, M., Lotfi, E. M., Maziane, M., Hattaf, K., & Yousfi, N. (2017). Stability Analysis for Stochastic Differential Equations in Virology. *Journal of Advances in Mathematics and Computer Science*, 1-12.

Marbouh, D., Abbasi, T., Maasmi, F., Omar, I. A., Debe, M. S., Salah, K., Jayaraman, R., & Ellahham, S. (2020). Blockchain for COVID-19: Review, Opportunities, and a Trusted Tracking System. *Arabian Journal for Science and Engineering*, *45*(12), 1–17. doi:10.100713369-020-04950-4 PMID:33072472

Mettler, M. (2016, September). Blockchain technology in healthcare: The revolution starts here. In *2016 IEEE 18th international conference on e-health networking, applications, and services (Healthcom)* (pp. 1-3). IEEE.

Phillips-Wren, G., & Ichalkaranje, N. (Eds.). (2008). *Intelligent decision making: An AI-based approach* (Vol. 97). Springer Science & Business Media. doi:10.1007/978-3-540-76829-6

Ranjan, J. (2009). Data mining in pharma sector: Benefits. *International Journal of Health Care Quality Assurance*, *22*(1), 82–92. doi:10.1108/09526860910927970 PMID:19284173

Riche, N. H., Hurter, C., Diakopoulos, N., & Carpendale, S. (Eds.). (2018). *Data-driven storytelling*. CRC Press. doi:10.1201/9781315281575

Schurink, C. A. M., Lucas, P. J. F., Hoepelman, I. M., & Bonten, M. J. M. (2005). Computer-assisted decision support for the diagnosis and treatment of infectious diseases in intensive care units. *The Lancet. Infectious Diseases*, 5(5), 305–312. doi:10.1016/S1473-3099(05)70115-8 PMID:15854886

Singh, R. P., Javaid, M., Haleem, A., & Suman, R. (2020). Internet of things (IoT) applications to fight against COVID-19 pandemic. *Diabetes & Metabolic Syndrome*, 14(4), 521–524. doi:10.1016/j.dsx.2020.04.041 PMID:32388333

Vaishya, R., Javaid, M., Khan, I. H., & Haleem, A. (2020). Artificial Intelligence (AI) applications for COVID-19 pandemic. *Diabetes & Metabolic Syndrome*, 14(4), 337–339. doi:10.1016/j.dsx.2020.04.012 PMID:32305024

Xie, X., Zhong, Z., Zhao, W., Zheng, C., Wang, F., & Liu, J. (2020). Chest CT for typical coronavirus disease 2019 (COVID-19) pneumonia: Relationship to negative RT-PCR testing. *Radiology*, 296(2), E41–E45. doi:10.1148/radiol.2020200343 PMID:32049601

ENDNOTE

[1]   WHO | World Health Organization.

APPENDIX

AI: Artificial Intelligence
IoT: Internet of Things
IoIT: Internet of Intelligent Things
BD: Big Data
ML: Machine Learning
IoMT: Internet of Medical Things
CDS: Clinical Decision Support
WHO: World Health Organisation
MRI: Magnetic Resonance Imaging
CT: Computed Tomography
EHRs: Electronic Health Records
COVID-19: Coronavirus disease 2019
ANN: Artificial Neural Network

Chapter 2
Overview of IoT and Machine Learning for E–Healthcare in Pandemics and Health Crises

Mohsin Raza
Edge Hill University, UK

Muhammad Awais
Edge Hill University, UK

Imran Haider
Capital University of Science and Technology, Pakistan

Muhammad Usman Hadi
University of Aalborg, Denmark

Ehtasham Javed
University of Helsinki, Finland

ABSTRACT

The outbreak of COVID-19 has severely affected the healthcare infrastructure. The limitations of conventional healthcare urge the use of the digital technologies to lessen the overall load on the healthcare infrastructure and assist healthcare workers/staff. This chapter focuses on digital technologies to enable smart healthcare solutions to sustain and improve health services. The chapter focuses on two main driving technologies (internet of things [IoT] and artificial intelligence [AI]), pioneering automation and digitalization of healthcare. The enabling technologies possess the potential to transform the healthcare with emergence of new and novel research directions to realize and address healthcare needs. Therefore, it is essential to focus on key driving and complementing technologies to establish multidisciplinary research solutions with cross-platform design coupled with translational learning to unlock the potentials of next generation healthcare.

DOI: 10.4018/978-1-7998-6736-4.ch002

HEALTH CRISIS IN PANDEMICS

Pandemics

Pandemic is a globally popular term for contagious infectious diseases that spreads among the people due to physical interaction between them. The outbreak of such diseases cross boundaries of the countries through infected carriers. These carriers are people mostly unfamiliar about their infectious state due to no visible symptoms. They travel to other countries becoming a source of infection, spread by direct or indirect contact, sneezing, and coughing in close vicinities (Manning, 2001)

Contagious diseases like influenza, cholera, dengue, respiratory infections, Ebola, AIDS, etc. have devastated human societies more than fifteen times since the 6th Century. The worst impacts of the pandemic are the crisis in the healthcare system, financial meltdown due to the loss in business activities, joblessness, social insecurity, and most importantly, the loss of worthy human lives (Qiu, 2017).

In the 20th century, influenza related diseases hit massive populations of the major countries across the globe. The origin of Spanish flu (1918-19) could not be confirmed but it was another variant of the H1N1 virus which spread among one-third of the world's population including people in countries like Spain, the USA, EU, etc. killing more than 20 million (Qiu, 2017). Hong Kong virus was caused by influenza, a combination of various genes from H2N2 and H3N2 viruses. The estimated deaths due to this pandemic were around one million people in China, EU, UK, USA, etc (CDC, 2019a). The wave of Asian flu originated from Singapore in 1957 and spread from Hong Kong to USA within months causing more than one million deaths (CDC, 2019b).

In the 21st century, the outbreak of the new virus gene H1N1 also called "Swine flu" started in the year 2009 in United States of America. H1N1 gene had unique properties that in past were neither observed in humans nor in animals. The virus penetrated the boundaries of countries and reached New Zealand, Israel, and many counties in the Europe where it resulted in deaths of over two hundred thousand people with majority comprising of elderly population.

The outbreak of pandemic called COVID-19 is the recent and ongoing contagious disease that is believed to be originated from China in 2019 and has infected almost 37.4 million people around the world, whereas more than 1 million people have lost their lives till now. COVID-19 is a novel variation in the family of Coronaviruses which can harm both humans as well as animals (WHO, 2020).

History of various pandemics observed in 19th and 20th century is presented in Table 1.

Table 1. History of the most Contagious Diseases spread worldwide during 19th & 20th Centuries

Disease	Timeline	Geographic Spread	Reported Deaths
COVID-19	2019 - to date	More than 200 countries, including USA, EU, Asia, Middle East, etc	1 million
H1N1 Swine Flu	2009-10	USA, EU, UK, Mexico, Israel, NZ	0.2 million
Asian Flu	1957-58	China, US, UK	1.5Million
Hong Kong Flu	1968-69	China, HK, UK, USA, EU	10Million
Spanish Flu	1918-19	Spain, USA, EU, UK	>20Million

The upcoming sections describe the impact of Covid-19 on healthcare, GDP, education and tourisms. These sections also discuss the limitations in the conventional healthcare systems and its inability to cope with pandemics.

Impact of Covid-19

COVID-19 is an extremely infectious respiratory disease that can be transmitted from one person to another in close contact through tiny droplets (microdroplets). Experts have referred to COVID-19 as the biggest emergency since World War II. The negative impacts of COVID-19 can be witnessed in almost every sector globally including, healthcare facilities, educational systems, tourism, gross domestic products (GDP) of countries, entertainment, and sports, etc as depicted in Figure 1 (Hiscott, 2020).

Healthcare Crisis

The infection also deteriorates the function of lungs by damaging its tissues while in some cases it also caused harm to the other body organs. The degree of impairment to the organs is higher in elderly population and those with a weak immune system. The elderly and vulnerable patients suffering from other diseases if infected with COVID-19 are likely to be hospitalized for medical care. Medical facilities available in the hospitals for routine healthcare problems is no way near to meet the needs of number of patients infected due to the spread of COVID-19 (Raza, 2021). The consistently growing number of infected people can trigger a healthcare crisis.

Figure 1. Impacts of COVID-19

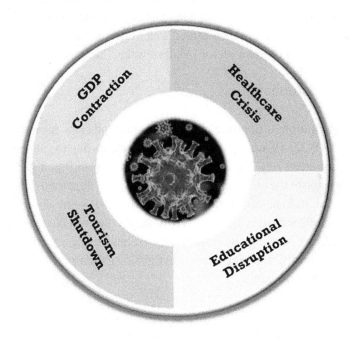

GDP Contraction

The GDP of developing countries is expected to fall by 2.5% whereas an overall global decline of 2.1% is expected due to COVID-19. The reduction in production of goods due to low demand and resultantly decreased exports affects the GDP of every country (Boatwright, 2020). The import capacity of countries has also been decreased as the income earned from exports is contracted. The closure of factories has resulted in significant rise in unemployment. The containment measures through social distancing have also left many workers to lose their jobs. The demand for goods reduced which resulted in a significant percentage of workers becoming jobless or forced to unpaid leaves. The severity of joblessness varies from country to country due to the degree of strictness in containment policies.

Tourism Shutdown

Travel agents are associated with recreational tours with opportunities of earning huge profits by arranging accommodation, lodging in hotels. The cost of global imports and exports has raised by almost 25% as transportation of goods becomes very challenging with road closures and reduction in other means of transport.

The high cost of transport due to less operating labor hours has also contributed along with the limited flight schedules at national and international airports social distancingas social distancing took effect. The unprecedented loss of about 75% is suffered by the global tourism sector (Maliszewska, 2020).

Educational Disruption

Educational institutions around the globe had to suspend class-room lectures to stop the spread of COVID-19 among the on-campus students due to gathering in classes and other study areas etc. The quality of education has suffered greatly (Karalis, 2020). While some of the universities, colleges and schools started delivering online lectures, yet the sudden transformation in medium of communication between students and tutors, was insufficient to replicate the desired outcomes. The online system of education, developed on ad-hoc basis, has raising frustration among the students and caused difficulty for teachers to transform their methodologies to online teaching/learning paradigm.

LIMITATIONS OF CONVENTIONAL HEALTHCARE SYSTEMS FOR PANDEMICS

People suffering from any type of illness need proper medical care, which may include radio imaging (Raza, 2019), pathological lab tests through blood and urine samples. Such test outcomes are interpreted by physicians through consultations at hospitals/clinics for proper diagnosis. Treatment plans and any prescribed medicines by the physician are conveyed to the patient through consultation.

The conventional healthcare system is organized in a way that bounds a patient to rely on availability of healthcare services within the boundary walls of hospitals/clinics (Raza, 2017b). Limited ICU services available at hospitals are normally adequate for incoming patients as it is not normally expected that everyone will require same type of medical care at same time. The number of incoming patients to the hospital are random which can be modeled as normally distributed random variable. However, the overall facilities available in the hospitals become very insufficient if a contagious disease starts spreading among people rapidly triggering a healthcare crisis. A graphical representation of such scenario is presented in Figure 2 whereas the list of required resources and their limitations are covered in Table 2.

The treatment capacity of hospitals/clinics becomes quite narrow compared to the number of incoming patients in case of exceptional demands due to the outbreak of epidemic or pandemic (Khalid, 2020). Hospital beds and intensive care units become completely occupied and more patients are seen lying on the hospital floors or even outside the premises. Healthcare professionals, like doctors, nurses who are responsible to treat the infected patients in case of a pandemic like, COVID-19 are also at greater risk of getting infected due to the prolonged direct contact with patients and in some cases, lack of protective clothing and Personal Protective Equipment (PPE). If number of frontline healthcare professionals starts decreasing due to lack of adequate PPEs then such deficit has a potency of turning health crisis into a disaster.

Figure 2. Depiction of healthcare crisis due to inadequate resources

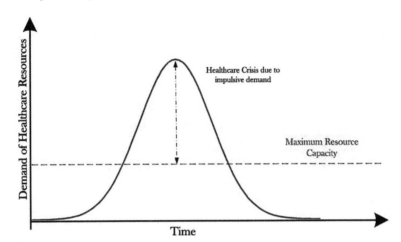

Table 2. List of Required resources and their limitation in conventional healthcare system

Resource	Limitation
Hospital Beds and ICUs	Hundreds of beds / ICUs for thousands of severe patients
Doctors, Nurses and Paramedics	24 Hrs. take care of admitted patients
Personal Protective Equipment (PPEs)	Production in massive Qty daily use of fresh pieces
Rapid test and diagnostic facility	Exponential rise of patients but linear testing facilities
Vaccine development and production	Longer trial times and limited production facilities

Viruses that have novel genes cause a real challenge for the medical experts to understand its properties, devise methodologies for its testing & diagnostics. The conventional healthcare system takes a lot of time to respond in setting up lab facilities for sample collection, it's processing and diagnostics due to limited resources. Unfortunately, the time elapsed in the deployment of large-scale testing facilities adds to ignorance of infected people regarding their infection status and they unintentionally become the reason for rapid disease spread. The development of vaccines becomes an essential requirement of countries to raise immunity against infectious disease (like COVID-19) in the bodies of citizens. However, the process of vaccine development and it's testing on volunteers, observation of future side effects take years. In the meantime, millions of lives are lost and billions of people suffer from disease itself.

It is quite evident that the current healthcare infrastructure is incapable to facilitate the rising demands amid pandemics due to limited resources such as medical staff, PPEs, in-patient medical facilities etc. Therefore, is it vital to explore information and communications technology (ICT) in healthcare to meet the rising demands and to develop more innovative and intelligent solutions for healthcare. The potential technologies for next generation healthcare are covered in the following section.

POTENTIAL TECHNOLOGIES AND FUTURE OF HEALTHCARE INFRASTRUCTURE

Medical and Technological advancements, like telecommunication networks, Artificial intelligence, Bigdata, cloud services have enabled health experts to bring revolution in the healthcare facilities for the betterment of patients by replacing the conventional ways of testing, diagnosis, and treatment methods. The architectural design of future healthcare facilities will be allowing most medical care services to give high quality healthcare within and away from the hospital. Some of the prominent technologies are explained below.

Telemedicine

Sharing medical data between the patients and medical consultants/specialists is possible using remote telemedicine services while both parties remain at different places even thousands of miles away (Raza, 2017b). Telemedicine services enable expert advice through two-way interactive audio/video communications through computers and network support. It also reduces the significant time for critical pediatric patients to reach directly to the Neonatal Intensive Care (NICU) service bypassing the process of consultation. Similarly, Telecare services are medical services provided at home for the physically challenged and old age patients. In this service, the Patient has to wear small-sized body sensors that gather biodata like, heart rate, blood pressure, ECG, and other vitals and sends it to the medical network after regular intervals. The data is monitored and analyzed to estimate the overall health status of the patient and the Remote patient management system can detect hazardous symptoms at an early stage. It is also essential for minimizing the contact and chances of further spread of contiguous outbreaks.

Artificial Intelligence

Artificial intelligence (AI) is capable of performing tasks like classification, detection, and even decision making in complex situations, replacing the need of thinking abilities of trained human resources (Awais, 2018). AI can be deployed into healthcare tasks to evaluate or reconstruct the available images from X-rays, CT and MRI scans, tumor detection, toxicity prediction, diagnose the diseases, and even to take critical decisions for the treatment plan. AI involvement in healthcare services is still in the early stages but it can still be used in diagnosis or detection of breast and skin cancers, tumors, diagnosis of heart and Alzheimer diseases, etc. These attributes of AI can offer exceptional support in pandemics and can off-load vital tasks in healthcare to reduce the burden on healthcare workers and medical experts.

Robotic Surgeries

The idea of using robots in surgical procedures at hospitals is innovative in healthcare systems. Surgeons can use robots in operations for better accuracy. The effective control and accuracy of robots will enable more minimally invasive surgeries being performed entirely by robots. Robots can be controlled by surgeons from a remote location for operations while the patient is admitted into hospital which is situated miles away, thus minimizing the risks in treating contiguous patients and safeguarding medical staff. Use of microrobots and nanorobots has shown great performance in minimizing surgical procedures. The results of abdominal surgeries show that the progression-free survival rate of robot-assisted surgeries are nearly similar to surgeries performed by humans (Vatandoost, 2019).

Internet of Things (IoT)

Internet of things (IoT) can be described as a network of tiny devices that exchange data with specific nodes through a short-range communication network to form mass storage of information gathered for specific goals (Awais, 2020). Those goals can be avoiding traffic accidents, reporting emergencies, minimizing health disasters etc. to make efficient healthcare solutions. IoT healthcare systems can be comprised of the following basic components.

Body Sensors

These are wearable sensors placed at various body parts to sense the vital parameters of the body, like temperature, pulse rate, blood pressure, etc. They all share data with a central device that is placed at a distance not greater than the length of the body (Baker, 2017).

Central Device

Data from all body sensors are taken by the central device and it is forwarded to the external network. The power bank of the central device (gateway) has a comparatively much longer operational capacity than other body sensors in order to communicate with an external network which may be miles away using narrow band IoT (NB-IoT) or similar technologies (Baker, 2017).

Figure 3. Taxonomy of technologies for future Healthcare system

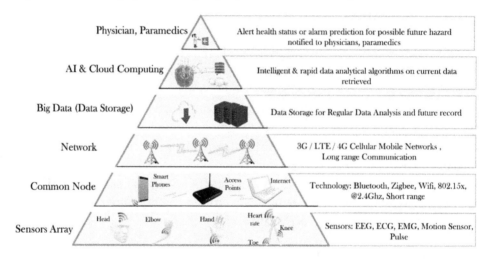

Short-Range Communication

Body sensors share data with the central device by following a standard protocol for short-range communications (e,g Bluetooth, Zigbee 802.15x) (Raza, 2017a). Transmission of radio signals from sensors mounted on the body parts must have SAR (specific absorption rate) impact lower than FCC guidelines to avoid health hazards (Baker, 2017).

Long-Range Communications

The central device combines the data acquired from body sensors and transmits it towards the database or cloud where the physicians can have access. Long-range communication takes place according to network standards such as 3G, LTE/4G, 5G, Microwave links etc (Baker, 2017).

Cloud Storage and Data Analytics

Health information of patients is saved in a secure manner into mass cloud storage. The stored data can be accessed by machine learning (Awais, 2016) and data mining solutions to consistently process and analyze the data as well as keep track of incoming patients' health status and raise an alarm if there is a chance of some hazard (Baker, 2017).

The advancements in the field of IoT, AI, robotics, communications, cloud services, fog, data analytics, body sensors and telemedicine has opened new venue for exploration. A taxonomy of these technologies within the healthcare is presented in Figure 3.

ROLE OF IoT IN PANDEMICS AND HEALTHCARE CRISIS

Internet of things can play a key role in managing the pandemics. Contagious diseases can spread very quickly among the people in communities, cities, and even countries to take shape of a pandemic. The outbreak of disease can infect millions so the essential goal of the healthcare system is to respond quickly and control the spread of infection. The use of latest technologies like IoT as part of 5G telecommunication network combined with artificial intelligence (AI) can help deploy a response system much faster than the conventional techniques. These technologies can provide a suitable and long-lasting system for screening, monitoring, and prevention of the infection by using machine learning, neural networks, cloud computing, data analytics, and deep learning (Swayamsiddha, 2020).

Cognitive Internet of Things (CIoT) is a variant of IoT network for device-to-device data exchange with less latency, timely channel access, and bandwidth availability for essential applications. The task of providing enough bandwidth is achieved by avoiding the wastage of available bandwidth. This means that the radio spectrum available for exchange of data among the interconnected nodes is limited and the static allocation of frequency bandwidth might result in wastage. Therefore, an efficient scheme is employed to allocate the bandwidth to the demanding applications according to their varying needs. The scheme is called dynamic allocation of spectrum.

This technique uses search and hunt strategy to identify allocated radio resources which are not currently loaded. Frames of shorter durations are sent over the entire spectrum in an opportunistic manner to find out the radio channels which are not being used for data exchange. The unused channels are put into the available pool of channels to be used by another demanding application (Swayamsiddha, 2020).

Figure 4. Internet of Things (IoT) extends specialized class of CIoMT for Medical Industry

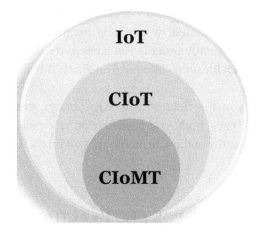

CIoMT and Its Application in Pandemics

Cognitive Internet of Medical Things (CIoMT) is a variant of CIoT with a focus on medical services while eliminating the conservative medical procedures for better healthcare. CIoMT empowers healthcare authorities to control the outbreak by gathering real-time data of infected patients with their GPS locations. Automated processing of sensors acquired data is communicated through base stations of 5G network for proper monitoring of patients and tracing of other people who had contact with the infected patients. CIoMT is involved to carry out numerous tasks for control of the pandemic (Swayamsiddha, 2020). A hierarchical presentation of IoT, CIoT and CIoMT is presented in Figure 4 whereas the significant components of CIoMT is presented in Figure 5.

Tracking of Infected Patients

Real-time updates of new patients suffering from the disease and their locations are tracked through CIoMT network. AI is used to predict the overall situation due to pandemic by analyzing death counts, people who have cured through treatment along with active patients under treatment. The predicted result is available to the health authorities for rethinking measures taken to control the spread of disease (Swayamsiddha, 2020).

Monitoring of Infected Patients

The front-line team of healthcare professionals, like doctors, nurses, paramedic staff members cannot maintain distance while treating infected patients. Therefore, they are at high risk to acquire the disease. The 5G based CIoMT network enables the medical staff to remotely monitor the vital parameters (like BP, HR, ECG, EMG, EED, temperature, pulse, etc.) of the infected patients. Wearable sensors attached to relevant body parts of the patients constantly send data to CIoMT network entities (Swayamsiddha, 2020).

Testing and Diagnosis

People tracked by the CIoMT network for having in contact with the infected patients are also advised to remain in isolation even if they do not exhibit any clinical symptoms. The testing procedures are imitated with the suspected patients immediately after tracking to rule out infection. CIoMT enables medical experts with remote access to the results of X-rays and CT scans through live data sharing. The results can be fed to the AI-engines for confirmation of interpreted results (Swayamsiddha, 2020).

Tracking Contacts and Grouping

Travel locations of the infected patients are stored in the database. This location information is used to track down the suspected patients, quarantine and test them. CIoMT allows the interconnection of healthcare units to collect real-time locations of infected patients and put them in a separate category of the containment region. The area map is marked with unique identification of zones to separate regions of infections, suspects, and healthy areas in a city or overall country. Health teams can be directed to the marked regions to secure the suspected areas, start testing people for possible infection. The AI-assisted bordering of the areas is quite helpful in the speedy response by government authorities. The area-wise lockdown and social distancing can be implemented in infected zones and to some extent in suspected zones also (Swayamsiddha, 2020).

Figure 5. Significant components of Cognitive Internet of Medical Things

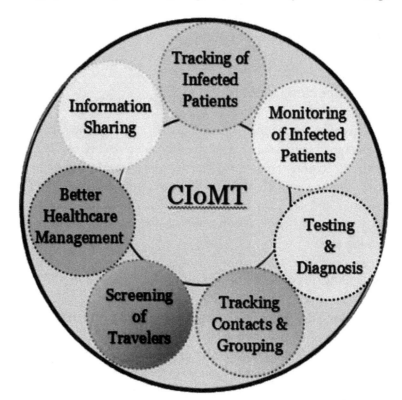

Screening of Travelers

The outbreak of any contagious disease spreads beyond boundaries of cities and countries after infected patients travel to other destinations and they unintentionally transfer the infection to the local people through close contact. Common entry and exit points used by travelers are airports, seaports, train and bus stations. People gather in the close proximity of each other to attend concerts, sports matches, etc. and become the reason for the spread of the virus. Each attendee is more likely to touch the next one or sneeze or cough and infect the people in the close vicinity. All the airports, train stations, entry/exit points of public gathering can be screened through surveillance imaging devices which takes the thermal impression of the incoming person to check their body temperature level. The data screened by the imaging devices is shared remotely with the healthcare authorities through CIoMT network. Remote access enables the healthcare authorities to run AI analytic algorithms on the stored data or visually observe for the identification of possible infection carriers (Swayamsiddha, 2020).

Better Healthcare Management

Normally, hospitals have limited staff, doctors with limited bed capacity, and ICU services. The outbreak of a pandemic can result in chaos for healthcare professionals to deal with an abrupt rise in the incoming patients. Moreover, the massive process of testing, isolation of suspected patients, diagnosis, monitoring, and treatment engages all health workers in 100% capacity. Despite utilizing all the available resources, still large proportion of patients remain unattended because of limited capacity of the overall conventional healthcare system. Therefore, CIoMT provides solutions to remotely observe and diagnose all the patients by its network of interconnected devices while patients do not need to leave home. The medical instructions can also be generated by medical experts combined with AI-based decisions on acquired sensors' data. Consultation can also be provided through telemedicine, telecare at the patient's door-step and with the automated delivery of drugs (Swayamsiddha, 2020).

Information Sharing

Citizens must be aware of the current situation of the pandemic in the local area to stay alert and plan their actions accordingly. People need to leave their homes to perform some tasks which are essential for their and their family's survival. Therefore, people need to get out of their houses, no matter the situation outside. It is therefore government's responsibility to have the area-specific information regarding virus outspread and density infected people shared. If people are aware of the red zones and green zones within the town then they can easily make safe choices about which grocery stores to visit and refill the home supplies. CIoMT can play a major role in gathering area-specific information about virus spread, and trace and track. Gathered data can be communicated to cloud/fog servers where AI-based algorithms, data mining techniques and intelligent analysis can be regularly performed. The same information can be shared with the locals through applications that can maintain anonymity and are accessible through handheld devices (smart phones) (Swayamsiddha, 2020).

Challenges for CIoMT

5G network infrastructure, CIoMT, AI, and data analytics have provided a robust system to the healthcare authorities to perform overall management of pandemic in real-time. However, the 5G network combined with the CIoMT is also an evolving technology which show great potential for improvement. are being researched and improved day by day. There is some weakness of the CIoMT like, data privacy protection while being shared from multiple entities in CIoMT network. There are also health issues regarding the army of sensors mounted on the body parts of the infected patients (Swayamsiddha, 2020). The sensors use short-range communication protocols to transmit data to a data sink/data hub. The communications may take place using Bluetooth, Zigbee, ISA100.11a, OpenHART, or similar open source frameworks which operate in the licensed free frequency band called ISM band (Raza, 2017a). Security of the data is a major challenge while communicating the personal/medical information of the patients. The data acquired by the body sensors of the infected regarding his blood pressure, pulse rate, electrocardiogram (ECG), electroencephalogram (EEG), electromyography (EMG), Oxygen saturation through a sensor, etc. is being transferred to the central node at carrier frequencies. The same data can be received by another node with malicious intent and will exploit the patient's privacy (Swayamsiddha, 2020). Wearable body sensors have a significant effect on the overall effectiveness of CIoMT. The human body is composed of sensitive tissues that absorbed the electromagnetic (EM) energy generated by the array of sensors mounted on key body parts. The overall absorption of the EM energy into the body tissues is called the Specific Absorption Rate (SAR). The maximum allowable exposure limits of SAR for human tissues are specified by the American and European standards (FCC & IEC) (Swayamsiddha, 2020).

AI DRIVEN SMART HEALTHCARE ENVIRONMENTS

In the past decade, AI has received unprecedented interests in every domain including healthcare due to the ever increasing 1) amount of the data generated by the devices and 2) the computational power available. The use of AI has become more dominant quite recently due to the Covid-19 which has affected the whole worlds badly ranging from economy, education, tourism, social and personal life and more importantly healthcare. Therefore, the AI can be utilized in a variety of different ways as shown in Figure 6. The following subsections will provide a detailed insight on how AI has been used in a variety of different application to assist the national as well as global healthcare infrastructure to better cope with pandemics.

Track and Trace

AI has helped significantly to track and trace the contacts who have recently got virus or were in contact with the patients having COVID -19. It is suggested that using AI for track and trace, countries like China, Singapore and South Korea have effectively reduced the infection rate since they have utilized location base app and services to gather data and trace people's movements (Afriyie, 2020). These apps

Figure 6. Role of AI in Developing Smarter Environment to Cope with Pandemic

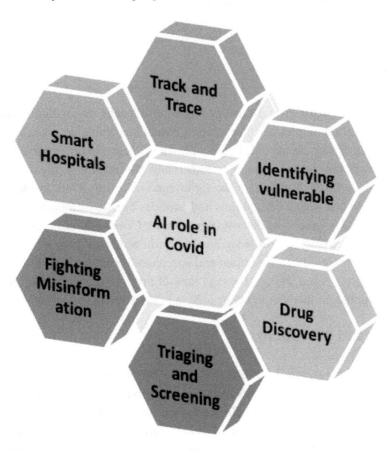

coupled with AI can effectively track and track the location an individual have visited such as restaurants, trains stations, hospitals, airports, shopping malls etc.

Identifying Vulnerable

AI based predictive analytics can been used effectively to identify vulnerable individuals using a variety of different data sources such as electronic health records (EHR) comprised of general health history, blood screening, BMI, medical imaging and other heartcare data sources. More recently, Israel (Heaven, 2020) have incorporated AI in its existing system to identify the vulnerable population to Covid. The system has used variety of medical data records such as person's visit to hospital, their BMI, diabetic or heath conditions etc. The system identified a total of 2% (40,000) individuals in the medical records as vulnerable which were then tested for Covid on fast-track. This could have been cumbersome if any manual process has been followed to identify the vulnerable individuals. Similarly, AI can be used to identity key workers who are vulnerable to receive Covid, which can then be moved to a work areas with less exposures to Covid.

Drug Discovery

AI is used actively for drug discovery in the past decade by predicting the target biomolecule using complex machine learning based algorithms. However, discovering the right drug or vaccine can only be possible if sufficient amount of data is available to train the machine learning models which is now possible due to big data. Arshadi et al. (Arshadi, 2020) highlighted the significance of using AI to develop vaccine for Covid and provided a compounds and peptides based "CoronaDB-AI" dataset that can be used to excel drug discovery process for Covid. Moreover, a recent study (Zhou, 2020) provides a detailed guideline on how AI can help accelerate drug repurposing for Covid in an efficient and accelerated manner. In addition to faster vaccine generation and starting testing phase of drug, repurposing drugs using AI can save significant that would occur in case of discovering new drugs.

Triaging and Screening

AI can help direct patients in pre-hospital and hospital triage in an efficient and better way. For instance, in US, Partners healthcare (Wittbold, 2020) in Boston launched an online healthcare assistance helpline for the public to meet the rising demands of public getting assistance regarding Covid by providing pre-triage assistance. The aim was to assist the most critical and vulnerable patients in-hospital and to provide remote care to less vulnerable and less critical through the medical staff. However, soon after the launch, the helpline went overwhelmed and the wait time went over half an hour causing callers to give up before they have had received any medical advice. The company start developing AI chatbot based Covid screening utilizing US center for disease control and prevention (CDC) guidelines. The AI bot is up and running while serving enormous number of patients simultaneously remotely to direct them towards appropriate healthcare including the vulnerable and in critical condition requiring urgent healthcare.

Recently, Computerized Tomography (CT) scan-based triage screening tool is developed in China which uses deep learning-based AI algorithm to differentiate between individuals with and without Covid (Vardhanabhuti, 2020). The screening tool has been tested in several fever clinics and provides good accuracy in detecting the patients with and without Covid

Fighting Misinformation

Amid pandemic, it is very essential to get control of the misinformation, false and illegitimate news spreading over social media platforms such as Facebook and Twitter. Recent study (Benson, 2020) suggested that around one quarter of the misinformation on Twitter is flooded by its own chatbots and the information is misleading and of low credibility. Facebook which is the world largest social media platform also suffered from misinformation and misleading facts about Covid shared in enormous amount every day. As a consequence, social media companies designed AI based tools to combat with Covid misinformation and label or flag sources with misleading information. However, still a lot more to be done as the current tools are not capable enough to label the misleading information since not only the misinformation related to Covid is often overlooked but also the legitimate information is also labelled as illegitimate.

Smart Hospitals

AI can help hospitals to work in a smart and efficiently way through better screening, resource allocation and protecting workforce. The AI chatbot can screen patients upon their arrival using a variety of different Covid related questionnaires in addition to temperature and other health checks which will accelerate the screening process. Moreover, the medical staff and keyworkers in hospital can utilize wearables that will show vital signs using AI enable data analytics to identify the health status of the whole staff instead of performing manual health checks costing significant time and resources. The hospital resource allocation such as beds and health medical supplies including personal protective equipment (PPE) can also be tracked and managed using AI in order to keep up with the supply (Raza, 2021). The AI can in this way can form smart hospitals which can communicate with each other to observe how much resources are being utilized in a particular hospital. This will help hospital to avoid overwhelming and directing patients to those hospitals which have plenty of free resources available.

ENABLING TECHNOLOGIES FOR SMART HEALTHCARE

Enabling technologies can help healthcare infrastructure to better cope with pandemics alike Covid. The enabling technologies to produce smart healthcare are shown in Figure 7 and further details are provided in the following subsections.

Figure 7. Enabling Technologies for Smart healthcare

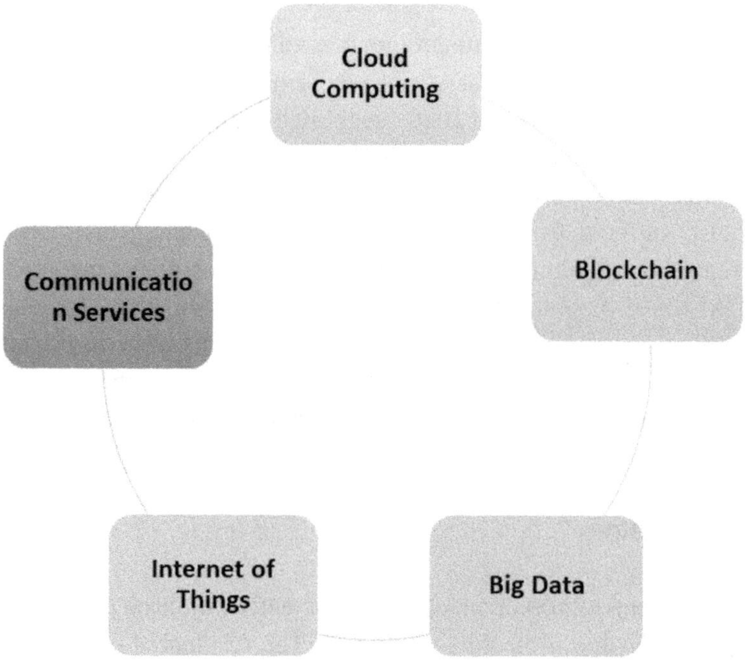

Cloud Computing

Cloud computing can help healthcare infrastructure to better prepare for pandemics by providing 1) data storage scalability, 2) data sharing ease 3) high computational power 4) better management of medical records, 5) drug discovery. Data scalability in pandemics alive Covid is very important since the huge amount of data is generated in a very short span. Cloud computing in this regard can help to save data in an efficient and reliable way, which would have very difficult to perform otherwise in a paper-based form or without the availability of such huge data storage capacity (Kirsal, 2021). Data sharing is another benefit of cloud computing amid pandemic since organizations often shared data with each other which would been very resource consuming and slow if imagined without cloud computing. This also enable multiple healthcare providers to use the patients' data and share knowledge more rapidly when patient's transfer from one to another healthcare facility.

Cloud computing is also equipped with high performing processing units which enable big data analytics to utilize these resources in order to extract meaningful information and patterns from data. Better and efficient management of data in pandemics also becomes possible through cloud computing in the form of EHR without losing any health-related information which is quite probable if data would have stored locally. The healthcare data availability on a single platform help assist drug discovery researchers and organizations to access the centralized patients' datasets, thus accelerating the discovery stage by knowing more about the pandemic characteristics.

Blockchain

Block chain is very reliable mean of providing reliable, secure and efficiently data sharing. This becomes very significant amid pandemic with enormous amount of misinformation and lack of trust raising between organizations and countries worldwide. The transactions in blockchain are recorded through block technology using shared and protected database. The blockchain technology can be used in a variety of ways i.e., 1) patients privacy protection 2) medical staffing, 3) providing secure EHR, 4) medical supply chain management, 5) handling false information. Patient privacy is always the primary concern of every healthcare infrastructure during pandemic and in normal circumstances, which can easily be implemented possible through blockchain technology (Moschou, 2020). Block chain also helps to regulate the General Data Protection Regulation (GDPR) guidelines more effectively which is quite essential to implement in Europe in order to enable data sharing. The national health services (NHS), UK and also worldwide, healthcare infrastructure experiences medical staffing crisis during pandemic as the staffing process itself can take from several months to sometime year or so due to the variety of verifications organizations have to do before hiring someone. Block chain in this regard can help health care infrastructure to excel the staffing process by providing end to end verification of the academic, professional and other personal documents through its reliable resources centralizing all stakeholders. Blockchain also enable secure transmission of EHR between organizations without any data loss of issues of tempering data while sharing. Medical supply chain management can also be better equipped using blockchain technology since it can ease the validation process by connecting all stakeholders ensuring transparency and authenticity of the information provided. This will also eliminate any dependences on third party organizations thus reducing order generation and validation time, operational cost and by providing faster deliveries. Misinformation can spread chaos amid pandemic and its spread should be avoided at the best possible way. Blockchain in this regard can provide health organizations, social media companies and other stakeholders a reliable platform to validate the information and to stop the spread of unauthentic information.

Big Data

Big data analytics has helped significantly the world to accumulate and synthesize the disease and incident related information of Covid patients worldwide in an efficient and reliable way (Ting, 2020). Moreover, big data has helped the global community to better understand the novel Covid-19 by exchanging the symptomatic information, the progression of disease, its transmission and contagious nature, incubation period and the possible diagnosis that can be used to identify patients. Big data helped to diagnose patients faster and in accurate manner using AI enabled analytics. Its also assisted medical practitioners to excel in the drug discovery domain by collating all the data of patients under trials which enabled faster decision making to decide if a particular therapy is useful or not. Big data also assisted healthcare organizations to track and trace through tracking their travel records and other location based geographical information. Big data through communication technologies has got the potential to store information related to patients' mobility which can help the healthcare infrastructure and local enforcement authorities to investigate if individuals are adhering to self-isolation rules and regulation or not.

Internet of Things

Internet of things (IoT) can play a vital role in helping healthcare to better fight with pandemic (Ting, 2020) in several domains: 1) Identifying the pandemic epicenter-IoT comprised of mobile devices coupled with geographical information system (GIS) can help to trace the origination and spread of the virus alike Covid, 2) Smart factory – IoT can provide better coordination between the supply chain trail by using the RFID or other sensing methodologies to keep track of the available medical supplies and their demand and supply, 3) in-hospital resourcing – IoT devices can track and manage the availably of life saving equipment such as oxygen cylinders, ICU beds and other supplies (PPEs, drugs, sanitizers, masks, consumables etc.) to assist hospital management in making informed decisions, 4) identifying vulnerable: IoT ambient and wearable sensors (Awais, 2019) deployed in domestic environment can track occupants' vital signs and inform healthcare services accordingly if there are any vulnerable individuals living inside a particular vicinity.

Communication Services

The communication services have played vital role in connecting world since the dependency on the digital infrastructure has received unprecedented increase due to significant amount of population working from home (Saeed, 2020). Without communication services, it would have been nearly impossible for the healthcare services to send updates about the pandemic to all public in timely and accurate manner. Communication technologies provided such means to healthcare infrastructure in the form of voice and text messages, emails and websites to send frequency updates in order to keep people informed about the emerging situation. Moreover, the people suffering from mental health issues would have much larger during lockdown and self-isolation restrictions, if there were no communication services to connect with relatives, friends and beloved ones remotely via voice or video conferencing platforms. Moreover, such services enabled Covid-19 patients to communicate and get assistance of emergency services such as mobile health teams or ambulances. Telecommunication services also helped public health departments to track and trace the individuals who had close contact with a patient tested positive for Covid-19.

CASE STUDIES

Human Emotion Detection

Amid pandemic, physical and mental health have been significantly affected. More recently, IoT based human emotion detection was proposed which used AI algorithm on human physiological descriptors (Awais, 2020). The physiological descriptors used to detect human emotions were electromyogram (EMG), electrocardiogram (ECG), blood volume pressure (BVP), galvanic skin response (GSR) and respiration sensors (RSP) and skin temperature (SKT). The basic objective of the work was to offer a remote emotion detection solution to assist in analyzing the emotions and communicate these to relevant personnel in near real time to assist in a variety of healthcare and learning situations. The work proposed long short-term memory (LSTM) based emotion detection system which classified human emotions with very high performance of 95%. In addition, ultra-low latency communication was achieved to enable near real-time communications. An IoT framework was proposed to achieve ultra-low-latency communications to transmit the physiological sensors data to IoT hub.

Monitoring of Parkinson Disease Patients Using IoT Framework

Parkinson disease (PD) is one of the leading neurological disorder with high treatment cost posing significant burden in term of requirements and resources in conventional healthcare system. Raza et al (Raza, 2020) proposed a IoT based framework to monitor the progression of PD patients remotely. The proposed IoT framework offered priority enabled communications with both static as well as dynamic scheduling to offer on-demand communication of the physiological and environmental sensory data. The findings suggested that the proposed framework in capable to offer effective communications with very low latency and high number of users. In addition, a machine learning based paradigm was also proposed which computed several features from auditory inputs obtained from PD patients and applied these to extreme gradient boosting (XGB) classifier to predict PD progression. The study concluded that the machine learning based PD progression evaluation is capable to predict the PD progression using auditory sensors.

LIMITATIONS OF SMART HEALTHCARE SOLUTIONS AND FUTURE RESEARCH DIRECTIVES

Smart healthcare solution, though promising alternative for the conventional healthcare, these are nowhere near the intended smart healthcare solutions. The vision of smart healthcare solutions is still long way from becoming a reality. Achieved outcomes and healthcare solutions, though impressive, yet, pose several limitations. Continuous improvement is needed in consistent research and

Over the years, the smart healthcare has transformed significantly. Several new research driven healthcare solutions and transformation of conventional healthcare to more diverse and technology driven digital healthcare systems has been witnessed. While a notable improvement in the proposed smart healthcare solutions offered promising results, yet, the outbreak of Covid-19 has changed the perception held for smart healthcare. The developments in the recent years, while promising, are in no position to overtake the conventional healthcare services. This has become abundantly evident during Covid crisis where new challenges have emerged which transformed the long-held vision for smart healthcare systems. While the smart healthcare solutions involving IoT, machine intelligence, decision support systems, diagnosis and analysis, rescue and emergency services, patient monitoring and artificial care services offer great potential there are certain limitations within the existing solutions which need thorough analysis and benchmarking. The main limitations of existing solutions can broadly be divided in four categories and evidently these are also the key aspects where the future research need to be directed for envisioned impact.

Policy Implementation and Legislations

Policies and legislations have a great significance in the healthcare sector. The role out of the new smart healthcare technologies cannot take place unless the stakeholders, social societies and governments play their part. The necessary evaluation of the liabilities, threats, limitations and legal standings is essential in any intelligent healthcare initiative implemented on large scale. While the governing bodies are taking different proposal under consideration. It is also important that the technology aspect is perfected before it is eligible to be used in healthcare. Due to the critical nature of the healthcare and high risks involved if something goes wrong, the job of the researchers/scientists is to maintain highest quality of work with absolute certainty of promised outcomes to be replicated in each consequent study.

Cross Platform/Technology Development

The healthcare solutions inherently require a multitude of technologies to solve any problems. While there are many individual proposals which use single technology to offer a solution in one aspect. It is the need of the time to bring into use all the technologies available and aim for a cross platform solution to be able to resolve more complex conventional healthcare problems. Cross platform smart healthcare solutions which may use, IoT, AI, cloud, edge services, decision support system, fog, software defined networking, blockchain, big data, deep neural networks and digital twins can only deem as a suitable and sustainable solution capable to sustain healthcare infrastructure in post Covid crisis.

Standardization and Benchmarking

It is vital that any healthcare solution follows specific evaluation as well as experimental similarity to benchmark various studies carried out. Currently, while the proposals are in abundance with very promising outcomes, however, lack of similar laboratory/ simulation parameters results in highly diverse results. Thus, it is hard to find out the ideal solution in the plethora of new proposals. Standardization and benchmarking is therefore necessary to introduce real impact with smart healthcare solutions.

Technology Resilience Enhancement in Pandemics

The current outbreak of Covid-19, while devastating, also offers an insight into potential health crisis of the future. Most of the smart healthcare solutions proposed in past few years do not envision the unpredictable and dynamic nature of healthcare needs and thus lack resilient solutions to cope with the changing healthcare needs. It is, therefore, highly desired to aim for the smart solutions capable of adopting with the needs. It is of utmost importance to improve resilience of the technology solutions to be able to help and support in wide range of health situations and needs. While the direct and dedicated solutions have played an important part in addressing specific problems, it is high time to investigate possibilities to introduce translational research solutions capable to transform and adapt with changing needs to offer desired resilience.

CONCLUSION

The healthcare infrastructure has been severely affected by the pandemics. The outbreak of Covid-19 has resulted in the worldwide impact unseen in the past pandemics. It highlighted the need for resilient healthcare solutions which bring technology to forefront of rescue efforts. In the quest for technology driven smart healthcare solutions, IoT and machine intelligence along with other enabling technologies can play a vital role. There are several aspects of healthcare where the technology driven solutions can make a real difference. Especially, IoT and machine learning can play an important role in enabling smart healthcare solutions whether it is diagnosis, tracking of infected patients, monitoring the vulnerable, testing, diagnosis, healthcare management, track and trace, smart healthcare facilities development or information sharing. In addition to these certain enabling technologies such as cloud, fog, blockchain, big data, etc. also offer potential to develop suitable solutions to ease the load from conventional healthcare infrastructure.

While there is great potential of developing smart healthcare solutions by using the state-of-the-art and enabling technologies there are certain limitations and emerging needs which need to be considered. There is an absolute need for the cross-platform development which benefits from diverse technologies to offer a substantial alternate to the conventional healthcare services. It is also needed that the resilience of the proposed healthcare solutions to be explored and new strategies are devised to enable transfer learning and translational research to cope with the changing healthcare needs. The benchmarking is also important in order to benefit from the developments across the globe and make use of the existing proposals and evaluate suitability of these for standardization.

REFERENCES

Afriyie, D. K., Asare, G. A., Amponsah, S. K., & Godman, B. (2020). COVID-19 pandemic in resource-poor countries: Challenges, experiences and opportunities in Ghana. *Journal of Infection in Developing Countries*, *14*(08), 838–843. doi:10.3855/jidc.12909 PMID:32903226

Arshadi, A. K., Webb, J., Salem, M., Cruz, E., Calad-Thomson, S., Ghadirian, N., ... Yuan, J. S. (2020). Artificial Intelligence for COVID-19 Drug Discovery and Vaccine Development. *Front. Artif. Intell*, *3*, 65. doi:10.3389/frai.2020.00065

Awais, M., Chiari, L., Ihlen, E. A. F., Helbostad, J. L., & Palmerini, L. (2018). Physical activity classification for elderly people in free-living conditions. *IEEE Journal of Biomedical and Health Informatics*, *23*(1), 197–207. doi:10.1109/ JBHI.2018.2820179 PMID:29994291

Awais, M., Palmerini, L., Bourke, A. K., Ihlen, E. A., Helbostad, J. L., & Chiari, L. (2016). Performance evaluation of state of the art systems for physical activity classification of older subjects using inertial sensors in a real life scenario: A benchmark study. *Sensors (Basel)*, *16*(12), 2105. doi:10.339016122105 PMID:27973434

Awais, M., Raza, M., Ali, K., Ali, Z., Irfan, M., Chughtai, O., Khan, I., Kim, S., & Ur Rehman, M. (2019). An Internet of Things based bed-egress alerting paradigm using wearable sensors in elderly care environment. *Sensors (Basel)*, *19*(11), 2498. doi:10.339019112498 PMID:31159252

Awais, M., Raza, M., Singh, N., Bashir, K., Manzoor, U., ul Islam, S., & Rodrigues, J. J. (2020). LSTM based Emotion Detection using Physiological Signals: IoT framework for Healthcare and Distance Learning in COVID-19. *IEEE Internet of Things Journal*.

Baker, S. B., Xiang, W., & Atkinson, I. (2017). Internet of things for smart healthcare: Technologies, challenges, and opportunities. *IEEE Access: Practical Innovations, Open Solutions*, *5*, 26521–26544. doi:10.1109/ACCESS.2017.2775180

Benson, T. (2020), *Twitter Bots Are Spreading Massive Amounts of COVID-19 Misinformation.* URL: https://spectrum.ieee.org/tech-talk/telecom/internet/twitter-bots-are-spreading-massive-amounts-of-covid-19-misinformation

Boatwright, A., & Wynne, W. A. (2020), *Record Global GDP Contraction Indicative of COVID-19's Cross-Country Effect.* https://www.dallasfed.org/research/ economics/2020/1006

Centers for Disease Control and Prevention. National Center for Immunization and Respiratory Diseases (NCIRD). (2019b) *Pandemic (H2N2 virus) 1957-1958.* https:// www.cdc.gov/flu/pandemic-resources/1957-1958-pandemic.html

Centers for Disease Control and Prevention (CDC). National Center for Immunization and Respiratory Diseases (NCIRD). (2019a) *Pandemic (H3N2 virus) 1968.* Available: https://www.cdc.gov/flu/pandemic-resources/1968-pandemic.html

Heaven, W. D. (2020). *Israel is using AI to flag high-risk covid-19 patients.* https:// www.technologyreview.com/2020/04/24/1000543/israel-ai-prediction-medical-testing-data-high-risk-covid-19-patients/

Hiscott, J., Alexandridi, M., Muscolini, M., Tassone, E., Palermo, E., Soultsioti, M., & Zevini, A. (2020). The global impact of the coronavirus pandemic. *Cytokine & Growth Factor Reviews*, *53*, 1–9. doi:10.1016/j.cytogfr.2020.05.010 PMID:32487439

John, M. L. (2001). *A dictionary of epidemiology*. Oxford university press.

Karalis, T., (2020). Planning and evaluation during educational disruption: Lessons learned from COVID-19 pandemic for treatment of emergencies in education. *European Journal of Education Studies*.

Khalid, M., Awais, M., Singh, N., Khan, S., Raza, M., Malik, Q. B., & Imran, M. (2021). *Autonomous Transportation in Emergency Healthcare Services: Framework, Challenges and Future Work. IEEE Internet of Things Magazine*.

Kirsal, Y., Ever, Y. K., Mapp, G. E., & Raza, M. (2021). *3D Analytical Modelling and Iterative Solution for High Performance Computing Clusters. IEEE Transactions on Cloud Computing*.

Lepan, N. (2020). *Visualizing the History of Pandemics*. URL: https://www.visualcapitalist.com/history-of-pandemics-deadliest/

Maliszewska, M., Mattoo, A., & Van Der Mensbrugghe, D. (2020). *The potential impact of COVID-19 on GDP and trade: A preliminary assessment*. Academic Press.

Moschou, K., Theodouli, A., Terzi, S., Votis, K., Tzovaras, D., Karamitros, D., & Diamantopoulos, S. (2020). Performance Evaluation of different Hyperledger Sawtooth transaction processors for Blockchain log storage with varying workloads. In *2020 IEEE International Conference on Blockchain (Blockchain)* (pp. 476-481). 10.1109/Blockchain50366.2020.00069

Qiu, W., Rutherford, S., Mao, A., & Chu, C. (2017). The pandemic and its impacts. *Health, Culture and Society (Pittsburgh, Pa.)*, *9*, 1–11. doi:10.5195/HCS.2017.221

Raza, M., Aslam, N., Le-Minh, H., Hussain, S., Cao, Y., & Khan, N. M. (2017a). A critical analysis of research potential, challenges, and future directives in industrial wireless sensor networks. *IEEE Communications Surveys and Tutorials*, *20*(1), 39–95. doi:10.1109/COMST.2017.2759725

Raza, M., Awais, M., Ellahi, W., Aslam, N., Nguyen, H. X., & Le-Minh, H. (2019). Diagnosis and monitoring of Alzheimer's patients using classical and deep learning techniques. *Expert Systems with Applications*, *136*, 353–364. doi:10.1016/j.eswa.2019.06.038

Raza, M., Awais, M., Singh, N., Imran, M., & Hussain, S. (2020). Intelligent IoT framework for indoor healthcare monitoring of Parkinson's disease patient. *IEEE Journal on Selected Areas in Communications.*

Raza, M., Le, M. H., Aslam, N., Le, C. H., Le, N. T., & Le, T. L. (2017b). Telehealth technology: Potentials, challenges and research directions for developing countries. In *International Conference on the Development of Biomedical Engineering in Vietnam* (pp. 523-528). Springer.

Raza, M., Singh, N., Khalid, M., Khan, S., Awais, M., Hadi, M.U., Imran, M., Islam, S., & Rodrigues, J.J.P.C. (2021). Challenges and limitations of Internet of Things enabled Healthcare in COVID-19. *IEEE Internet of Things Magazine.*

Saeed, N., Bader, A., Al-Naffouri, T. Y., & Alouini, M. S. (2020). When Wireless Communication Responds to COVID-19: Combating the Pandemic and Saving the Economy. *Frontiers in Communications and Networks*, *1*, 3. doi:10.3389/frcmn.2020.566853

Swayamsiddha, S., & Mohanty, C. (2020). Application of cognitive Internet of Medical Things for COVID-19 pandemic. *Diabetes & Metabolic Syndrome*, *14*(5), 911–915. doi:10.1016/j.dsx.2020.06.014 PMID:32570016

Ting, D. S. W., Carin, L., Dzau, V., & Wong, T. Y. (2020). Digital technology and COVID-19. *Nature Medicine*, *26*(4), 459–461. doi:10.103841591-020-0824-5 PMID:32284618

Vardhanabhuti, V. (2020). CT scan AI-aided triage for patients with COVID-19 in China. *The Lancet. Digital Health*, *2*(10), e494–e495. doi:10.1016/S2589-7500(20)30222-3 PMID:32984793

Vatandoost, M., & Litkouhi, S. (2019). The Future of Healthcare Facilities: How Technology and Medical Advances May Shape Hospitals of the Future. *Hospital Practices and Research*, *4*(1), 1–11. doi:10.15171/hpr.2019.01

Wittbold, K., Carroll, C., Iansiti, M., Zhang, H. M., & Landman, A. B. (2020). How Hospitals Are Using AI to Battle Covid-19. *Harvard Business Review*, 3.

World Health Organization. (2020). *World Coronavirus Disease (COVID-19) Dashboard.* https://covid19.who.int/

Zhou, Y., Wang, F., Tang, J., Nussinov, R., & Cheng, F. (2020). Artificial intelligence in COVID-19 drug repurposing. *The Lancet. Digital Health*, *2*(12), e667–e676. doi:10.1016/S2589-7500(20)30192-8 PMID:32984792

Chapter 3
Data Analytics Epidemic Modelling and Human Dynamics Approaches for Pandemic Outbreak

Marcello Trovati

ⓘD https://orcid.org/0000-0001-6607-422X
Edge Hill University, UK

ABSTRACT

A pandemic is a disease that spreads across countries or continents. It affects more people and takes more lives than an epidemic. Examples are Influenza A, HIV-1, Ebola, SARS, pneumonic plague. Currently, the ongoing COVID-19 pandemic is one of the major health emergencies in decades that has affected almost every country in the world. As of 23 October 2020, it has caused an outbreak with more than 40 million confirmed cases, and more than 1 million reported deaths globally. Also, as of 23 October 2020, the reproduction number (R) and growth rate of coronavirus (COVID-19) in the UK range is 1.2-1.4. Due to the unavailability of an effective treatment (or vaccine) and insufficient evidence regarding the transmission mechanism of the epidemic, the world population is currently in a vulnerable position. This chapter explores data analytics epidemic modelling and human dynamics approaches for pandemic outbreaks.

DOI: 10.4018/978-1-7998-6736-4.ch003

1. INTRODUCTION

Pandemic outbreaks refer to diseases that spread across countries or continents. They affect more people and take more lives than epidemics. Examples are Influenza A, HIV-1, Ebola, SARS, pneumonic plague (Gatherer, 2009). Currently, the ongoing COVID-19 pandemic is one of the major health emergencies in decades that has affected almost every country in the world. As of 23 October 2020, it has caused an outbreak with more than 40 million confirmed cases, and more than 1 million reported deaths globally. Also, as of 23 October 2020, the reproduction number (R) and growth rate of coronavirus (COVID-19) in the UK range is 1.2-1.4 (GOV. uk, 2020a). Due to the unavailability of an effective treatment (or vaccine) and insufficient evidence regarding the transmission mechanism of the epidemic, the world population is currently in a vulnerable position (Ghosh and Chakraborty, 2020).

Data Analytics models for epidemic and the human dynamics of such approaches are becoming increasingly important for global health policy makers and for the research community. These epidemiology models are aimed at understanding the spread of the disease and the impacts of different interventions. This is an important endeavour, especially as the world is currently witnessing a pandemic that has changed the landscape of events across the world. There is urgent need for global public health policy makers and researchers to design and develop strategies and models that can potentially help to control and contain existing and future pandemic outbreaks.

Many data analytics models have been applied to model epidemic. These models are aimed at predicting the number of new cases and for identifying the best measures to reduce transmission. Important challenges often faced by researchers that analysis epidemic data are that the data are inherently dependent and are usually incomplete in the sense that the actual process of infection is not observed (O'Neill, 2002). However, these challenges are often overcome by using stochastic models to describe the key features of epidemic spread and then use classical or Bayesian inference to estimate the parameters of the model and subsequently provide quantities of interest. This chapter presents a review of data analytics epidemic modelling and human dynamics approaches for pandemic outbreaks.

The chapter is organised as follows: In Sect. 2, we present a background and literature review and categorised them into a) Epidemic models approaches b) Human dynamics models of pandemic outbreaks. In Sect. 3, we present a discussion of the integration of the approaches. In Sect. 4, we conclude our work.

2. BACKGROUND AND LITERATURE REVIEW

Epidemic models have been categorised into Discrete event simulation (DES), Agent-based modelling (ABM), system dynamics (SD) and hybrid simulation (Currie et al, 2020). SD models are based on differential equation that represent real world systems in terms of material resources, knowledge, people, money, flows between them as well as the information that determines the values of the flows (Borshchev and Filippov, 2004). ABMs use stochastic models to address the human dynamics component of a pandemic outbreak. More specifically, they are used to model the interactions of individuals within a population thereby allowing a decision-maker to determine how changes in behaviour and interaction may influence population level outputs. In fact, the modelling of social networks and spatial movements are vital for accurately describing transmission. The use of stochastic models enables the variability of human behaviour to be incorporated and this helps to understand the variability in the likely effectiveness of proposed interventions. DES are stochastic models that consider the variability in the time taken to carry out activities and the times between arrivals into the hospital system. In fact, it is used to determine the impact of essential service resource availability (doctors; nurses), on waiting times and the number of entities waiting in the queues or going through the system. In fact, it helps to address the availability of such resources on the waiting queues in Intensive care Unit (ICU), while HS models are used to represent a complex system behaviour where different parts of the system can be better captured by two or more simulation methods. In this study we use this category to classify each of the models described.

Some models of the spread of epidemics are based on compartmental models that assume individuals are classified into non-intersecting sets. Moreover, some models have been specifically focused on flattening the growth curve of epidemic in order to reduce the burden on the healthcare system. The SEIR is an epidemic model that reflects the flow of people between four states: susceptible (S), infectious (I), and recovered (R) (Kermack and McKendrick, 1927). It is used at a population level to describe the proportion of the population in each state at any given time. Typically, in this model, individuals in S state would be infected by the I state individuals with probability β, whereas the I state individuals would recover to R state with a recovery probability γ. Thus, this produces a differential equations of SIR model. Various modification and extension of the SIR model have been used in the modelling of pandemic outbreaks. An example is the SEIR where the E represent exposed individual. In what follows, we describe each of the approaches and categorise them accordingly

In the remaining part of this section, the authors present approaches related to models for pandemic outbreaks. The authors have categorised the models into a) Epidemic models approaches b) Human dynamics models of pandemic outbreaks.

2.1. Epidemic Models Approach

O'Neill (2002) showed some Bayesian methods for the analysis of infectious disease outbreak data using stochastic epidemic models. Here the population consist of *N* households labelled *1, ..., N* and each containing individuals of whom certain numbers are initially infectious and the rest susceptible. Within the household *J,* an infected individual has a probability 1 - *qj* of being able to independently infect each other individual in the household. Newly infected individuals can then try to infect remaining susceptible individual sin the same manner, and the process continues until there are no more active infectives left. It used network inference techniques for learning the relevant epidemic parameters. These methods rely on Markov chain Monte Carlo methods that considered temporal and non-temporal data to perform the inference. The drawback of the model is that the available data do not explicitly contain the real-time progress of the epidemic. The result is an aggregate representation of the network and cannot distinguish among individuals with the same node degrees. Thus, the central properties of the individuals are ignored.

Das et al (2008) presented a simulation-based model that considered the demographic dimension of pandemic outbreaks. The approach mimics stochastic propagation of an influenza pandemic controlled by mitigation strategies. They modelled the problem of mitigating a pandemic outbreak as a Markov decision process (MDP). The model was tested on a hypothetical community with over 1.1 million people. They posit that their simulation-based framework can serve as the foundation for developing dynamic mitigation strategies and can be applied to other types of infectious disease outbreaks.

Youssef and Scoglio (2011) provided an individual-based approach to model the spread of epidemics in a network. The approach is based on continuous time Markov chain SIR model. In the model, the network is composed of nodes and edges where the node represents an individual and the edge represent the contact between a pair of individuals. Each individual can be in the S, I or R state with a given probability for each state. The approach used continuous-time Markov chain SIR model to decrease the complexity of the solution from exponential $O(3^N)$ to polynomial $O(N)$. Hence, each individual is studied specifically by decomposing $Q_3N \times_3 N$ matrix to *N* infinitesimal matrices, with three states: contact level between individual *v* and individual *z* in a weighted or unweighted network, and the Kronecker delta function 1 that represents the event that individual *z* is infected and zero otherwise. Thus, this evaluates the probability of infection of every individual, separately considering the probability of infection of the individual's neighbours. They performed Monte Carlo (MC) simulation to evaluate the accuracy of the approach. An important advantage of this model is that they provided individual-based approach which help to overcome the drawback of the models that only provide aggregate representations of the network.

Uribe-Sánchez et al (2011) provided simulation-based optimization methodology for generating dynamic predictive mitigation strategies for pandemic outbreaks. The methodology combines a cross-regional simulation model, a set of single-region simulation models, and a dynamic optimization control. They classified the regions as unaffected, ongoing outbreak and contained. These regions are interconnected by air and land travel, which is emulated by the cross-regional model. They used the single region model to mimic the population and disease dynamics inside each ongoing region, impacted by available pharmaceutical and non-pharmaceutical prevention and intervention. They simulated a mock outbreak of the pandemic from the ongoing regions to unaffected regions by infectious travelers who pass through regional border control. The cross-regional model invokes the optimization control which uses measures of morbidity, mortality, and social distancing, which are translated into the costs of lost productivity and medical services. They showed a simulation optimization algorithm and trained their model on pandemic data from four major population centers in USA of over 4 million. Finally, they showed a sensitivity analysis that estimate the impact of changes in the budget availability and variability of some of the critical parameters of mitigation strategies.

Sharareh et al. (2016) adopted a system dynamics approach to study the relationships between spread of disease, public attention, situational awareness, and community's response to the Ebola epidemic. They used SusceptibleInfectedRecovered (SIR) model to define the mathematical equations for contagion and depletion flow rates for the Ebola epidemic. The model adopts a third and fourth order information delay structure to capture the changes in public attention and situational awareness. The model used data from WHO. Their study demonstrate that quarantine has a significant impact on the spread of Ebola. They noted that the simulation models that are used to estimate the impact of quarantine strategies at the global level require many simplifying assumptions such as perfect mixing (i.e. each individual has the same probability to be infected by anyone in the population). They concluded that the best fit to historical data are achieved when behavioral factors specific to West Africa like the Situational Awareness and Public Attention are included in the model

Fang et al (2020) showed a parameterized SEIR model that simulated the spread dynamics of the COVID-19 outbreak and impact of different control measures. They applied the warehouse model on the population to study the infection rate, probability of infection per exposure as well as the migration rate and recovery time. They conducted the sensitivity analysis to identify the key factor and then plotted the trend curve of effective reproductive number (R). Thereafter, they performed data fitting that showed the peak existing confirmed cases. The evidence from their study suggest that the optimization of therapeutic strategy and the development of specific drugs would be of more importance than quarantine and protective procedures as more cases accrue.

Tang et al (2020) provided a deterministic, compartmental SEIR model that is based on the clinical progression of the disease, epidemiological status of the individuals, and intervention measures. The study provided analytics of data from China and the simulation of the model showed that reducing the contact rate persistently by isolation and quarantine decreases the peak value but may either delay or accelerate the peak.

Peng et al, (2020) showed a generalized SEIR model by including the self-protection and quarantine to analyze epidemic. Using public data on the cumulative numbers of quarantined cases from China, they showed a simulation that estimate key epidemic parameters and make predictions on the inflection point and possible ending time of specified provinces in China. They argued that their predictions have been proven to be well in agreement with the real situation.

Similarly, Mangoni and Pistilli (2020) develop a generalised SEIR model based on Peng et al (2020). They train the model on the dataset made available by the Italian government about the COVID-19 and analyze the dynamic epidemic characteristics of the outbreak in Italy. They used the model to estimate the epidemic parameters and make predictions about the future evolution of the outbreak. More specifically they analyse the data from different regions and forecast the inflection point, ending time and total infected cases.

Ghosh and Chakraborty (2020) propose an integrated deterministic-stochastic approach to forecast the long-term trajectories of the COVID-19 curve for Italy and Spain. In this approach, the deterministic component of the daily-cases univariate time-series is assessed by an extended version of the SIR (SIRCX) model, whereas its stochastic component is modeled using an autoregressive (AR) time series model. here they used the AR to analyse the residuals' uncertain behavior produced by the compartmental SIRCX model. They stated that the experimental analysis of the model shows significant improvement in the long-term forecasting of COVID-19 cases for Italy and Spain in comparison to the ODE-based SIRCX model.

2.2. Human Dynamics Models for Pandemic Outbreaks

Human dynamics plays an important role in the spread of infectious diseases and understanding the influence of these dynamics on the spread of diseases can be key to improving control efforts (Funk et al., 2010). The human dynamics of pandemic outbreaks can be considered from the perspective of the total numbers of humans infected, dead, denied hospital admission and denied vaccine/antiviral drugs, and also through an aggregate cost measure incorporating healthcare cost and lost wages (Das et al, 2008). Moreover, the demographic dimension could consider the ethnic composition, human movements, human behavious within and outside communities, hospitalization as well as daily human activities. Essentially, some of the epidemiology models described in this chapter are ideal for predicting the number of new cases or for identifying the best measures to reduce transmission. However, they may not be sufficient to address the human dynamics perspectives that are intricately linked with the spread of infectious diseases. For example, the reactions of humans to the spread of the disease, the interplay of the impact of individuals' behavior on the capacity of every essential system such as the health care system and food supply chains system (Currie et al, 2020). Essentially these are the human behaviours that have historically been linked with the spread of the disease (McNeill, 1998).

As the information about the disease and its spread is diffused simultaneously, the individuals who know about the disease will change their behavior to avoid being infected or prevent infecting the others (Zhang et al, 2016). The individual behaviour components of the human dynamics of pandemic outbreak can be considered from two perspectives. Firstly, Self-initiated or voluntary behaviour such as the scenarios where people first assess a situation based on both the information available to them about the disease and their beliefs, attitudes and then make a personal decision about how to respond to the given situation (Funk et al, 2010). Secondly, imposed behaviour as a result of government-imposed regulations and recommendations such as keeping two meters apart, the wearing of masks and other imposed rules during lockdown (GOV.uk, 2020b).

In this section, we present some models that captures the human dynamics of pandemic outbreaks.

Meloni et al (2011) provide a metapopulation modelling framework of self-initiated individual behavioural responses to the mobility patterns of individuals during the pandemic outbreaks. They defined a population of size N and partitioned it into V subpopulation. Each of the subpopulations consist of individuals that are stratified based on their dynamical state with respect to whether they are susceptible, infected, removed. More specifically, they used the SIR model to model the epidemic dynamics of the population. The model uses the network approach where the subpopulations are spatially structured as a network of V nodes and the edges denote the mobility connections of individuals across subpopulations. With this they defined the probability that any given subpopulation is connected to k other subpopulations. They indicate the average number of individuals in a subpopulation with a degree N_k. They modelled the self-initiated behavioural changes by assuming the probability of individual travelling from subpopulation i to subpopulation j is related to the level of infection at the destination subpopulation so that the higher the incidence of the infection at the destination, the less likely the individual will engage in traveling. Therefore, if travel is not cancelled, the individual uses the shortest path to get to the destination, however this is dependent on the changes in the traveling routes through the nodes in the network. They provided a simulation of the metapopulation network and found that prevalence-based travel limitations do not alter the epidemic invasion threshold. They noted that when travellers decide to avoid locations with high levels of prevalence, this self-initiated behavioral change may enhance disease spreading.

Similarly, Apolloni et al. (2014) describe a spatially structured population with non-homogeneous mixing and travel behaviour through a multi-host stochastic epidemic metapopulation model. Here individuals are distributed in subpopulations and connected by a network of mobility flows. Epidemic dynamics occurs inside each subpopulation and is ruled by a transmission matrix that account for the population partitions, mixing patterns and mobility structures. In fact, the model put the individual into two types of groups, 1 and 2 differing in contact and travel behaviour. The interaction between groups is described by a 2 x 2 contact matrix encoding the average behaviour of the two groups. Disease transmission is then modelled with a SIR compartmental scheme. The susceptible individuals may contract the infection from infectious individuals and enter the infectious compartment; all infectious individuals then recover permanently and enter the recovered compartment. They showed a mathematical formulation of the model and derive a semi-analytical expression of the threshold condition for global invasion of an emerging infectious disease in the metapopulation system. They validated the model by presenting the comparison between the results recovered so far and the output of stochastic numerical simulations, where all processes are simulated explicitly. The authors argue that the model can account for two different layers of heterogeneity relevant for the propagation of epidemics in a spatially structured environment, namely contact structure and heterogenous travel behaviour.

Li et al, (2017) propose a nonlinear differential model for human dynamics on nationwide epidemic spreading in Côte d'Ivoire. The model incorporates human mobility networks and human interaction intensity and demographic features. The epidemic spreading dynamic of the model is based on the SIR model. The model network consists of 255 nodes corresponding to 255 sub-prefectures in Côte d'Ivoire and the individual populations are allocated within these nodes. The connection between the sub-prefectures is characterised by the human mobility volume which they denoted as a matrix $A = [A_{ij}]$ where A_{ij} is the number of people moving from sub-prefecture i to j. The model uses local basic reproductive number (BRN) R_0 to indicate the number of infected cases that one case generates on average over the course of his infectious period such that When R0 < 1, the infection will die out in the long run in that region; if $R_0 > 1$, the infection will be able to spread among the population. More so, they used a weighted kshell method to detect the potential regions based on the human mobility matrix. The model was validated on a Call Detailed Record (CDR) data and an estimated population distribution based on the census in 1989. They showed a result that suggest that the impacts caused by human mobility on epidemic dynamics are strong. They posit that the combining the human interactions and weighted k-shell results, can identify critical paths for preventing nationwide epidemic outbreaks in the future.

Lin et al. (2020) adopted the SEIR framework and proposed a conceptual model that considered individual behavioural reaction and governmental actions. In the approach, they employed the estimates of individual behaviours and governmental actions from the 1918 influenza pandemic in London and incorporated zoonotic introductions and the emigration. With these they then computed future trends and the reported ratio. They used data from Wuhan, China to model the epidemic and assess the impact of mass social isolation policies. Their work is focused on the transmission of COVID-19 in Wuhan, China and they argued that their conceptual framework can be applied to other countries or be built into one (multiple-patched) model for multiple cities/countries.

Wang et al, (2020) employed Markov Chain Monte Carlo algorithm to propose a dynamical transmission model with contact tracing and quarantine for COVID-19. They simulate the data on the number of cumulative confirmed cases and used that to predict the trend of the infection. They estimate the basic reproductive number of COVID-19 and posit that reducing contact and increasing trace about the risk population are likely to be effective measures for the pandemic.

Hellewell et al. (2020) use a stochastic transmission model, parameterised to the COVID-19 epidemic to assess the effectiveness of contact tracing and isolation of cases. The model considered scenarios that varied in the number of initial cases, the basic reproduction number (R0), the delay from symptom onset to isolation, the probability that contacts were traced, the proportion of transmission that occurred before symptom onset, and the proportion of subclinical infections. They used the model to simulate outbreaks using disease transmission characteristics specific to the pathogen and give the best available evidence if contact tracing and isolation can achieve control of outbreaks. The study concludes that the effectiveness of isolation of cases and contacts to control outbreaks of COVID-19 depends on the precise characteristics of transmission.

Wells et al. (2020) and Gostic et al. (2020) provides models to determine the impact of international travel on epidemic. Wells et al. (2020) trained their model on incidence data and global airport network connectivity data and used Monte Carlo simulations to estimate exported cases with and without measures of travel restriction and screening. They validated estimates of importation risk using data from 21 countries reporting the arrival date of the first imported case. However, while Wells et al. (2020) focused on how limiting international travel will impact the course of the epidemic, combining data on the probability of transmission with data on global connectivity, Gostic et al. (2020) estimate the effectiveness of screening of travellers. Gostic et al. (2020) argue that their work underscores the need for measures to limit transmission by individuals who become ill after being missed by a screening program. They stated that their findings can support evidence-based policy to combat the spread of COVID-19 pandemic, and prospective planning to mitigate future emerging pathogens.

Disaster operations management (DOM) framework (Altay and Green, 2006) specifies the set of activities that are performed before, during, and after a disaster with the goal of preventing loss of human life, reducing its impact on the economy, and returning to a state of normalcy as disaster operations. DOM is split into four phases, mitigation, preparedness, response and recovery. Mitigation are the activities to prevent the onset of disaster or reduce its impact; Preparedness are the plans to handle an emergency; Response are the implementation of plans, policies and strategies from the preparedness phase while recovery are the long-term planning actions to bring the community back to normality. However, we note that these phases may not be as distinct in a pandemic situation as in other types of disaster because of the volatile and evolving nature of a pandemic as suggested by the current COVID-19 pandemic. Nonetheless, this framework will be used to classify each of the phases the models described in this work addressed.

3. DISCUSSION OF THE APPROACHES AND MOTIVATION FOR A HOLISTIC MODEL

In this chapter, the authors have presented and discussed various data analytics epidemic modelling for pandemic outbreaks. The models considered and addressed the human dynamics components to pandemic. Importantly, the models of human movements and behaviours were described. Moreover, a brief discussion of the categories of epidemic modelling techniques was presented. Most of the modelling techniques are based on stochastic and SEIR models. Some of the models described are ideal for predicting the number of new cases and best measures to reduce transmission while the others addressed the human dynamics perspectives of pandemic outbreaks. Essentially, the use of stochastic models enables the variability of human behaviour to be incorporated and this helps to understand the variability in the likely effectiveness of proposed interventions.

We argue for a comprehensive and a holistic model for pandemic outbreak that must take into consideration the integration of models from these categories. In particular, this integration would also need to consider the misinformation regarding public health, which mass media and social networks have shared and disseminated (Tagliabue, et al, 2020). The compartmental models described can be used to estimate the infection parameters given the number of confirmed infected cases during pandemics and epidemics. They can also be used to predict the peak of the infected cases and to define and test efficient mitigation strategies. However, a drawback of some of these compartmental models is that they are aggregate representations of the network, as they cannot distinguish among individuals with the same node degrees and ignores the central properties of the individuals (Zhang et al, 2016). However, the models provided by Youssef and Scoglio, (2011); Meloni et al (2011); Apolloni et al. (2014) overcome these drawbacks by providing individual-based approach. While Youssef and Scoglio (2011) considered the evaluation of the state probability for every individual in the spread of the disease, Meloni et al (2011) and Apolloni et al. (2014) considered the specific self-initiated individual behaviours changes that have impact on the spread of the pandemic. Therefore, we argue for a framework for the integration of these models. The model must incorporate the impact of isolation, quarantine and human behaviours that mediates spreading of disease (Sharareh et al., 2016, Tang et al 2020, Peng et al, 2020); therapeutic strategy and the development of specific drugs (Fang et al, 2020); individual behaviour and government actions (Lin et al. 2020); and models that provides evidence for contact tracing, which is the main determinant of the disease transmission (Wang et al, 2020, Hellewell et al, 2020). Moreover, models that considers human movements by limiting international travels and screening of travelers (Li et al, 2017, Wells et al. 2020, Gostic et al., 2020) as well as models that takes into account the mobility pattern of individual triggered by Self-initiated behavioural changes (Meloni et al 2011; Apolloni et al. 2014) can also be incorporated to provide holistic framework for evidence-based policy for pandemic outbreak.

The aim of this chapter is to provide a description of the main frameworks related to epidemic modelling and human dynamics. As a consequence, a detailed discussion on the technical aspects (including their implementation) of the different approaches is not included. For a review on this area, refer to Giordano at al. (2020) and Mata (2021).

Table 1. Evaluation of Epidemic modelling approaches

Author	Modelling Technique	Category of Modelling Technique	DOM Phase Addressed	Result and Implication for Pandemic Outbreak
O'Neill (2002)	Bayesian methods/ stochastic epidemic models	Agent-based modelling (ABM), Discrete event simulation (DES)	Mitigation, Preparedness, Response, recovery	Developing Bayesian inference for large population models is important for developing models for pandemic outbreaks
Das et al (2008)	Stochastic model	Agent-based modelling (ABM), Discrete event simulation (DES)	Preparedness, Response	Simulation-based framework that can serve as the foundation for developing dynamic mitigation strategies for shortage of vaccines/ antiviral drugs and costs during pandemic outbreaks.
Youssef and Scoglio (2011)	Markov chain stochastic model/SIR model	Discrete event simulation (DES)	Preparedness, Response,	Provided individual-based approach to model the spread of epidemics in a network. Model can be used to evaluate the probability of infection of every individual separately considering the probability of infection of the individual's neighbours
Meloni et al (2011)	metapopulation approach based on SIR model	Agent-based modelling (ABM), Discrete event simulation (DES)	Mitigation, Preparedness	Formulated and analysed a metapopulation model that incorporates several scenarios of self-initiated behavioral changes into the mobility patterns of individuals. Model can provide guide on government-imposed regulations that triggers individual behavioural changes
Li et al. (2017)	metapopulation approach based on SIR model	Agent-based modelling (ABM), Discrete event simulation (DES)	Mitigation, Preparedness	Provides human mobility and human interaction intensity on epidemic dynamics. the model identifies critical paths of human mobility for preventing nationwide epidemic outbreaks in the future.
Apolloni et al. (2014)	Stochastic model	Agent-based modelling (ABM)	Mitigation, Preparedness	Model can be used for pandemic preparedness to identify adequate interventions and quantitatively estimate the corresponding required effort to assess the pandemic potential of the pathogen from population and early outbreak data.
Uribe-Sánchez et al (2011)	simulation-based optimization methodology	Agent-based modelling (ABM), Discrete event simulation (DES)	Preparedness, Response	Provides a model for developing dynamic strategies for allocation of limited resources during a pandemic outbreak involving multiple regions.
Sharareh et al. (2016)	System dynamics, causal loop diagram and SIR model	System Dynamics	Response, recovery	Increase of quarantining rate over time and understanding behaviour of communities had a significant impact on the control of epidemic

continues on following page

Table 1. Continued

Author	Modelling Technique	Category of Modelling Technique	DOM Phase Addressed	Result and Implication for Pandemic Outbreak
Lin et al. (2020)	SEIR	Agent-based modelling (ABM),	Preparedness, Response, recovery	Has implication for individual behavioural reaction and governmental actions such as hospitalisation and quarantine intervention for pandemic outbreak. Model can be used for modelling multiple cities/countries context.
Fang et al (2020)	SEIR	Agent-based modelling (ABM),	Preparedness, Response, recovery	Provides evidence for intervention for early detection, early isolation, early treatment and comprehensive therapeutic strategy
Tang et al (2020)	SEIR	Agent-based modelling (ABM),	Response, recovery	Provides evidence on estimating the basic reproduction number (r) for determining the potential and severity of an outbreak and for providing critical information for identifying the type of disease interventions and intensity
Peng et al, (2020)	SEIR	Agent-based modelling (ABM),	Preparedness, Response, recovery	Provides evidence on estimating key epidemic parameters that can serve as cue for making predictions on the inflection point and possible ending time
Mangoni and Pistilli (2020)	Generalised SEIR model	Agent-based modelling (ABM),	Response, recovery	Provides evidence on forecasting the potential trajectory of pandemic outbreak that can inform appropriate measures by policy makers
Ghosh and Chakraborty (2020)	Deterministic SIRCX/Stochastic model	Hybrid simulation (HS)	Response, recovery	Model provides evidence on long-term forecasting of pandemic outbreak
Wang et al, (2020)	SEIR	Agent-based modelling (ABM)	Mitigation, Preparedness, Response, recovery	Provides evidence on using contact tracing and quarantine to predict the peak time and final size for daily confirmed infected cases
Hellewell et al. (2020)	Stochastic model	Agent-based modelling (ABM), Discrete event simulation (DES),	Preparedness, Response, recovery	Provides evidence that highly effective contact tracing and case isolation is enough to control a new outbreak of pandemic within 3 months

4. CONCLUSION

In this chapter, we have provided a review of data analytics epidemic and human dynamics modelling approaches for pandemic outbreaks and how these may affect the relevant mitigation measure. These models are based on various parameters, which can potentially influence the decision-making process in investigating, assess and contain disease transmission and interventions, resource management. From our discussion, it is clear that an integration of these models can provide a holistic framework for interventions for pandemic outbreaks, so that their limitations can be minimized, whilst enhancing their predictive capabilities. Furthermore, an integrated approach of these models has significant potential to inform large-scale anti-contagion policies that are required for pandemic outbreaks.

REFERENCES

Altay, N., & Green, W. G. III. (2006). OR/MS research in disaster operations management. *European Journal of Operational Research*, *175*(1), 475–493. doi:10.1016/j.ejor.2005.05.016

Apolloni, A., Poletto, C., Ramasco, J. J., Jensen, P., & Colizza, V. (2014). Metapopulation epidemic models with heterogeneous mixing and travel behaviour. *Theoretical Biology & Medical Modelling*, *11*(1), 3. doi:10.1186/1742-4682-11-3 PMID:24418011

Borshchev, A., & Filippov, A. (2004, July). From system dynamics and discrete event to practical agent based modeling: reasons, techniques, tools. In *Proceedings of the 22nd international conference of the system dynamics society* (*Vol. 22*). Academic Press.

Currie, C. S., Fowler, J. W., Kotiadis, K., Monks, T., Onggo, B. S., Robertson, D. A., & Tako, A. A. (2020). How simulation modelling can help reduce the impact of COVID-19. *Journal of Simulation*, *14*(2), 1–15. doi:10.1080/17477778.2020.1751570

Das, T. K., Savachkin, A. A., & Zhu, Y. (2008). A large-scale simulation model of pandemic influenza outbreaks for development of dynamic mitigation strategies. *IIE Transactions*, *40*(9), 893–905. doi:10.1080/07408170802165856

Fang, Y., Nie, Y., & Penny, M. (2020). Transmission dynamics of the COVID-19 outbreak and effectiveness of government interventions: A data-driven analysis. *Journal of Medical Virology*, *92*(6), 645–659. doi:10.1002/jmv.25750 PMID:32141624

Funk, S., Salathé, M., & Jansen, V. A. (2010). Modelling the influence of human behaviour on the spread of infectious diseases: A review. *Journal of the Royal Society, Interface, 7*(50), 1247–1256. doi:10.1098/rsif.2010.0142 PMID:20504800

Gatherer, D. (2009). The 2009 H1N1 influenza outbreak in its historical context. *Journal of Clinical Virology, 45*(3), 174–178. doi:10.1016/j.jcv.2009.06.004 PMID:19540156

Ghosh, I., & Chakraborty, T (2020). *An integrated deterministic-stochastic approach for forecasting the long-term trajectories of COVID-19.* Academic Press.

Giordano, G., Blanchini, F., Bruno, R., Colaneri, P., Di Filippo, A., Di Matteo, A., & Colaneri, M. (2020). Modelling the COVID-19 epidemic and implementation of population-wide interventions in Italy. *Nature Medicine, 26*(6), 855–860. doi:10.103841591-020-0883-7 PMID:32322102

Gostic, K., & Ana, C. R. (2020). Estimated effectiveness of symptom and risk screening to prevent the spread of COVID-19. *eLife, 9*, e55570. doi:10.7554/eLife.55570 PMID:32091395

GOV.uk. (2020a). *Guidance: The R number and growth rate in the UK.* Online available at: https://www.gov.uk/guidance/the-r-number-in-the-uk

GOV.uk. (2020b). *Guidance New National Restrictions from 5 November.* Online available at: https://www.gov.uk/guidance/new-national-restrictions-from-5-november

Hellewell, J., Abbott, S., Gimma, A., Bosse, N. I., Jarvis, C. I., Russell, T. W., ... Flasche, S. (2020). Feasibility of controlling COVID-19 outbreaks by isolation of cases and contacts. *The Lancet. Global Health, 8*(4), e488–e496. doi:10.1016/S2214-109X(20)30074-7 PMID:32119825

Kermack, W. O., & McKendrick, A. G. (1927). A contribution to the mathematical theory of epidemics. *Proceedings of the Royal Society of London. Series A, Containing Papers of a Mathematical and Physical Character, 115*(772), 700–721. doi:10.1098/rspa.1927.0118

Li, M. Y., Smith, H. L., & Wang, L. (2001). Global dynamics of an SEIR epidemic model with vertical transmission. *SIAM Journal on Applied Mathematics, 62*(1), 58–69. doi:10.1137/S0036139999359860

Li, R., Wang, W., & Di, Z. (2017). Effects of human dynamics on epidemic spreading in Côte d'Ivoire. *Physica A, 467*, 30–40. doi:10.1016/j.physa.2016.09.059

Lin, Q., Zhao, S., Gao, D., Lou, Y., Yang, S., Musa, S. S. & He, D. (2020). A conceptual model for the outbreak of Coronavirus disease 2019 (COVID-19) in Wuhan, China with individual reaction and governmental action. *International Journal of Infectious Diseases.*

Mangoni, L., & Pistilli, M. (2020). *Epidemic analysis of Covid-19 in Italy by dynamical modelling.* Academic Press.

Mata, A. (2021). An overview of epidemic models with phase transitions to absorbing states running on top of complex networks. *Chaos (Woodbury, N.Y.), 31*(1), 1. doi:10.1063/5.0033130

McNeill, W. H., & McNeill, W. (1998). *Plagues and peoples.* Anchor.

Meloni, S., Perra, N., Arenas, A., Gómez, S., Moreno, Y., & Vespignani, A. (2011). Modeling human mobility responses to the large-scale spreading of infectious diseases. *Scientific Reports, 1*(1), 62. doi:10.1038rep00062 PMID:22355581

O'Neill, P. D. (2002). A tutorial introduction to Bayesian inference for stochastic epidemic models using Markov chain Monte Carlo methods. *Mathematical Biosciences, 180*(1-2), 103–114. doi:10.1016/S0025-5564(02)00109-8 PMID:12387918

Peng, L., Yang, W., Zhang, D., Zhuge, C., & Hong, L. (2020). *Epidemic analysis of COVID-19 in China by dynamical modeling.* arXiv preprint arXiv:2002.06563. doi:10.1101/2020.02.16.20023465

Sharareh, N., Sabounchi, N. S., Sayama, H., & MacDonald, R. (2016). The ebola crisis and the corresponding public behavior: A system dynamics approach. *PLoS Currents*, 8. PMID:27974995

Tagliabue, F., Galassi, L., & Mariani, P. (2020). The "Pandemic" of Disinformation in COVID-19. *SN Comprehensive Clinical Medicine, 1–3*(9), 1287–1289. Advance online publication. doi:10.100742399-020-00439-1 PMID:32838179

Tang, B., Wang, X., Li, Q., Bragazzi, N. L., Tang, S., Xiao, Y., & Wu, J. (2020). Estimation of the transmission risk of the 2019-nCoV and its implication for public health interventions. *Journal of Clinical Medicine, 9*(2), 462. doi:10.3390/jcm9020462 PMID:32046137

Uribe-Sánchez, A., Savachkin, A., Santana, A., Prieto-Santa, D., & Das, T. K. (2011). A predictive decision-aid methodology for dynamic mitigation of influenza pandemics. *OR-Spektrum, 33*(3), 751–786. doi:10.100700291-011-0249-0 PMID:32214571

Wang, K., Lu, Z., Wang, X., Li, H., Li, H., Lin, D., & Ji, W. (2020). Current trends and future prediction of novel coronavirus disease (COVID-19) epidemic in China: A dynamical modeling analysis. *Mathematical Biosciences and Engineering, 17*(4), 3052–3061. doi:10.3934/mbe.2020173 PMID:32987516

Wells, C. R., Sah, P., Moghadas, S. M., Pandey, A., Shoukat, A., Wang, Y., & Galvani, A. P. (2020). Impact of international travel and border control measures on the global spread of the novel 2019 coronavirus outbreak. *Proceedings of the National Academy of Sciences of the United States of America, 117*(13), 7504–7509. doi:10.1073/pnas.2002616117 PMID:32170017

Youssef, M., & Scoglio, C. (2011). An individual-based approach to SIR epidemics in contact networks. *Journal of Theoretical Biology, 283*(1), 136–144. doi:10.1016/j.jtbi.2011.05.029 PMID:21663750

Zhang, Z. K., Liu, C., Zhan, X. X., Lu, X., Zhang, C. X., & Zhang, Y. C. (2016). Dynamics of information diffusion and its applications on complex networks. *Physics Reports, 651*, 1–34. doi:10.1016/j.physrep.2016.07.002

Section 2
Data Science Practices in Pandemic Management

Chapter 4
The Importance of Big Data Metadata in Crisis Management

Bill Karakostas
Independent Researcher, UK

ABSTRACT

Big data have the potential to change the way responders make sense of crisis situations, respond, and make decisions concerning the crises. At the same time, however, the explosion to the amount of crisis-related data can create an information overload to the crisis responders, and a challenge for their efficient management and utilisation. Crisis big data streams for epidemics may lack, for instance, key demographic identifiers such as age and sex, or may underrepresent certain age groups as well as residents of developing countries. Relevant metadata information needs therefore to be obtained and validated in order to trust make predictions and decisions based on the big data set. Crisis-related big data must be meaningful to the responders in order to form the basis of sound decisions. The aim of the chapter is to review all issues pertaining to the use of metadata for big data in emergency/ crisis management situations.

1. INTRODUCTION

1.1 The Rise of 'Big Data'

A recent IDC study titled "Discover the Digital Universe of Opportunities" states that from 2013 to 2020, the digital universe grew by a factor of 10, i.e. from 4.4

DOI: 10.4018/978-1-7998-6736-4.ch004

trillion gigabytes to 44 trillion. In particular, due to proliferation of technologies such as the Internet of Things (IoT), it is becoming easier and cheaper to capture ('Big') data from a variety of physical entities and processes, such as the natural environment. This provides tremendous opportunities to enhance our situation awareness under different circumstances, such as emergencies and crises, for instance, natural disasters, pandemics and other outbreaks. However, a mental leap is required to convert the captured Big Data into useful *information* that can enhance our understanding of the crisis in order to make better decisions. The gap between (Big) data and information needs to be bridged by technologies that augment the Big Data with additional (meta) data that make them meaningful in a particular context, and transform them into actionable *information*. One mechanism for data augmentation through metadata is *tagging*. However, the above mentioned IDC study estimates that only 3% of potentially useful data will be tagged (IDC, 2012).

There is general consensus, amongst researchers and practitioners alike, that metadata are paramount to Big Data success (Schmarzo, 2018). According to a Gartner blog, unstructured data content were estimated to represent as much as eighty percent of an organisation's total information assets (Stewart, 2013). Tapping on this ever-growing volume of unstructured data in an effective manner can create a competitive advantage, or alternatively, failure to exploit such data can ultimately cost the organisation lost market share. Being able to effectively organize and categorize such information assets ultimately deliver more intelligence into the business by enabling better and faster decision-making. A major problem is the vast volume of these information assets and the associated number of disparate information sources that can extend across multiple business units. In particular, semi-structured and unstructured data content spread across many internal IT systems and business applications, makes their cataloguing, retrieval and analysis hard.

1.2 Metadata and the 'Big Data Gap'

According to a report published by IDC (IDC, 2011), metadata is one of the fastest-growing sub-areas of enterprise data management. The IDC report emphasises that while metadata use is growing, it is not keeping pace with the rapid increase in Big Data projects, something referred to by IDC as the 'Big Data gap'. Metadata can greatly streamline and enhance processes to collect, integrate, and analyse Big Data sources. Without metadata, organisations may fail to gain from the deep insights that Big Data can yield. Metadata can capture and record the entire data life cycle, processes, procedures and customers or users affecting specific business information and can provide an audit trail that can be essential, especially for regulated businesses. Big Data metadata is the foundation for harnessing vast amounts of data from disparate data sources and information repositories before they become unmanageable.

With the increase of Big Data initiatives the value of metadata is therefore, quickly coming to the forefront and is surfacing as a critical priority for Big Data success. The most important characteristic of Big Data processing platforms such as Hadoop is that they are schema-agnostic. This means that the onus is on the platform users to understand what the data truly is. This can only be achieved if the data is supported by metadata, and for large scale process this requires support from a comprehensive metadata management infrastructure. Thus, the importance of metadata for Big Data cannot be underestimated.

1.3 Big Data Metadata and Crisis Management

Crisis information management includes the processing and use of Big Data by crisis responders in order to control the crisis situation (Boersma & Fonio, 2019). In crisis management, data generated by official organisations, administrations, media and ordinary citizens, can be collected and shared by social media platforms to provide effective response to the crisis. For this however, a crisis information management system is required, i.e. a system of hardware, software and networks to create, collect, filter, process and distribute data. Crisis information management means that data can be translated into actionable information to improve the quality of response (Boersma et al 2012). Although, traditionally, crisis responders relied on official crisis information systems for their information, the explosion of digital data, mainly due to the widespread use of mobile phones, represent additional sources of dynamic real time information about the crisis. This means that potentially new sources and streams of crisis data need to be dynamically added to the crisis information management system.

For instance, in pandemic crises, new Big Data sources must be considered, that include not only the passively observed Big Data streams from mobile phones, but also detailed environmental data and local sensor information from distributed devices, internet search information, and pathogen genomic data (Buckee, 2020). During epidemics and pandemic crises, decisions must be made quickly and situations monitored continuously for rapidly evolving emergencies. Additionally, new streams of Big Data must be transferred rapidly and communicated between geographically disparate teams of crisis responders.

Big data therefore, have the potential to change the way responders make sense of the crisis situation, respond to it and make decisions concerning the crisis. At the same time however, the explosion to the amount of crisis related data can create an information overload (Hiltz & Plotnick, 2013) to the crisis responders, and a challenge for their efficient management and utilisation.

Crisis Big Data streams, for epidemics, may lack, for instance, key demographic identifiers such as age and sex, or may underrepresent certain age groups as well as residents of developing countries (Potash, 2017). Relevant metadata information needs therefore to be obtained and validated in order to trust make predictions and decisions based on the Big Data set.

As with Big Data for other domains, therefore, crisis related Big Data must be meaningful to the responders in order to form the basis of sound decisions. In fact, as such data originate in multiple sources of unknown provenance, it becomes more important to obtain additional information about their content as well as the context in which they originated, i.e. metadata.

1.4 Chapter Objectives and Organisation

The aim of the chapter is to review all issues pertaining to the use of metadata for Big Data in emergency/crisis management situations. The Chapter reviews the current State of the Art and identify gaps in Big Data metadata management, particularly in epidemic and pandemic crises. Finally, it outlines the characteristics for a framework for effective management of Big Data metadata in a crisis management context.

The organisation of the chapter is as follows:

The next section defines the concept of Big Data metadata, and their significance and role in Big Data projects.

Section 3 reviews techniques and technologies for Big Data metadata management (governance) and recent initiatives towards metadata standardisation.

Section 4 discusses common types of metadata of importance to crisis management, such as geospatial metadata and mobile call records (CDRs).

Section 5 outlines a framework of key tenets of metadata management in a crisis context.

Finally, Section 6 summarises the findings of this Chapter and makes recommendations for further research needed

2. BIG DATA AND METADATA

2.1 What Is Metadata?

Metadata can be defined as '*a set of data that describes and gives information about other data',* according to the Oxford Dictionary. Metadata are critical items of information that enhances our understanding about properties of the Big Data such as provenance *(lineage)* and, ultimately, quality. Quality in turn, determines the trustworthiness of the Big Data. For instance, if the data quality is poor, the emergency response organisation that utilises such data to make decisions will suffer from the results of inconsistent or inaccurate analyses and will as a result, make bad decisions. The representational/selectivity property of the captured Big Data needs to be ascertained. Because the majority of Big Data is unstructured, it requires a lot of effort to transform unstructured types into structured types and further process the data, without the use of metadata. In addition, the diversity of Big Data sources with voluminous data types and complex data structures increases the difficulty of data integration. This represents a significant challenge to the existing Big Data management technologies.

Important types of metadata include:

- lineage (provenance) information, i.e. –how, when and by whom a dataset was created
- summary description, contact and resource information, themes and keywords
- metadata that describes the age, accuracy, content, currency, scale, reliability, authorship and custodianship of an individual dataset
- standards used in the creation of the dataset.

Although metadata management approaches exists for traditional structured information systems such as data warehouses and normalized relational databases, this is not the case for Big data sets as these are often unstructured. Big Data processing systems such as Hadoop, do not require the description of metadata at the time of Big Data capture, as only a unique identifier of the data is required. However, for effective analytical processing such metadata will have to be eventually defined. Once identified such metadata can be correlated to other metadata defined for traditional (structured) data sources in providing an overall comprehensive metadata model.

There are several types of Big Data metadata, such as:

Descriptive metadata that contains additional information to identify a Big Data set.

Structural metadata that depicts how information items such as records are related in the Big Data set.

Administrative metadata that provides information used to operationally manage the Big Data set (e.g. author, creation time, and so on).

However, as metadata are also data themselves, they can suffer from the same quality problems as the Big Data, namely incompleteness, incorrectness and ambiguity. For this purpose, Big Data metadata description standardisation and formal ontologies can play a positive role.

Completeness in terms of coverage and sampling that are representativeness of selectivity in the Big data capture process needs to be described through metadata. If, for instance, the subset of the population captured by the Big Data is representative of the general population with regard to a given variable, the Big data set is complete, otherwise it is selective. Sparsity is another relevant Big data quality dimension, impacting the informativeness of the Big Data set. Properties such as selectivity are of particular importance for epidemic related Big Data, as the impact of the epidemic on the different population subsets must be understood.

Metadata also help to create and maintain data consistency. Concepts and entities represented by the Big Data must have a common definition across the different applications and business units that utilise the Big Data. Often, the semantics of the same data entity may change in different application areas, affecting the integrity of the Big Data processing results. Approaches to resolve this issue includes the tagging of application terms or names with the help of domain specific ontologies that help to achieve semantic consensus. Often, lack of consistency in Big Data for crisis management results from infrastructure failures and malfunctions such as unreliable wireless communications. Metadata ensures a more accurate picture of data across your enterprise, further ensuring this level of data consistency for Big Data analytics and business applications. For instance, metadata can be used to monitor the consistency of Big Data streams, which can depict the trend of the parameters being monitored, or report a complex event.

2.2 The Value of Big Data Metadata

Metadata can help to make Big Data identifiable, discoverable, usable and ultimately, useful . This is especially valuable in crisis situations where diverse data sources and formats need to be handled. In general, the ability to collect and analyse internal and external data can dictate how well an organization such as a crisis responder will generate knowledge and understanding.

Big Data metadata can help to identify patterns that ultimately provides structure and meaning to the Big Data. Patterns help individual Big Data users to achieve their particular goals. In this respect, the focus of Big Data is to advance wide organizational goals, while patterns help individuals achieve personal goals. Patterns can help users get a better overview of the Big Data, i.e. situation awareness.

Metadata therefore can assist with data discovery and allows a way to interpret and use Big Data in an accurate manner. Metadata can link the disparate data assets by using different association criteria. The incorporation of meaningful metadata attributes into semi-structured or unstructured Big Data makes these data assets more valuable when searching for relevant information. Search algorithms can utilise metadata to yield high confidence results. This is particularly beneficial in Big Data initiatives whereby keyword based search can retrieve vast amounts of data. In contrast, by leveraging associations defined by metadata, Big Data analytics can quickly retrieve the right information across several and disparate Big Data sets.

2.3 Big Data Analytics and Metadata

Big Data analytics is a field that combines methods and technologies from computer science, statistics, signal processing, data mining, and machine learning (including, geospatial technologies, and visual analytics which are of interest in crisis management), to mine insights.

Big crisis data analytics, aims to leverage big data analytics techniques, along with digital platforms (such as mobile phones/Internet), for efficient humanitarian response to different crises (Quadir et al, 2016). There are many application areas of Big data for crisis response, including data-driven digital epidemiology (in which public health research is conducted using CDRs and social media) (Salathe et al. 2012), population surveillance and urban analytics (Boulos et al. 2011) (in which data is used to track the movement of population during a crisis), and crisis informatics and sociology (Palen et al. 2007) (in which data, along with participatory mapping and crowdsourcing technology, is used for analysing the sociological behaviour of the affected community through behavioural inference and '*reality mining*').

NLP (Natural Language Processing) and Machine Learning (ML) technologies that provide either visual analytics to prioritise information, or threat detection, have emerged as crisis management tools in recent years. The drivers for NLP and ML have been the increasing use of social media data and crowdsourcing in crisis situations, with social media in particular starting to become a major channel to disseminate and share crisis related information. The vast amount of information on social media makes the discovery of relevant information in an effective manner particularly hard, creating information overload and inability to separate relevant information from noise. Machine Learning and Information Extraction techniques are used to extract information from social media streams and use that information to learn patterns and trends (Lanfranchi, 2017) .

3. TECHNOLOGIES AND STANDARDS FOR BIG DATA METADATA MANAGEMENT

3.1 Metadata Governance

Metadata governance refers to approaches that establish stewardship for metadata. Governance of metadata further ensures data consistency and supports accurate Big Data driven analytics decisions. Stewardship is necessary for the implementation of metadata governance practices, as it provides the users with value and a context for understanding the Big Data. Some of the major responsibilities of the metadata governance includes documenting the context of the metadata (heritage and lineage), and the definitions of data entities and attributes, as well as of the relationships between such entities. Governance requires the existence of procedures for the validation of data timeliness, accuracy and completeness. Metadata governance can also assist in the development of data compliance and associated legal and regulatory controls. Proper metadata governance can contribute to the success of Big Data initiative success and further ensure complete and full realization of an organisation's information assets.

As Big Data utilisation increases, new types of metadata arise to address the special requirements of specific domains. Metadata governance can accommodate new types of metadata and leverage faster access to large diverse Big Data stores across the various repositories such as data lakes, data warehouses and relational databases.

Recent standardisation effort by organisations such as ISO and IEC target the formal and precise description of metadata as well as the transfer of such metadata between information systems. These standards utilise formal description languages (*ontologies*) such as the Basic Formal Ontology (BFO). BFO is a top-level ontology with the purposes of promoting interoperability among domain ontologies. The ISO/IEC 11179-1:2015 standard is used for the formulation of data representations, concepts, meanings and relationships to be shared among people and machines, independent of the organization that produces the data. The ISO/IEC 21838-2* Part 2, Basic Formal Ontology (BFO), standard provides definitions of its terms and relational expressions and formalizations in Web Ontology Language (OWL) and in Common Logic (CL).

The purpose of the ISO/IEC TR 19583-1 Part 1, standard is to:

- define metadata concepts
- provide the means for understanding the concept of metadata
- explain the kind and quality of metadata necessary to describe data, and
- specify the management of that metadata in a metadata registry (MDR).

Another relevant data representation standard for Big Data metadata management is the Resource Description Framework (RDF) model (Ducharme, 2013). The RDF model decomposes data into triples which are of subject, predicate and object type. RDF allows to describe both data and metadata in a common language. RDF query languages such as SPARQL which has syntax similar to SQL can be used to search through metadata.

3.2 Metadata Repositories

Metadata repositories are essential for effective metadata governance. They are used to store, curate and process metadata. The management of stored metadata, ensures consistency across the whole organisation. Design tools can greatly help to visualize the entities and relationships described in metadata. Data mapping can connect data visually between the source and destination attributes and define the Big Data processing logic. Business Process Execution Language (BPEL) is an example of a process description language that utilises a metadata visualization approach to define the logic of a data flow diagram.

Metadata repository functionality allows searches across both structured data and unstructured content repositories. Metadata can link all of the content related to one or more metadata attributes regardless of locality or format, for example, to provide information about a data item. A metadata attribute can also be used to link disparate Big Data sources, for cross-data integration purposes.

In general, there are three approaches to building a metadata repository. A central metadata repository, most prevalent today, that provides managed scalability for new metadata to be captured and allows access with high performance. In contrast, distributed metadata repositories have evolved over the years, enabling users to retrieve metadata from disparate repositories. Finally, a hybrid approach utilises characteristics of the prior two types of repositories, by supporting both real-time access across disparate repositories as well as providing a centralised location for maintaining metadata definitions. All of these approaches require the semantic integration of the different metadata sets, something exacerbated by Big Data that introduce further diversity of data content. Once the metadata repository is established, however, it can provide benefits such as comprehensive traceability, logical as well as physical data definitions and links between data model elements.

4. IMPORTANT TYPES OF BIG DATA METADATA FOR CRISIS MANAGEMENT

To recap the previous discussion, metadata is the information that describes other data – 'data about data'. Metadata comprises all the descriptive, administrative and structural data that defines a firm's data assets. Yet, as metadata specifically identifies the attributes, properties and tags that will describe and classify information, they could be more appropriately defined as 'information about data'. Metadata contain descriptions of characteristics associated with the Big Data information asset such as type of asset, author, date originated, workflow state, and usage within the organisation. Once defined, metadata provides the value and purpose of the data content, and thus becomes an effective tool for quickly locating information and supporting Big Data analytics.

Big Data under a crisis response context shares the characteristics of Big Data in general (McAffee et al, 2012), i.e. it is characterised by the dimensions of volume, velocity and variety. More specifically:

The large volumes of crisis data is caused by the proliferation of devices that generate such velocity, mainly the mobile devices as well as handheld and body sensors, cameras etc, used by the crisis responders as well as by ordinary citizens.

Velocity refers to the timeliness of the data. Timeliness is particular important in crisis situations due the dynamic nature of many such situations which means that old data may be irrelevant or potentially misleading.

Variety refers to the characteristics of Big Data such as structure (structured, semi-structured and unstructured data). Variety is characterised by the source (audio, video, web, text) of Big Data and the level of pre-processing (e.g. raw versus formatted data).

Most types of crises involve the understanding of certain variables (context parameters) that relate to location ('where'), time ('when') and agents ('who'). Consequently, this section discusses the types of metadata that address the above dimensions.

4.1 Spatial Metadata

Spatial data in general refers to the location, shape and size of an object in space (ANDS, nd). Geospatial data is a subset of spatial data that pertains to objects on Earth. Data that is created or captured with an associated geographic component is known as geospatial or spatial data. This means geospatial metadata represent the location, size, and shape in space of an object. This information is managed by Geographical Information Systems (GIS).

Geospatial metadata are crucial in emergency crisis management, as many types of Big Data may have a geospatial component in their metadata even though the Big Datum itself may not considered to be geospatial data. For example, health related captured Big Data may contain locational metadata such as geographic data in the form of coordinates, address, city, or postal code. This can be encoded in a range of formats such as static maps, aerial images and satellite/sensor data, GIS layers, and tabular data. Spatial and temporal consistency of geospatial data i.e. the consistency among several versions of the data at different locations and at different times, is essential. In this context, the quality of the geospatial data is an important consideration. Several standards focusing on maps quality, such as the ISO 19100 series of geographic information standards (with a specific focus on the

19107 Geographic information – Spatial schema standard) as well as the Spatial Data Transfer Standard, have been proposed to address quality issues.

Relevant to both geospatial metadata and crisis management, are the approaches of crisis mapping and visual analytics discussed below.

Crisismapping

Crisis mapping (Ziemke, 2012) is a recent interdisciplinary research field. The crisis maps contain up-to-date satellite imagery that are often collected and annotated using crowd computing and crowdsourcing techniques. These maps are used as real-time source of information and provide effective situational awareness with respect to spatial and temporal dimensions by giving a dynamic bird's-eye view to guide the crisis response efforts.

The process of crisis mapping is overseen by dedicated organizations such as the International Network of Crisis Mappers and managed through Crisis Mappers Humanitarian Technology Network.

Visual Analytics and Neo-geography

Visual analytics is Big Data exploration method that borrows techniques from computer vision and geospatial technologies. The aim of visual analytics is to support analytical reasoning through visual interfaces. As geospatial data can be critical for disaster response, visual analytics of Big Data such as images and videos can help to enhance situation awareness in crisis situations.

4.2 CDR

Call Detail Records (CDR), are attributes of phone calls that include connection time, duration, source and destination number, and respective cell-tower identifiers for both caller and callee, providing location information on both. CDR can be used to collect location information (Vaanhoof et al, 2012). This makes CDR metadata very attractive for largescale analysis of location and movement patterns. In the context of epidemiology, the attraction of CDR metadata lies in the fact that they are routinely recorded, network-wide and as such provide direct access to localization data for large samples of populations.

In a study reported in (Jones et al, 2018), the authors conclude that, there are possibilities for the wider use of CDR data in health research, but there are also major challenges to be addressed. In particular, the authors highlighted questions about the suitability of CDRs for wider use in health research and particularly as part of data-intensive infrastructures for population-scale studies.

5. CRITICAL EVALUATION, GAPS ANALYSIS AND FRAMEWORK PROPOSAL

This section provides a critical evaluation of Big Data metadata standards and technologies regarding their suitability in crisis management environments, and a gap analysis. As argued earlier, a metadata representation and management approach is essential in order to define the structure and the relations (i.e., the connections) between the heterogeneous Big Data sources, provided by sensors, mobile devices, medical devices and other information systems, to the crisis management decision makers.

One of the promises of Big Data analysis is to make sense of data by detecting meaningful patterns and trends that help the responders to better understand the crisis and therefore manage it. For instance, spatiotemporal data analysis promises to have great potential to transform the fields of epidemiology (Tang, 2021). Big Data holds promise to identify population health intervention targets through analysis of high volume and high variety data, and to target and refine ensuing interventions using high velocity feedback mechanisms (Mooney et al, 2015).

However, this is not possible without the use of additional descriptions about the data themselves, i.e. metadata. A metadata management framework needs to be generic, reusable and responsive to adapt to changes in the crisis situation, and able to accommodate new types of Big Data, thus keeping the decision makers up-to-date and ensuring the validity of the analysis results. As the data volumes involved can be vast, and responses must be made quickly, there is the need to judge the data quality of the different Big Data sets within a reasonable amount of time. Furthermore, this information has to be integrated and/or reconciled with other available data obtained through alternative methods, in order to have a more integrated picture of the crisis situation. For instance in (Jones et al, 2018), it is suggested to investigating the augmentation of call detail records (CDR) type metadata with geolocation data. However, this is not possible without the use of additional descriptions about the data themselves, i.e. metadata.

In that sense, the contribution of metadata is invaluable, as they can provide the necessary information to ascertain the required qualities of the Big Data, such as provenance, lineage, consistency, timeliness and others, as reviewed in Section 3 of the chapter.

Additionally, privacy of personal data must be maintained, even in crisis situations. Towards meeting privacy constraints, special types of metadata such as sensitive content indicators – flagging files that contain items of sensitivity and their location, can be utilised.

A metadata framework for crisis related Big Data, needs therefore to non-intrusively collect critical and relevant metadata, generate metadata where existing ones are missing (by attaching for example time or location metadata to Big Data records), pre-process, normalise, analyse, store, and presents metadata in an interactive, dynamic interface.

To conclude, the Big Data processing environment used in emergency crises needs to have governance processes in place, to ensure that Big Data metadata are captured recorded and curated in a meaningful, complete, unambiguous, and consistent manner. We also propose that for crisis management, the metadata governance framework needs to include both IT as well as field experts such as epidemiologists.

6. CONCLUSION

This Chapter discussed the role of metadata for the effective utilisation of Big Data in an emergency/crisis context. Metadata provide definition, description, and context for Big Data. This is of particular importance for crisis management, especially pandemics(Anderson, 2020). During pandemics, routine data collection and flows can rapidly become overwhelmed with massive amounts of structured and unstructured Big Data, from existing and new sources. Such data refer to a variety of sociological and physiological concepts and have underlying geographical and temporal dimensions. The pandemic response teams must have confidence in the quality and accuracy of collected data, in order to make the right decisions. Wrong decisions caused by incorrect understanding of the Big Data can lead to inadequate decisions, and consequently, to public- trust issues, ineffective acquisition and allocation of medicine, medical and testing equipment, and so on.

Such problems can largely be avoided by a Big Data metadata management framework such as the one outlined in this chapter. The framework needs to include processes for documenting the context of the Big Data (heritage and lineage), the key entities, attributes, and relationships between them, as well as validation of data timeliness, accuracy and completeness. For sharing the meaning of crisis data among the crisis responders, suitable open source crisis management ontologies (Omitola & Wills, 2019) may be utilised.

It is important also that, due to the nature of the pandemic crises, a Big Data metadata framework is based on open standards (DiMaio, 2008), to address any interoperability issues.

REFERENCES

Anderson M R. (n.d.). Data is King for Government Crisis Response. *Informatica*.

ANDS. (n.d.). *Geospatial data and metadata.* Retrieved from https://www.ands.org.au/working-with-data/metadata/geospatial-data-and-metadata

Batini, Rula, A., Scannapieco, M., & Viscusi, G. (2015, January). From Data Quality to Big Data Quality. *Journal of Database Management, 26*(1), 60–82. doi:10.4018/JDM.2015010103

Boersma, F. K., Passenier, D. F., Mollee, J. S., & van der Wal, C. N. (Eds.). (2012). *Proceedings of the 26th European Conference on Modelling and Simulation, ECMS2012.* Koblenz: ECMS.

Boersma, K., & Fonio, C. (2019). *Big data, surveillance and crisis management.* Routledge.

Boulos, K. M. N., Resch, B., & Crowley, D. N. (2011). Crowdsourcing, citizen sensing and sensor web technologies for public and environmental health surveillance and crisis management: Trends, OGC standards and application examples. *International Journal of Health Geographics, 10*(1), 67. doi:10.1186/1476-072X-10-67 PMID:22188675

Buckee, C. (n.d.). Improving epidemic surveillance and response: big data is dead, long live big data. *The Lancet Open Access.* doi:10.1016/S2589-7500(20)30059-5

Di Maio, P. (2008). *Ontology for ER: An open ontology for open source emergency response system abstract.* Retrieved from http://citeseerx.ist.psu.edu/viewdoc/summary?doi=10.1.1.93.1829

DuCharme, B. (n.d.). What Do RDF and SPARQL bring to Big Data Projects? *Big Data, 1*(1). doi:10.1089/big.2012.0004

Ereth, J. (2017). If Data is the New Oil, Metadata is the New Gold. *Cutting-Edge Analytics.* Retrieved from https://www.eckerson.com/articles/if-data-is-the-new-oil-metadata-is-the-new-gold

Hiltz, S. R., & Plotnick, L. (2013). *Dealing with information overload when using social media for emergency management: Emerging solutions.* ISCRAM.

IDC. (n.d.). The Digital Universe in 2020: Big Data, Bigger Digital Shadows, and Biggest Growth in the Far East. In *Big Data Governance and Metadata Management. Big data governance and Metadata management: Standards roadmap.* IEEE. Available from https://standards.ieee.org/industry-connections/BDGMM-index.html

IDC. (2011). *Leveraging Metadata Framework Technology to Take Control of the Information Explosion.* IDC Report.

ISO/IEC 11179-1:2015 Information technology — Metadata registries (MDR) — Part 1: Framework.

Jones, K. H., Daniels, H., Heys, S., & Ford, D. V. (2018, July). Challenges and Potential Opportunities of Mobile Phone Call Detail Records in Health Research [Review]. *JMIR mHealth and uHealth*, *6*(7), e161. doi:10.2196/mhealth.9974 PMID:30026176

Lanfranchi, V. (2017). Machine learning and social media in crisis management: agility vs ethics WiPe/CoRe Paper – T4 – Ethics Legal and Social Issues. *Proceedings of the 14th ISCRAM Conference.*

McAfee, A., Brynjolfsson, E., Davenport, T., Patil, D. J., & Barton, D. (2012). Big data: The management revolution. *Harvard Business Review*, *90*, 61–67. PMID:23074865

Mooney, S. J., Westreich, D. J., & El-Sayed, A. M. (2015, May). Commentary. *Epidemiology in the Era of Big Data Epidemiology.*, *26*(3), 390–394. doi:10.1097/EDE.0000000000000274 PMID:25756221

Omitola, T., & Wills, G. (2019). Emergency Response Ontology Informatics: Using Ontologies to Improve Emergency and Hazard Management. *International Journal of Intelligent Computing Research, 10*(3).

Palen, L., Vieweg, S., Sutton, J., Liu, S. B., & Hughes, A. (2007). *Crisis Informatics: Studying Crisis in a Networked World*. In Third International Conference on e-Social Science, Ann Arbor, MI.

Potash, S. (2017). *Focus: Big data for infectious disease surveillance, modelling*. NIH Fogarty International Center. Available from https://www.fic.nih.gov/News/GlobalHealthMatters/january-february-2017/Pages/big-data-infectious-disease-surveillance-modeling.aspx

Qadir, J., & Anwaar, A. (2016). Crisis analytics: Big data-driven crisis response. *Journal of International Humanitarian Action*, *1*(1), 12. doi:10.118641018-016-0013-9

Salathé, M., Bengtsson, L., Bodnar, T. J., Brewer, D. D., Brownstein, J. J., Buckee, C., Campbell, E. M., Cattuto, C., Khandelwal, S., Mabry, P. L., & Vespignani, A. (2012, July). Digital Epidemiology. *PLoS Computational Biology*, *8*(7), e1002616. doi:10.1371/journal.pcbi.1002616 PMID:22844241

Schmarzo, B. (2018). *Importance of Metadata in a Big Data World*. Data Science Central. Available from https://www.datasciencecentral.com/profiles/blogs/importance-of-metadata-in-a-big-data-world

Stewart, D. (2013). *Big Content: The Unstructured Side of Big Data.* Gartner. Available from https://blogs.gartner.com/darin-stewart/2013/05/01/big-content-the-unstructured-side-of-big-data/

Tang, C. (2021). The Intersection of Big Data and Epidemiology for Epidemiologic Research. *The AMIA 2021 Virtual Clinical Informatics Conference.*

Vanhoof, M., Reis, F., Smoreda, Z., & Plötz, T. (2012). Detecting Home Locations from CDR Data: Introducing Spatial Uncertainty to the State-of-the-Art. *Journal of Map & Geography Libraries: Advances in Geospatial Information. Collections & Archives, 8*(2), 101–117.

Ziemke, J. (2012). Crisis Mapping: The Construction of a New Interdisciplinary Field? International Network of Crisis Mappers, John Carroll University & the Harvard Humanitarian Initiative, University Heights, OH, USA. *Journal of Map & Geography Libraries: Advances in Geospatial Information. Collections & Archives, 8*(2), 101–117.

Chapter 5
Pandemic Management With Social Media Analytics

Ibrahim Sabuncu

https://orcid.org/0000-0001-8625-9256
Yalova University, Turkey

Mehmet Emin Aydin

https://orcid.org/0000-0002-4890-5648
University of the West of England, UK

ABSTRACT

Social media analytics appears as one of recently developing disciplines that helps understand public perception, reaction, and emerging developments. Particularly, pandemics are one of overwhelming phenomena that push public concerns and necessitate serious management. It turned to be a useful tool to understand the thoughts, concerns, needs, expectations of public and individuals, and supports public authorities to take measures for handling pandemics. It can also be used to predict the spread of the virus, spread parameters, and to estimate the number of cases in the future. In this chapter, recent literature on use of social media analytics in pandemic management is overviewed covering all relevant studies on various aspects of pandemic management. It also introduces social media data sources, software, and tools used in the studies, methodologies, and AI techniques including how the results of the analysis are used in pandemic management. Consequently, the chapter drives conclusions out of findings and results of relevant analysis.

DOI: 10.4018/978-1-7998-6736-4.ch005

INTRODUCTION

This chapter introduces a review on approaches and applications of social media analytics used for pandemic management in a wider respect.

Technological developments such as the Internet, mobile applications, and social media have led to the emergence of large amounts of data and the development of data-driven management models. Business analytics turns to be more popular with the discovery of the internet and related emerging technologies including mobile application development, social media platforms and facilitated data handling technologies, which leads to the development of data-driven management and decision-making models. Business analytics is known to be the use of information technology, statistical analysis, quantitative methods, mathematical or computer-based models to help managers better understand their operations and make fact-based decisions (Evans, 2017)., which helps an organisation improve performance and efficiency by exploiting of all relevant emerging technologies (Bag, 2016).

An important subfield of business analysis methods is Social Network Analytics (Shmueli et al., 2017) also known as Social Media Analytics, which is known as the process of generating useful information by collecting data from social media, analysing, and evaluating them (Chatterjee & Krystyanczuk, 2017).

Within its scope, the aim is to derive useful knowledge and information by analysing data collected from social media applications such as Facebook, Twitter, Instagram, YouTube, and TripAdvisor (W. Y. Wang et al., 2016). The data produced/collected from social media is large and mostly in unstructured nature. Therefore, more sophisticated methods are required to process these data than classical statistical analyses. The advancement in facilities and technological infrastructure such as enlarging data storage and increasing compute and processing power, further developments and enhancements in artificial intelligence and machine learning helped facilitate and widespread. Likewise, progressing natural language processing (NLP) technologies, data mining, and subject modelling can be utilised to handle and process unstructured data.

Businesses can utilise Social Media Analytics in a variety of areas; from marketing to finance including understanding customer demand and expectations, tracking brand image (Culotta & Cutler, 2016), (Pournarakis et al., 2017), financial risk management (Cerchiello & Giudici, 2016), estimating the value of a stock (X. Zhang et al., 2011), (Goel & Mittal, 2012), (Attigeri et al., 2016).

Public organizations, on the other hand, use social media analytics, understanding public opinion on important issues (Ravi & Ravi, 2015), following political trends (Chauhan et al., 2020), predicting election results (Makazhanov et al., 2014), (Burnap et al., 2016), (Grover et al., 2018), (Singh et al., 2020) and disaster management (Luna & Pennock, 2018; Ragini et al., 2018; Rexiline Ragini et al., 2018; Squicciarini et al., 2017). For example, it can be used to identify the needs of individuals in disaster areas with social media analytics in disasters and to support the disaster area in line with these needs (Ragini et al., 2018). Similarly, information obtained from social media can be used in pandemic management.

USE OF SOCIAL MEDIA ANALYTICS (SMA) IN PANDEMIC MANAGEMENT

As in all management activities, data, and information-driven decision making in pandemic management helps improve the success of the administration. Acquisition and timely use of up-to-date pandemic information can be achieved via SMA, which is expected and observed helping understand public perception of pandemic, public concerns on the pandemic, emerging needs and expectations, and public demands from managing bodies, e.g. national and local governments (Ordun et al., 2020), (Wicke & Bolognesi, 2020), (Park et al., 2020), (Sha et al., 2020), (Han et al., 2020), (Depoux et al., 2020), (L. Li et al., 2020), (Cinelli et al., 2020). Besides, it can help predict where the virus has spread, the rate and speed of spread, and the number of future cases. On the other hand, SMA can be utilised for identifying and resolving many social issues such as detecting false and misguiding news and information and their originators (C. Li et al., 2020), (Jahanbin & Rahmanian, 2020), (Alkouz et al., 2019). In the following section, several studies on pandemics for various purposes will be presented.

Symptom Detection

Symptom detection is one of the challenging issues faced during the early stages of COVID-19 pandemic, which was known very little about by medical experts. Symptom-wise and treatment-related information shared by experts over social media such as Twitter has been observed that helps achieve the quickest awareness about the disease. Medical experts, e.g. doctors and drug-developers, would benefit from this shared information in any regard to fighting the pandemic, timely developing treatments to cure patients, and stopping the spreading disease. Sarket et al.(2020) have achieved to determine what symptoms were seen in the people who identified themselves as infected by COVID-19 by analysing the words used in their Twitter posts. They were able to identify the symptoms associated with COVID-19 and which of these were more common. Conducting such studies periodically is important in monitoring the emergence of different symptoms as a result of the mutation of the relevant virus or bacteria in Pandemics such as COVID-19.

Information Management

Another important element in pandemic management is information management. The needs and demands of people subject to pandemics can be discovered by analysing the data shared on social media, and then, it can be reported to the local or national authorities to tackle and meet the needs. In a study, Shen et al.(2020), have analysed the data collected from Sina-Weibo, a popular Chinese social media platform equivalent to Twitter, and achieved identifying the burning issues and most emerging discussion topics using Latent Dirichlet Allocation (LDA) method. The study has discovered the changes in circumstances overtime. The results and recommendations have been reported to authorities to tackle emergencies, solve the burning problems, and help avoid post-disaster problems. The study concludes that using SMA would help discover the emerging problems to be timely tackled by authorities and identify the public moods and morale due to the pandemics, e.g. COVID-19, to be considered for support and post-disaster management.

In another study (L. Li et al., 2020), in which SMA techniques applied the data collected from the Sina-Weibo social media platform, only situational information was proposed to be valuable and useful for the public and authorities to respond to the epidemic. Natural language processing techniques (NLP) were used to classify collected posts about COVID-19 according to seven types of state information. These seven types of situations are listed as follows: 1) attention and advice; 2) notifications and measures taken; 3) donations of money, goods or services; 4) emotional support; 5) seeking help; 6) raise suspicion and criticize, and 7) counterargument/rumour. The main theme proposed imposes that the authorities' decision-making based on this situation information will be useful for pandemic management.

Studies including Zhao et al.(2020), and Yin et al.(2020) have concluded that social media is beneficial for pandemic management and turned to be a major source of information for public management as well as pandemic management, through their topic modelling analysis approach applied to the data collected from Sina Weibo, the Chinese social media platform. It is stated that it is an important data source that can generate information.

Santis et al.(2020) have analysed Twitter data collected from people under quarantine due to COVID-19 pandemics concluding that people under quarantine communicate over social media. The purpose of this analysis was to monitor pandemic measures and identify emerging issues using natural language processing (NLP) and visual analytics techniques. They calculated the frequencies of the words, term frequencies (TF), used in the tweets (Grimaldi et al., 2020), and the social impact of those who shared the tweets and identified the prominent issues from the discussions.

SMA has also been used to monitor public opinion and reaction to imposed pandemic measures. For instance, the public response to Covid19 social distance measures and quarantine practices has been investigated by Saleh et al.(2020). In this study, tweets containing keywords related to the measures (#socialdistancing and #stayathome) were collected, analysed using NLP and machine learning models, and sentiment analysis was performed to determine the emotions it contained. In the study, they evaluated the subjectivity of Tweets, estimated the frequency of discussing social distance rules, and determined discussion clusters using topic modelling and related emotions. As a result, they concluded that Twitter users supported social distance in the early stages of implementation.

One more interesting area of use for SMA happened to identify and monitor the trends in national news channels. A study conducted in Spain (Yu et al., 2020) reports their findings through LDA topic modelling applied on the posts of two mainstream newspapers of Spain on Twitter, which are resulted in eight different categories. Then, the changes in these issues over the three periods of pandemics (pre-crisis, quarantine, and recovery period) were evaluated. It is concluded that the information they obtained would be useful in understanding the attitude of the media towards the pandemic.

Another study (Abd-Alrazaq et al., 2020) used Twitter data, which stated that analysing the issues that appeared on social media platforms regarding the pandemic can help policymakers and healthcare organizations assess the needs of their stakeholders and address them appropriately. The word frequencies (in the forms of unigram and bigram) in the tweets collected using keywords related to COVID-19 were calculated. LDA topic modelling method was used to identify the topics discussed in the tweets. Also, sentiment analysis was performed, the average number of retweets, likes, and followers for each topic was extracted, and the interaction rate per topic was determined. As a result, the public attitude on 12 different issues regarding Covid19 was evaluated and recommendations were made.

Park et al.(2020) have conducted an SMA study in Korea revealing that real-time analysis of social media data can help serve as a starting point for creating bespoke strategic messages for serving health organizations and for establishing an effective communication system during Pandemic periods. The study has applied content analysis of tweets collected from Korean users of Twitter about Covid19 and identified emerging topics within the public. A network analysis has also been applied to the same data to determine the speed of information spread and distribution. The study has concluded that the determined spread speed and distribution of pandemic information within the public and the identified emerging topics can offer support to health professionals to make a fast and timely decision within unclear and complicated circumstances.

Twitter has been defined by a study (Medford et al., 2020) as a medium in which public perception and sensitivities about the pandemic can be identified in real-time, and as an enabling tool to shape personalised public health messages users interests and emotional status. The study was conducted using collected tweets with all hashtags related to COVID-19 and analysed the data to determine the frequency of themes and keywords relevant to infection prevention and avoidance. Sensitivity analysis was performed to determine the emotion polarity and dominant emotions in the tweets, and topic modelling was implemented to determine the trends of emerging topics and subjects of discussions. The emotions and topics of the most popular tweets defined by the number of retweets were compared. As a result of the analysis, the most discussed issues related to the pandemic were unveiled. A correlation between the increase in the number of tweets and the growth of COVID-19 cases has been concluded.

Glowacki et al.(2020) have investigated the impact of pandemics on combat with addictions. Tweets containing the words "addiction" and "COVID-19" were collected and analysed to reveal the feelings and thoughts of individuals, who are in combat with addictions such as alcohol, smoking, drug, or gambling addiction during the Covid19 quarantine periods. The emerging topics in the tweets have been identified using a text miner tool (Chakraborty et al., 2014). As a result, it was suggested that the information concluded/obtained was found helpful for health authorities to identify public concerns about addiction during the COVID-19 outbreak. It has also been concluded that such findings of text mining studies addressing health issues can serve as preliminary analysis to go for more comprehensive models to generate recommendations for larger audiences and inform decision-makers.

Wang et al.(2021) have studied if SMA can also be used to analyse the dissemination of accurate information and the effectiveness of communication between public institutions involved in pandemic management. The study reports that risk and crisis communication between public health agencies and federal stakeholders in the early stages of the Covid19 pandemic has been analysed in terms of competence, timeliness, compliance, consistency, and coordination.

For this analysis, tweets sent by the official accounts of the World Health Organization (WHO), 12 federal agencies, six official stakeholders, and 50 state-level public health agencies were collected. First, tweets were filtered using keywords related to COVID19, including "coronavirus", "corona", "sars-cov-2", "ncov" and "covid". These tweets were, then, manually divided into 16 categories following the study by Wukich(2016), which suggested 22 types of social media messages for emergency management. Using Gephi software (Bastian et al., 2009), communication networks between these agencies were estimated by using retweeting (RT) and mentioning @ relationships. It is reported and revealed by dynamic network analysis, that a changing communication model was observed with an increasing level of connection and coordination between institutions and stakeholders related to the pandemic during the study period.

Misinformation Distribution; "Infodemic"

Social media analytics can also be used to detect misinformation about pandemics spread within the public, which can make matters in pandemic management. Cinelli et al.(2020) have tried to determine misinformation and wrong procedures spread among people used to prevent or treat COVID-19. In addition, it was attempted to determine how the spread of false information can cause panic within the public and how much such information was spread and how serious it has been taken. It demonstrates that, by analysing the spread of such misinformation, the authorities can be advised of the seriousness of the situations and let them take initiative and relevant action to guide public awareness correctly.

Sear et al.(2020) have studied the level of communication and discussions among pro-vaccine and anti-vaccine user groups, which can easily cause, create spread misinformation. They have automatically classified Facebook pages and relevant contents of pro and anti-vaccination groups to reveal the impact of each party. It is thought that the information they have obtained may be effective in combating false thoughts such as anti-vaccination that may make pandemic management difficult.

Predicting the Number of Cases

The number of cases can be estimated with SMA applied to the data collected of monitoring the increase and decrease in the numbers of social media posts. Also, depending on the locations where the posts are fired, the heath-map of levels of the cases can reflect the density of the cases over the regions, which would help authorities take precautions in advance. Culotta(2010) has conducted one of the earlier studies with the purpose analysing Twitter data to estimate the number of cases of influenza outbreaks. The data has been collected using symptoms (flu, cough, sore throat, headache) as keywords to filter in relevant tweets. Then, it is looked for correlations between the most frequently repeated words in the tweets, manually collected, and the number of cases to identify new keywords to deepen the investigations. As a result, a correlation of 0.78 between the number of tweets containing the keywords identified and the number of cases was found.

Another study (Alkouz et al., 2019) was conducted in the United Arab Emirates (UAE) to estimate the number of cases in influenza outbreaks using Twitter data. The tweets collected in this study are filtered and divided into two categories as case reporting and non-reporting. By using case reporting tweets, it was tried to predict the number of future flu cases with a linear regression model. The estimated results are compared with actual hospital visits recorded by the UAE Ministry of Health. As a result, they found a high correlation between the predictions with Twitter data on influenza and visits to hospitals due to influenza.

Recently, social media and search engine indexes have been used to estimate the number of COVID-19 cases. Qin et al.(2020), social media search for the keywords of "dry cough", "fever", "chest pain", "coronavirus", and "pneumonia" in the Baidu Index, (a popular search engine in China) and all relevant social media search indexes (SMSI) have been collected. Analysis has been done to determine if there is any correlation between the number of COVID-19 cases and the daily frequency of search with the above-mentioned keywords, which seems to happen significantly as suggested. It is concluded that by using such analysis with SMSI data, the number of COVID-19 cases can be predicted accurately 6-9 days in advance.

In another study (C. Li et al., 2020) it is attempted to predict the number of cases with the searches related to the pandemic using both search engine indexes and social media posts, where Sina Weibo Index, a social media platform widely used in China, Trends and Baidu Index were used. They determined the frequency of search for two keywords, "coronavirus" and "pneumonia", in search engines and the number of posts containing these words on the Sina Weibo social media platform. Their analysis demonstrated and determined a high correlation ($r > 0.89$) between the number of cases and the internet searches and collected social media data. Through delayed correlation analysis, the maximum correlation was observed between the frequency of internet search and social media posts with corresponding keywords and laboratory-confirmed cases and suspected cases appeared the 8-12 days and 6-8 days prior to search and sharings, respectively. They concluded that social media and internet search data can provide an accurate, timely, and cost-effective forecast of the COVID-19 pandemic progression.

Jahanbin & Rahmanian(2020) have analysed the relationship between Twitter data and the estimation of the number of cases. In this study, tweets containing the keywords #corona, #ncov, #wuhan, #china, #2019-nCoV, #virus, #corona virus china, #coronavirus outbreak, #wuhan virus were collected and the counts by countries were calculated. The study suggests that there is a consistent relationship between the distribution rates of these tweets across countries and the distribution of case numbers by countries retrieved from the World Health Organization (WHO). As a result, it is concluded that Twitter social media sharing data was an effective tool to track the spread of the Pandemic.

THE PROCESS, METHODS AND TOOLS OF SOCIAL MEDIA ANALYTICS

It is beyond the scope of this section to describe in detail how to use social media analytics tools. For detailed information, the readers are referred to North (2012), Chatterjee & Krystyanczuk (2017), Evans (2017), and Shmueli et al. (2017) as relevant resources. It is aimed to provide rather general information in this emerging field to brief novice researchers and encourage them to pay attention to the field.

Social media analytics is basically a three-phase process: (i) data collection from social media, (ii) data analysis with best bespoke methods and tools, and (iii) driving conclusions from analysis. Once data is collected, it should be cleaned of unnecessary contents to make it fit the purpose of the analysis, where the aim and objectives set for the research play a crucial role in the goodness of fit. If unnecessary data is not cleaned or filtered out, the analysis may be diverted unintentionally. The analysis approaches prominently emerge in social media analytics are found to be content analysis by 15.4%, NLP by 15.3%, and sentiment analysis by 13.4% (Misirlis & Vlachopoulou, 2018), while both content analysis and sentiment analysis techniques have notably been used in researches on COVID-19 pandemics. Additionally, it is observed that predicting the number of cases over social media data has been an overwhelming hot topic. Throughout this section, methods and software that can be used to realise the three-phase process, as indicated in Figure 1, will be introduced.

Data Collection From Social Media

This subsection introduces data sources of social media for pandemic management, data collection, relevant methods for analysis, and the tools used, which are mainly known to be R, Python, and RapidMiner. The prominent analysis methods are known as sentiment analysis, topic modelling, and predictive analytics, which are used to dive into the data to retrieve useful information and derive conclusions to be used for pandemic management purposes.

There are companies that help gather data from Social Media providing services for a price, which can be used to collect social media data for pandemic management. For example, Hootsuite, Brand24, and Sprout Social are just a few of the many companies that collect data from different social media platforms such as Facebook, Instagram, Twitter. These companies are able to collect social media data with pre-determined keywords and store data in useful formats, such as CSV, etc., for analytical studies, and to visualize the data and apply sentiment analysis towards a purpose. Alternatively, companies can take-action and collect social media data directly from social media platforms using provide APIs, where it is known that each social media platform has relevant API provided to developers and professionals for this purpose, which helps implement and develop data analysis approaches and apply the data in this regard. APIs are compatible with major programming languages such as Python and specialised languages such as R. Besides, specialised data mining packages such as RapidMiner can also be used to perform all relevant analytical methods to derive useful knowledge throughout of collected data. R language and

Figure 1. Social Media Analytics Process Steps

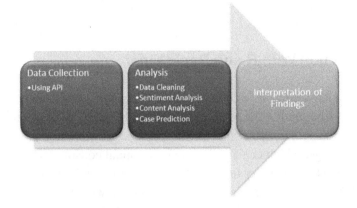

RapidMiner package will be paid attention to in upcoming sections and Python will be slightly touched with this respect.

The first stage of data collection form social media is to identify related keywords, and then the collection can be actioned from Facebook (Ketter, 2016), (Sitta et al., 2018), Instagram (Kale, 2016), TripAdvisor (Chang et al., 2017), while Twitter appears to be the most used data source for SMA applications (Birjali et al., 2017), (Ahuja & Shakeel, 2017), (Öztürk & Ayvaz, 2018), (Kim et al., 2014), (Saif et al., 2016), (Culotta & Cutler, 2016), (Pournarakis et al., 2017),(X. Zhang et al., 2011), (Goel & Mittal, 2012), (Attigeri et al., 2016). Due to this fact, Twitter is considered as the prominent data source of social media analytics studies in this research.

The keyword identification process for the research can be done following some preliminary studies going through expert views, relevant literature review, prototypical research (Sarker et al., 2020). For instance, keyword determination for thorough research planned to reveal public opinion on vaccine development for COVID-19 can follow preliminary research is conducted using a much fewer number of tweets, which helped identify further keywords such as "pandemics" alongside "covid" and "treatment" besides "vaccine".

Researchers with a Twitter account need to apply for a developer account to gain access to Twitter data sources via Twitter API, which means Twitter account holders are allowed to use Tweeter API. Once a developer account application is submitted, and approval is gained, the access to data sources and use of API is authenticated through the provided access code, which is generated with relevant key and tokens. Typically, the *TwitteR* package of the R program or the *SearchTwitter* operator of the RapidMiner data mining software is used to gain access to Twitter data to search through, filter out and download the appropriate posts following the authentication operation mentioned above as a necessary pre-process of Twitter API application. It is paramount to indicate that access gain to Twitter data and other associated sources and use it is subject to a price, which is scalable with the size of data per time window.

Data Collection With R and RapidMiner

To use the open-source R programming language to extract and analyse data from Twitter, first the R (The R Foundation, 2020) then R studio (RStudio PBC., 2020b) program is needed, which is an open-access software. R language is a scripting language, which can also be run on terminal consoles. The coding starts by downloading the necessary library files/packages (RStudio PBC., 2020a) for the functions to be used. These packages can be directly downloaded and installed from the R program using the install.packages("package to be downloaded") statement. For example, with the code install.packages('twitteR'), the twitteR package, which enables to search on Twitter and download data, is downloaded and installed in the program. library() is used in the software to activate the downloaded packages and use the functions in its content. For example, library(twitteR).

The next step is to gain access to the Twitter account via R software by using the setup_twitter_oauth function with the keys and tokens of the API application. The following codes can be written for this:

```
consumer_key <- '8kmONz7G5MYVBh***'
consumer_secret <- 'vORYByyR9it4m9tEq1lVDN9jlZHVGsgCPt3dnwf***
**3J9'
access_token <-
'1158143544-A4xVk7iCqdeD7eEWmW8CtOwg0ifKk8DW****'
access_secret <- 'reBZWrtVA02awxpVjmgLM5qyyhfRVDE2K****'
setup_twitter_oauth(consumer_key, consumer_secret, access_
token, access_secret)
```

Then, by using the Twitter search function *searchTwitter* in the twitteR package, tweet messages containing the searched expressions in the desired language can be downloaded in the desired amount (this amount constitutes the upper limit)(Shmueli et al., 2017):

```
datafilename <- searchTwitter("searched_word", lang='en', n =
the upper limit of the number of tweets to be downloaded)
```

These tweet messages can be transformed into a variable, a multidimensional array, or a table and saved. The data collected in this way includes not only the tweet messages containing the sought expressions, but also a total of 16 different characteristics for every tweet such as who shared this tweet (account name), how many times it was retweeted, and the date it was created. Each attribute creates a separate column of the file (*datafilename*).

RapidMiner (RapidMiner Inc., 2020b) is a software platform developed for machine learning, data mining, text mining, predictive analysis, and business analysis purposes. Although the software is often used in business and commercial applications, it can also be used for research purposes. It can provide a free license for academic research and educational use purposes (RapidMiner Inc., 2020c). "*Search Twitter*" operator is used for data retrieval from Twitter with RapidMiner. To use this operator, it is necessary to connect with a Twitter account first. For this process, the "*Create Connection*" option under the RapidMiner Connection menu is selected, Twitter is selected as the connection type and a name is given to the connection. On the next screen, click the *OAuth* icon next to the Access token option and click the "*Request Access Token*" option from the menu that appears. This button allows opening your Twitter account in the internet browser after logging in with username and password authentication. Following that, access authorisation to the Twitter account is required to be granted to the RapidMiner application. Once permission is granted, the connection is created by using the given code. The developer account, API application, and access codes required for R and Python programs are not required for this connection and for operations such as searching on Twitter with RapidMiner and downloading data. In this respect, it is observed easier to collected data RapidMiner.

Once the Twitter connection is established, the following parameters of the "*Search Twitter*" operator are adjusted according to the purpose of the study:

- *Connection Entry*: The Twitter connection created in this field is selected for use.
- *Query*: The keywords to be searched on Twitter put together to go for search. Logic operators are used to composing queries for multiple keywords; the "OR" operator is the most used one, while different queries can be composed using other logic operators.
- *Result Type*: This parameter specifies the preferred type of search result. A choice between the most recent tweets, the most popular tweets, or the most recent or popular tweets containing the specified keywords.
- *Language*: This field is to specify if the search is to be applied to tweets in a particular language or languages. Once is left blank, tweets from all languages will be collected. A language can be specified with the ISO 639-1 code to only collect the tweets posted in that language.

Data Cleaning

Review studies indicate that pre-processing tweets helps increase the success of the analysis. Removal of punctuation marks, numbers, web page links / URLs, extra spaces (Singh et al., 2020), numbers, dates (Grimaldi et al., 2020), unused words, special characters, repetitive tweets (Budiharto & Meiliana, 2018), emojis, symbols (e.g. $, &, +) and conjunctives/stopwords (e.g. the, from, and, or, in) (Castro et al., 2017) from tweet-data would be useful. Also, converting all letters to lowercase (Bansal & Srivastava, 2018) and reducing words to their roots (stemming using Porter Stemmer algorithm) (Wicaksono et al., 2017) can be beneficial for better processing.

The str_replace_all function can be used in the R programming language to purify tweets from unnecessary symbols and expressions, which removes them by replacing each with blank values. This necessitates writing the cleaning statements one-by-one. On the other hand, RapidMiner uses the following operators to clean tweeters from unwanted expressions an easier way:

- *Extract content*: HTML cleaning can be done.
- *Transform cases*: converts all to lower case.
- *Filter Stop Words*: removes stopwords like "*in, and, or*" from the text.
- *Filter tokens*: This operator can filter words that are smaller or larger than a certain number of letters. It can be used to delete single letter characters or symbols etc.
- *Stemming*: reducing to the root of words. In topic modelling, all of the words with various suffixes will be evaluated as a different word and their frequencies will be calculated as a separate word. For this reason, reducing the words to their roots will enable more accurate term frequency calculations.

Sentiment Analysis

Sentiment analysis is a text analysis approach that helps automatically determine the emotion/ mood (anger, joy, sadness, etc.) and polarity (negative, positive, neutral) contained in a text using artificial intelligence techniques. The approaches for sentiment analyses are mainly developed with either machine learning techniques or dictionary-based ones, while there are hybrid methods used for this purpose, too. (Valdivia et al., 2018):

Lexicon-Dictionary-based (LD) method works with dictionaries to break down emotional expressions. The dictionaries used in this approach are generally composed of core words and their synonyms and antonyms. On the other hand, Machine Learning-based (ML) methods use a number of approaches to training models with pre-tagged sentences so as to predict, evaluate and classify upcoming sentences. The hybrid approach imposes combining LD and ML methods to avoid the shortcomings of each standalone approach and benefit of advantages.

The following studies present the most frequently used sentiment analysis approaches. *Bing* is one of the first dictionary-based methods used for sentiment analysis, which scores relevant expressions sentences with -1 (negative), 0 (neutral), or 1 (positive) (Hu & Liu, 2004). SentiWordNet (Esuli, 2019) is another dictionary-based approach marking the sentences with a scale between -1 and +1 (Baccianella et al., 2010). The latest version exploits semi-supervised learning and random-walk steps to improve the sentiment scores.

AFINN is another earlier study bases on dictionary-based sentiment analysis scoring the words between -5 and +5 and demonstrates the sentiment identified, negative scores indicate negative emotions and positive scores indicate positive emotions (Nielsen, 2011). This study applied to messages obtained from social media such as Twitter (Choy et al., 2012), (Wicaksono et al., 2017).

Sentiments analysis with NRC (Mohammad, 2020) used dictionary-based tools in which sentiments of the words have been primarily identified using a manual crowdsourcing method with respect to the following emotion categories; "Anger", "Expectation", "Disgust", "Fear", "Joy", "Sadness", "Surprise", "Trust", "Positive" and "Negative" (Mohammad & Turney, 2013). On the other hand, Vader (Hutto, 2020) is a dictionary-based approach (Gilbert & Hutto, 2014), which is developed to conduct sentiment analysis of social media contents such as Twitter (Ramteke et al., 2016), (Anuta et al., 2017). It takes both the dictionary inputs and the characteristics of the sentence to determine emotional polarity in which the sentences are scored and scaled between -1 and +1 through normalising the cumulative scores calculated word-by-word. CoreNLP (Stanford NLP Group, 2020) is a machine learning-based approach developed by the Stanford NLP group using deep learning (Manning et al., 2014). The tool scores the sentiments between 0 (very negative) to 4 (very positive), and it supports 6 languages: Arabic, Chinese, English, French, German, and Spanish.

Aylien (Aylien Ltd., 2020a) is known to be a commercial text mining software, which can perform machine learning-based sentiment analysis calculating the sentiment scores entity-by-entity within the same single social media message (Aylien Ltd., 2020b). It may not be useful to come up with a more generalised cumulative sentiment for a data source, but it turns to be very useful to derive multiple sentiments from the same messages and generalise this across the whole data source using some supportive tools. For instance, it can help identify and catch up a positive statement about mask measures and a negative statement about curfew in a tweet as part of pandemic measures, if this is the case.

MeaningCloud (MeaningCloud LLC., 2020) is another commercial tool that performs machine learning-based sentiment analysis and other text mining operations. It can conduct subject-based sentiment analysis as in Aylien application renaming that subject-based sentiment analysis with aspect-based sentiment analysis.

Finally, two very prominent machine learning-based sentiment analysis approaches, namely *"Bidirectional Encoder Representations from Transformers (BERT)"* (Devlin, 2020), (Devlin et al., 2019) and *"Generative Pre-trained Transformer-2 (GPT-2)"* (OpenAI, 2019), (Radford et al., 2019), are pre-trained models with a huge amount of data with the proven success of sentiment analysis.

Sentiment Analysis With R, Python, and RapidMiner

Sentiment analysis with R, Python and RapidMiner tools can be done with built-in functionalities, which can be summarised in this section. R language offers a package called *"Syuzhet"* to conduct dictionary-based sentiment analysis. A number of getter methods including get_sentiment() help apply analysis to collected social media data to achieve pre-set targets such as understanding public opinion under pandemic circumstances . (Grover et al., 2018). Following example (Julia Silge & Robinson, 2020) provides various forms of get_sentiment() use (Jockers, 2017b):

```
get_sentiment(char_v, method = "syuzhet", path_to_tagger =
NULL, cl = NULL, language = "english", lexicon = NULL)
AFINN: get_sentiments("afinn"),
Bing: get_sentiments("bing"),
NRC: get_sentiments("nrc") or get_nrc_sentiment()(Jockers,
2017a)
CoreNLP: get_stanford_sentiment(text_vector, path_to_stanford_
tagger) Arguments
```

The same methods can also be used in the Python programming language as follows:

- AFINN (Nielsen, 2019):

```
from afinn import Afinn
afinn = Afinn()
afinn.score('Write your sentence here for calculating sentiment
score')
```

- CoreNLP (Angled, 2020)

```
import corenlp
text = "Write your sentence here for calculating sentiment
score"
with corenlp.CoreNLPClient(annotators="tokenize ssplit pos
lemma ner depparse".split()) as client:
ann = client.annotate(text)
```

Similar sentiment analysis can be done with RapidMiner (RapidMiner Inc., 2019) through in-built operators, e.g. "*Extract Sentiment*", that can be accessed for use once "*Operator Toolbox*" is installed and configured. "*Extract Sentiment*" operator can be pipelined to "*Search Twitter*" to streamline the tweet data acquisition with sentiment analysis, while it can also be applied to readily available other data sets. Meanwhile, it is beneficial to indicate that "*Extract Sentiment*" operator cannot only work with open-source sentiment analysis models such as *Vader* and *SentiWordNet 3.0* but also incorporate with models from commercial systems such as *Aylien* and *MeaningCloud*. In order to use commercial models, a charge will be applicable to create an account first and to establish a link to the corresponding API in a similar way to Twitter cases.

Data Visualisation

Data visualisation is one critical stage and a tool in the process of data analytics. This stage follows data cleaning and production of descriptive statistics, which is aimed to visualise the status of the data in many respects. Tools and instruments can be used to visualise data span form a very basic to very complicated, where relevant data sections or statistics can simply be tabulated or be plotted out in various types of figures and graphics. For instance, MS Excel spreadsheets can be used for these purposes by creating charts, diagrams, etc. with built-in tools; the number of daily messages, Twitter posts, referring to Covid-19 can be transferred to an Excel spreadsheet and daily changes can be observed. With such simple visualisation, it would not be difficult to conclude that an important development attracting public attention is happening or has happened with observing the peaked number of tweets. Of course, the content analysis would be needed to understand what is happening or has happened.

As reported in (Sabuncu & Atmis, 2020), Twitter data has been analysed for sentiments cleaning operations, where the score has been estimated for positive and negative polarities and 10 sentiments using the get_nrc_sentiment function of R programming language as explained below. The daily positive and negative tweet numbers are plotted in blue and red colours to visualise data.

```
Sentiment <- get_nrc_sentiment(purified$clean_text)
tweets<- cbind(purified, Sentiment)
tweetsPositive <- tweets[tweets$positive>tweets$negative,]
tweetsPositiveCopy <- tweetsPositive %>%
group_by(created=floor_date(created, "day")) %>%
summarize(positive=sum(positive))
barplot(tweetsPositiveCopy$positive, names.
arg=tweetsPositiveCopy$created, xlab="Date", ylab = "Number of
Tweets",col = "blue",
main = "Positive Sentiment Chart",border = "red", las=2)
```

The code in R language provided above downloads tweets into a file of 16 columns named "purified". Then, the data is cleaned of unnecessary expressions with *str_replace_all* function, added a new column to the same file - 17th column of "purified" file named as "clean_text". The estimated 12 sentiments, as mentioned above, from all cleaned tweets and copied into another file called "tweets". Afterward, all tweets have been compared with respect to the positive and negative sentiment scores, grouped based on the higher score, and the grouped of tweets are stored in two different files, either *"tweetsPositive"* or *"tweetsNegative"*. The corresponding cleaned and processed tweets have been plotted with *barplot* function to visualise them through days.

Social network analysis (SNA) can be considered as another way of data visualisation, where social networks are modelled and analysed with graph theory (Otte & Rousseau, 2002). The social networks are modelled with vertices connected with edges, where the relationships are characterised using individuals and group bodies as vertices while the connections as edges. Recent studies have used this approach successfully (Grandjean, 2016; Santis et al., 2020; Yu et al., 2020). This approach imposes changing visual representation of the vertices and edges in order to reflect the qualities and characteristics. Gephi (Gephi, 2020), (Bastian et al., 2009) is an open-source software to be used for social network analysis, which can be effectively used to identify the characteristics of the interactions among social media users.

Content Analysis by Topic Modelling

Content analysis is the process of identifying the categories or themes detected from the contents of the texts. There is a common presumption that topic modeling algorithms are suitable approaches for content analysis (Bakharia, 2019). This presumption is supported with the frequently use of topic modeling to conduct a content analysis of social media data by many studies (Abd-Alrazaq et al., 2020; Doogan et al., 2020; Medford et al., 2020; Odlum et al., 2020; Ordun et al., 2020; Sha et al., 2020; Yu et al., 2020).

Topic modeling is an unsupervised classification approach implemented for various application cases including document classification of blog posts, social media data, news articles, and grouping large numerical data sets (J Silge & Robinson, 2017). It helps determine which kind of topics have been mentioned within pandemics related social media posts.

Latent Dirichlet allocation (LDA) (Lda Project, 2020) is a popular subject modeling method (Ordun et al., 2020), (Abd-Alrazaq et al., 2020; Han et al., 2020), which treats each document as a mixture of topics and each topic as a mixture of words. That allows documents to be assessed with a level of "overlapping" in terms of content - rather the grouping the documents - which reflects typical use of natural language (J Silge & Robinson, 2017). Biterm Topic model (BTM) (Yan, 2018) is another topic modelling method that learns the topics in the text by modelling the words' co-occurrences (Yan et al., 2013). It is acclaimed to be more successful than LDA in processing short texts like Twitter messages (Bansal & Srivastava, 2019).

R programming language offers a number of functions and operators to perform topic modelling by accessing to the text mining libraries; "*tm*", "*topicmodel*", and "*dplyr*" (Grover et al., 2018). On the other hand, with RapidMiner, the tweets/expressions are tokenised into words with "*Tokenize*" operator (RapidMiner Inc., 2020d) to start topic modelling. Then, using the *Ngrams* operator, consecutive keywords, e.g. two-word (bigrams) or three-word (tri-grams), and expressions can be extracted. Thus, the expressions in the content of the tweets are detected and their frequencies are calculated. The most frequently mentioned expressions in tweets can be revealed. Finally, conclusions can be driven to unveil the topics included in the posts and determine the most attracting topics posted.

Geographical Analysis

Pandemic management requires regional data and relevant analysis for effective and efficient operations. However, collecting social media data including regional details is not always possible due to the fact that platforms such as Twitter do not impose location information to be shared. Once a location and positional data is set on, the posts would include latitude and longitude of the locations in which each individual post is fired. Both R language and RapidMiner tool would be able to help perform analysis including location and regional information.

A different method for determining the location posts is to access the location of the account details of the users, e.g. tweeter, any location information has publicly been provided as part of the account. The location information of the user account in this way would only consist of city or country names, not the exact location, but, the latitude and longitude of such location information can be converted to regional information through the Google Maps API (Google, 2020) for regional coordinates to some extent. For these operations, the location information of each Twitter user can be obtained through the *getUser ()* function of the *twitteR* package of the R programming language. It refers to the location attribute of the data obtained and the location (city and/or country information) of the user. The location information obtained can be converted into latitude and longitude information with the help of *geocode_helpers* and *modified_geocode* libraries (Puente, 2016) using the google maps API application. Using the open-source package, called *leaflet*, the visualisation process obtained and converted location data can be performed by positioning the markers at the locations corresponding to this latitude and longitude information on google maps.

Case Number Estimation With Predictive Analytics

The literature reviewed, rather a recent one, including (Culotta, 2010), (F. Zhang et al., 2014), (C. Li et al., 2020), (Qin et al., 2020), (Jahanbin & Rahmanian, 2020), (Alkouz et al., 2019), conclude that a relationship can be unveiled between the number of posts about the pandemic on social media and the number of cases. It means that the change in the number of cases within pandemic circumstances can be predicted with the change in social media posts related to pandemics. In order to improve the success rate of this method, the frequencies of the words in the posts/ tweets can be calculated (Grimaldi et al., 2020), and the words with a correlation between the daily frequency change of these words and the number of cases can be added to the keyword list (related to pandemic). Similar analyzes are made for existing search terms and words that do not show correlations can be removed from the search list. If word search is done by including location information, increase and decrease by region can also be estimated.

In addition to the number of posts about the pandemic on social media, the measure index (University of Oxford, 2020) related to the pandemic, the statistics of air pollution and exhaust amount, which can be a measure of the amount of travel of people, the rate of use of indoor spaces and other relevant parameters such as temperature, season, which may affect the ventilation of these spaces, to independent variables. Using a regression model with the number of dependent variables or RapidMiner Auto Model (RapidMiner Inc., 2020a) and machine learning models, it will be possible to establish a correlation and increase the success of case prediction.

CONCLUSION

Pandemic management requires effective ways to operate and efficiency in conduct so as to meet the public needs and effectively resolve the issues. That necessitates regular and timely public opinion and reaction about the policies and ongoing activities. The timeliness is crucial in this act and requires data to monitor public take. Regular public polls are the common and traditional ways to collect data for public view, but is very time-consuming. Social media analytics appears to be a new and innovative way to collect information on public views and emerging issues.

This chapter reviews and summaries how pandemic management for COVID-19 has been using social media analytics and how helpful the existing tools are in collecting the public perception for ongoing management policies, to determine the emerging issues, and to monitor the trend of the spreading pandemic. Social media analytics help fast data collection, effective analysis, and emergencies-driven policy-making and management. This can also help understand disinformation, mis-conceptualisation, and spread of social media abuse, which will not be in benefit of the public, and take relevant measures upon such cases.

A principle conclusion driven is that social media analytics is a useful and efficient tool to use to obtain important information such as the spread of the pandemic, the number of cases, and the number of future cases. In order to access such benefits, organisations take action to setup purpose-driven divisions and/or departments to help handle pandemic-related public concerns and problems. It is believed that social media data and its analytics will remain prominent too for pandemic management for public and local authorities and decision-makers. As a result, in this section, the reader is briefed on how to use social media, which is an important source of big data for risk identification, assessment, and management, during pandemic periods.

REFERENCES

Abd-Alrazaq, A., Alhuwail, D., Househ, M., Hai, M., & Shah, Z. (2020). Top concerns of tweeters during the COVID-19 pandemic: A surveillance study. *Journal of Medical Internet Research*, *22*(4), 1–9. doi:10.2196/19016 PMID:32287039

Ahuja, V., & Shakeel, M. (2017). Twitter Presence of Jet Airways-Deriving Customer Insights Using Netnography and Wordclouds. *Procedia Computer Science*, *122*, 17–24. doi:10.1016/j.procs.2017.11.336

Alkouz, B., Al Aghbari, Z., & Abawajy, J. H. (2019). Tweetluenza: Predicting flu trends from twitter data. *Big Data Mining and Analytics*, *2*(4), 273–287. doi:10.26599/BDMA.2019.9020012

Angled, L. (2020). *GitHub Stanford Corenlp*. https://github.com/stanfordnlp/python-stanford-corenlp

Anuta, D., Churchin, J., & Luo, J. (2017). *Election bias: Comparing polls and twitter in the 2016 us election*. ArXiv Preprint ArXiv:1701.06232.

Attigeri, G. V., Manohara Pai, M. M., Pai, R. M., & Nayak, A. (2016). Stock market prediction: A big data approach. *IEEE Region 10 Annual International Conference, Proceedings/TENCON*. 10.1109/TENCON.2015.7373006

Aylien Ltd. (2020a). *The News Intelligence Platform - AYLIEN News API*. https://aylien.com/

Aylien Ltd. (2020b). *Using Entity-level Sentiment Analysis to understand News Content - AYLIEN News API*. https://aylien.com/blog/using-entity-level-sentiment-analysis-to-understand-news-content

Baccianella, S., Esuli, A., & Sebastiani, F. (2010). SENTIWORDNET 3.0: An enhanced lexical resource for sentiment analysis and opinion mining. *Proceedings of the 7th International Conference on Language Resources and Evaluation, LREC 2010*, 2200–2204.

Bag, D. (2016). Business Analytics. In *Business Analytics* (2nd ed.). Routledge. doi:10.4324/9781315464695

Bakharia, A. (2019). On the Equivalence of Inductive Content Analysis and Topic Modeling. In Advances in Quantitative Ethnography (pp. 291–298). doi:10.1007/978-3-030-33232-7_25

Bansal, B., & Srivastava, S. (2018). On predicting elections with hybrid topic based sentiment analysis of tweets. *Procedia Computer Science*, *135*, 346–353. doi:10.1016/j.procs.2018.08.183

Bansal, B., & Srivastava, S. (2019). Lexicon-based Twitter sentiment analysis for vote share prediction using emoji and N-gram features. *International Journal of Web Based Communities*, *15*(1), 85–99. doi:10.1504/IJWBC.2019.098693

Bastian, M., Heymann, S., & Jacomy, M. (2009). Gephi: An open source software for exploring and manipulating networks. *BT - International AAAI Conference on Weblogs and Social. International AAAI Conference on Weblogs and Social Media*, 361–362.

Birjali, M., Beni-Hssane, A., & Erritali, M. (2017). Analyzing Social Media through Big Data using InfoSphere BigInsights and Apache Flume. *Procedia Computer Science*, *113*, 280–285. doi:10.1016/j.procs.2017.08.299

Budiharto, W., & Meiliana, M. (2018). Prediction and analysis of Indonesia Presidential election from Twitter using sentiment analysis. *Journal of Big Data*, *5*(1), 51. doi:10.118640537-018-0164-1

Burnap, P., Gibson, R., Sloan, L., Southern, R., & Williams, M. (2016). 140 characters to victory?: Using Twitter to predict the UK 2015 General Election. *Electoral Studies*, *41*, 230–233. Advance online publication. doi:10.1016/j.electstud.2015.11.017

Castro, R., Kuffó, L., & Vaca, C. (2017). Back to #6D: Predicting Venezuelan states political election results through Twitter. *2017 4th International Conference on EDemocracy and EGovernment, ICEDEG 2017*. 10.1109/ICEDEG.2017.7962525

Cerchiello, P., & Giudici, P. (2016). Big data analysis for financial risk management. *Journal of Big Data*, *3*(1), 18. doi:10.118640537-016-0053-4

Chakraborty, G., Pagolu, M., & Garla, S. (2014). *Text mining and analysis: practical methods, examples, and case studies using SAS*. SAS Institute.

Chang, Y.-C., Ku, C.-H., & Chen, C.-H. (2017). Social media analytics: Extracting and visualizing Hilton hotel ratings and reviews from TripAdvisor. *International Journal of Information Management*.

Chatterjee, S., & Krystyanczuk, M. (2017). *Python Social Media Analytics*. Packt Publishing Ltd.

Chauhan, P., Sharma, N., & Sikka, G. (2020). The emergence of social media data and sentiment analysis in election prediction. *Journal of Ambient Intelligence and Humanized Computing*, 1–27. doi:10.100712652-020-02423-y

Choy, M., Cheong, M. L. F., Ma, N. L., & Koo, P. S. (2012). US Presidential Election 2012 Prediction using Census Corrected Twitter Model. *Research Collection School Of Information Systems*, 1–12. https://arxiv.org/abs/1211.0938

Cinelli, M., Quattrociocchi, W., Galeazzi, A., Valensise, C. M., Brugnoli, E., Schmidt, A. L., . . . Scala, A. (2020). *The COVID-19 Social Media Infodemic*. https://arxiv.org/abs/2003.05004

Culotta, A. (2010). Towards detecting influenza epidemics by analyzing Twitter messages. *SOMA 2010 - Proceedings of the 1st Workshop on Social Media Analytics*, 115–122. 10.1145/1964858.1964874

Culotta, A., & Cutler, J. (2016). Mining Brand Perceptions from Twitter Social Networks. *Marketing Science*, *35*(3), 343–362. doi:10.1287/mksc.2015.0968

De Santis, E., Martino, A., & Rizzi, A. (2020). An Infoveillance System for Detecting and Tracking Relevant Topics from Italian Tweets during the COVID-19 Event. *IEEE Access: Practical Innovations, Open Solutions*, *8*, 132527–132538. doi:10.1109/ACCESS.2020.3010033

Depoux, A., Martin, S., Karafillakis, E., Preet, R., Wilder-Smith, A., & Larson, H. (2020). The pandemic of social media panic travels faster than the COVID-19 outbreak. *Journal of Travel Medicine*, *27*(3), 1–2. doi:10.1093/jtm/taaa031 PMID:32125413

Devlin, J. (2020). *GitHub Bert*. https://github.com/google-research/bert

Devlin, J., Chang, M. W., Lee, K., & Toutanova, K. (2019). BERT: Pre-training of deep bidirectional transformers for language understanding. *NAACL HLT 2019 - 2019 Conference of the North American Chapter of the Association for Computational Linguistics: Human Language Technologies - Proceedings of the Conference*, *1*(Mlm), 4171–4186.

Doogan, C., Buntine, W., Linger, H., & Brunt, S. (2020). Public Perceptions and Attitudes Towards COVID-19 Non-Pharmaceutical Interventions Across Six Countries: A Topic Modeling Analysis of Twitter Data (Preprint). *Journal of Medical Internet Research*, *22*(9), e21419. Advance online publication. doi:10.2196/21419 PMID:32784190

Esuli, A. (2019). *GitHub SentiWordNet*. https://github.com/aesuli/SentiWordNet

Evans, J. R. (2017). Business analytics (2nd ed.). Pearson Education Limited.

Gephi. (2020). *Gephi - The Open Graph Viz Platform*. https://gephi.org/

Gilbert, C. H. E., & Hutto, E. (2014). Vader: A parsimonious rule-based model for sentiment analysis of social media text. *Eighth International Conference on Weblogs and Social Media (ICWSM-14)*. http://comp. social. gatech. edu/papers/icwsm14

Glowacki, E. M., Wilcox, G. B., & Glowacki, J. B. (2020). Identifying #addiction concerns on twitter during the COVID-19 pandemic: A text mining analysis. *Substance Abuse*, *0*(0), 1–8. doi:10.1080/08897077.2020.1822489 PMID:32970973

Goel, A., & Mittal, A. (2012). *Stock prediction using twitter sentiment analysis*. Stanford University.

Google. (2020). *Get an API Key | Maps Embed API | Google Developers*. https://developers.google.com/maps/documentation/embed/get-api-key

Grandjean, M. (2016). A social network analysis of Twitter: Mapping the digital humanities community. *Cogent Arts & Humanities, 3*(1), 1–14. doi:10.1080/2331 1983.2016.1171458

Grimaldi, D., Diaz, J., & Arboleda, H. (2020). *Inferring the votes in a new political landscape. The case of the 2019 Spanish Presidential elections.* Research Square; doi:10.21203/rs.3.rs-16463/v1

Grover, P., Kar, A. K., Dwivedi, Y. K., & Janssen, M. (2018). Polarization and acculturation in US Election 2016 outcomes – Can twitter analytics predict changes in voting preferences. *Technological Forecasting and Social Change*, (September), 1–23. doi:10.1016/j.techfore.2018.09.009

Han, X., Wang, J., Zhang, M., & Wang, X. (2020). Using social media to mine and analyze public opinion related to COVID-19 in China. *International Journal of Environmental Research and Public Health, 17*(8), 2788. Advance online publication. doi:10.3390/ijerph17082788 PMID:32316647

Hu, M., & Liu, B. (2004). Mining and summarizing customer reviews. *Proceedings of the 2004 ACM SIGKDD International Conference on Knowledge Discovery and Data Mining - KDD '04*, 168. 10.1145/1014052.1014073

Hutto, C. J. (2020). *GitHub Vader Sentiment.* https://github.com/cjhutto/vaderSentiment

Jahanbin, K., & Rahmanian, V. (2020). Using twitter and web news mining to predict COVID-19 outbreak. *Asian Pacific Journal of Tropical Medicine, 13*(8), 378–380. doi:10.4103/1995-7645.279651

Jockers, M. (2017a). *Introduction to the Syuzhet Package.* https://cran.r-project.org/web/packages/syuzhet/vignettes/syuzhet-vignette.html

JockersM. (2017b). *Package 'syuzhet'.* https://github.com/mjockers/syuzhet

Kale, G. Ö. (2016). Marka İletişiminde Instagram Kullanımı. *The Turkish Online Journal of Design. Art and Communication, 6*(2), 119–127. doi:10.7456/10602100/006

Ketter, E. (2016). Destination image restoration on facebook: The case study of Nepal's Gurkha Earthquake. *Journal of Hospitality and Tourism Management, 28*, 66–72. doi:10.1016/j.jhtm.2016.02.003

Kim, E., Sung, Y., & Kang, H. (2014). Brand followers' retweeting behavior on Twitter: How brand relationships influence brand electronic word-of-mouth. *Computers in Human Behavior, 37*, 18–25. doi:10.1016/j.chb.2014.04.020

Lda Project. (2020). *GitHub LDA*. https://github.com/lda-project/lda

Li, C., Chen, L. J., Chen, X., Zhang, M., Pang, C. P., & Chen, H. (2020). Retrospective analysis of the possibility of predicting the COVID-19 outbreak from Internet searches and social media data, China, 2020. *Eurosurveillance*, *25*(10), 1–5. doi:10.2807/1560-7917.ES.2020.25.10.2000199 PMID:32183935

Li, L., Zhang, Q., Wang, X., Zhang, J., Wang, T., Gao, T. L., Duan, W., Tsoi, K. K. F., & Wang, F. Y. (2020). Characterizing the Propagation of Situational Information in Social Media during COVID-19 Epidemic: A Case Study on Weibo. *IEEE Transactions on Computational Social Systems*, *7*(2), 556–562. doi:10.1109/TCSS.2020.2980007

Luna, S., & Pennock, M. J. (2018). Social media applications and emergency management: A literature review and research agenda. *International Journal of Disaster Risk Reduction*, *28*, 565–577. doi:10.1016/j.ijdrr.2018.01.006

Makazhanov, A., Rafiei, D., & Waqar, M. (2014). Predicting political preference of Twitter users. *Social Network Analysis and Mining*, *4*(1), 193. Advance online publication. doi:10.100713278-014-0193-5

Manning, C. D., Bauer, J., Finkel, J. R., Bethard, S. J., Surdeanu, M., Bauer, J., Finkel, J. R., Bethard, S. J., & McClosky, D. (2014). The Stanford CoreNLP natural language processing toolkit. *Proceedings of 52nd Annual Meeting of the Association for Computational Linguistics: System Demonstrations*, 55–60. http://macopolo.cn/mkpl/products.asp

MeaningCloud LLC. (2020). *Sentiment Analysis API | MeaningCloud*. https://www.meaningcloud.com/developer/sentiment-analysis

Medford, R. J., Saleh, S. N., Sumarsono, A., Perl, T. M., & Lehmann, C. U. (2020). An "Infodemic": Leveraging High-Volume Twitter Data to Understand Early Public Sentiment for the Coronavirus Disease 2019 Outbreak. *Open Forum Infectious Diseases*, *7*(7), ofaa258. Advance online publication. doi:10.1093/ofid/ofaa258 PMID:33117854

Misirlis, N., & Vlachopoulou, M. (2018). Social media metrics and analytics in marketing – S3M: A mapping literature review. *International Journal of Information Management*, *38*(1), 270–276. doi:10.1016/j.ijinfomgt.2017.10.005

Mohammad, S. M. (2020). *NRC Emotion Lexicon*. http://saifmohammad.com/WebPages/NRC-Emotion-Lexicon.htm

Mohammad, S. M., & Turney, P. D. (2013). Crowdsourcing a word-emotion association lexicon. *Computational Intelligence*, *29*(3), 436–465. doi:10.1111/j.1467-8640.2012.00460.x

Nielsen, F. Å. (2011). *AFINN sentiment analysis in Python: Wordlist-based approach for sentiment analysis*. Technical University of Denmark. https://github.com/fnielsen/afinn

Nielsen, F. Å. (2019). *GitHub Afinn*. https://github.com/fnielsen/afinn

North, M. (2012). *Data mining for the masses* (Vol. 615684378). Global Text Project Athens.

Odlum, M., Cho, H., Broadwell, P., Davis, N., Patrao, M., Schauer, D., Bales, M. E., Alcantara, C., & Yoon, S. (2020). Application of topic modeling to tweetsas the foundation for health disparity research for COVID-19. In Studies in Health Technology and Informatics (Vol. 272). doi:10.3233/SHTI200484

Open, A. I. (2019). *Better Language Models and Their Implications*. https://openai.com/blog/better-language-models/

Ordun, C., Purushotham, S., & Raff, E. (2020). *Exploratory analysis of covid-19 tweets using topic modeling, umap, and digraphs*. https://arxiv.org/abs/2005.03082

Otte, E., & Rousseau, R. (2002). Social network analysis: A powerful strategy, also for the information sciences. *Journal of Information Science*, *28*(6), 441–453. doi:10.1177/016555150202800601

Öztürk, N., & Ayvaz, S. (2018). Sentiment analysis on Twitter: A text mining approach to the Syrian refugee crisis. *Telematics and Informatics*, *35*(1), 136–147. doi:10.1016/j.tele.2017.10.006

Park, H. W., Park, S., & Chong, M. (2020). Conversations and Medical News Frames on Twitter: Infodemiological Study on COVID-19 in South Korea. *Journal of Medical Internet Research*, *22*(5), e18897. doi:10.2196/18897 PMID:32325426

Pournarakis, D. E., Sotiropoulos, D. N., & Giaglis, G. M. (2017). A computational model for mining consumer perceptions in social media. *Decision Support Systems*, *93*(2016), 98–110. doi:10.1016/j.dss.2016.09.018

Puente, L. (2016). *Mapping Twitter Followers in R | Lucas Puente*. http://lucaspuente.github.io/notes/2016/04/05/Mapping-Twitter-Followers

Qin, L., Sun, Q., Wang, Y., Wu, K.-F., Chen, M., Shia, B.-C., & Wu, S.-Y. (2020). Prediction of Number of Cases of 2019 Novel Coronavirus (COVID-19) Using Social Media Search Index. *International Journal of Environmental Research and Public Health, 17*(7), 2365. doi:10.3390/ijerph17072365 PMID:32244425

Radford, A., Wu, J., Child, R., Luan, D., Amodei, D., & Sutskever, I. (2019). Language models are unsupervised multitask learners. *OpenAI Blog, 1*(8), 9.

Ragini, J. R., Anand, P. M. R., & Bhaskar, V. (2018). Big data analytics for disaster response and recovery through sentiment analysis. *International Journal of Information Management, 42*, 13–24. doi:10.1016/j.ijinfomgt.2018.05.004

Ramteke, J., Shah, S., Godhia, D., & Shaikh, A. (2016). Election result prediction using Twitter sentiment analysis. *2016 International Conference on Inventive Computation Technologies (ICICT), 1*, 1–5. 10.1109/INVENTIVE.2016.7823280

RapidMiner Inc. (2019). *Sentiment Analysis using the new Extract Sentiment operator — RapidMiner Community*. https://community.rapidminer.com/discussion/55251/sentiment-analysis-using-the-new-extract-sentiment-operator

RapidMiner Inc. (2020a). *Introducing RapidMiner Auto Model | RapidMiner*. https://rapidminer.com/resource/automated-machine-learning/

RapidMiner Inc. (2020b). *RapidMiner | Best Data Science & Machine Learning Platform*. https://rapidminer.com/

RapidMiner Inc. (2020c). *Rapidminer Educational License | RapidMiner*. https://rapidminer.com/get-started-educational/

RapidMiner Inc. (2020d). *Text and Web Mining with RapidMiner*. https://academy.rapidminer.com/courses/text-and-web-mining-with-rapidminer

Ravi, K., & Ravi, V. (2015). A survey on opinion mining and sentiment analysis: Tasks, approaches and applications. *Knowledge-Based Systems, 89*, 14–46. doi:10.1016/j.knosys.2015.06.015

Rexiline Ragini, J., Rubesh Anand, P. M., & Bhaskar, V. (2018). Mining crisis information: A strategic approach for detection of people at risk through social media analysis. *International Journal of Disaster Risk Reduction, 27*, 556–566. doi:10.1016/j.ijdrr.2017.12.002

RStudio PBC. (2020a). *R Packages - RStudio*. https://rstudio.com/products/rpackages/

RStudio PBC. (2020b). *RStudio - RStudio*. https://rstudio.com/products/rstudio/

Sabuncu, İ., & Atmis, M. (2020). Social Media Analytics for Brand Image Tracking: A Case Study Application for Turkish Airlines. *Yönetim Bilişim Sistemleri Dergisi, 6*(1), 26–41. https://dergipark.org.tr/tr/download/article-file/1104512

Saif, H., He, Y., Fernandez, M., & Alani, H. (2016). Contextual semantics for sentiment analysis of Twitter. *Information Processing & Management, 52*(1), 5–19. doi:10.1016/j.ipm.2015.01.005

Saleh, S. N., Lehmann, C. U., McDonald, S. A., Basit, M. A., & Medford, R. J. (2020). Understanding public perception of COVID-19 social distancing on twitter. *Infection Control and Hospital Epidemiology, 2019*, 1–8. doi:10.1017/ice.2020.406 PMID:32758315

Sarker, A., Lakamana, S., Hogg-bremer, W., Xie, A., Al-garadi, M. A., & Yang, Y. (2020). Self-reported COVID-19 symptoms on Twitter: An analysis and a research resource. *Journal of the American Medical Informatics Association: JAMIA, 27*(July), 1310–1315. doi:10.1093/jamia/ocaa116 PMID:32620975

Sear, R. F., Velasquez, N., Leahy, R., Restrepo, N. J., El Oud, S., Gabriel, N., Lupu, Y., & Johnson, N. F. (2020). Quantifying COVID-19 Content in the Online Health Opinion War Using Machine Learning. *IEEE Access: Practical Innovations, Open Solutions, 8*, 91886–91893. doi:10.1109/ACCESS.2020.2993967

Sha, H., Al Hasan, M., Mohler, G., & Brantingham, P. J. (2020). Dynamic topic modeling of the COVID-19 Twitter narrative among U.S. governors and cabinet executives. *ArXiv Preprint ArXiv:2004.11692, 2*, 2–7. https://arxiv.org/abs/2004.11692

Shen, C., Chen, A., Luo, C., Zhang, J., Feng, B., & Liao, W. (2020). Using Reports of Symptoms and Diagnoses on Social Media to Predict COVID-19 Case Counts in Mainland China: Observational Infoveillance Study. *Journal of Medical Internet Research, 22*(5), e19421. doi:10.2196/19421 PMID:32452804

Shmueli, G., Bruce, P. C., Yahav, I., Patel, N. R., & Lichtendahl, K. C. Jr. (2017). *Data Mining for Business Analytics: Concepts, Techniques, and Applications in R.* John Wiley & Sons.

Silge, J., & Robinson, D. (2017). *Text Mining with R: A Tidy Approach.* O'Reilly Media. https://books.google.com.tr/books?id=qNcnDwAAQBAJ

Silge, J., & Robinson, D. (2020). *2 Sentiment analysis with tidy data | Text Mining with R.* https://www.tidytextmining.com/sentiment.html

Singh, P., Dwivedi, Y. K., Kahlon, K. S., Pathania, A., & Sawhney, R. S. (2020). Can twitter analytics predict election outcome? An insight from 2017 Punjab assembly elections. *Government Information Quarterly, 37*(2), 101444. doi:10.1016/j. giq.2019.101444

Sitta, D., Faulkner, M., & Stern, P. (2018). What can the brand manager expect from Facebook? *Australasian Marketing Journal, 26*(1), 1–6. doi:10.1016/j. ausmj.2018.01.001

Squicciarini, A., Tapia, A., & Stehle, S. (2017). Sentiment analysis during Hurricane Sandy in emergency response. *International Journal of Disaster Risk Reduction, 21*(May), 213–222. doi:10.1016/j.ijdrr.2016.12.011

Stanford, N. L. P. Group. (2020). *Overview - CoreNLP*. https://stanfordnlp.github. io/CoreNLP/index.html

The R Foundation. (2020). *R: The R Project for Statistical Computing*. https:// www.r-project.org/

University of Oxford. (2020). *Coronavirus Government Response Tracker | Blavatnik School of Government*. https://www.bsg.ox.ac.uk/research/research-projects/ coronavirus-government-response-tracker

Valdivia, A., Luzón, M. V., Cambria, E., & Herrera, F. (2018). Consensus vote models for detecting and filtering neutrality in sentiment analysis. *Information Fusion, 44*, 126–135. Advance online publication. doi:10.1016/j.inffus.2018.03.007

Wang, W. Y., Pauleen, D. J., & Zhang, T. (2016). How social media applications affect {B2B} communication and improve business performance in {SMEs}. *Industrial Marketing Management, 54*, 4–14. doi:10.1016/j.indmarman.2015.12.004

Wang, Y., Hao, H., & Platt, L. S. (2021). Examining risk and crisis communications of government agencies and stakeholders during early-stages of COVID-19 on Twitter. *Computers in Human Behavior, 114*(June), 106568. doi:10.1016/j.chb.2020.106568

Wicaksono, Suyoto, & Pranowo. (2017). A proposed method for predicting US presidential election by analyzing sentiment in social media. *Proceeding - 2016 2nd International Conference on Science in Information Technology, ICSITech 2016: Information Science for Green Society and Environment*. 10.1109/ ICSITech.2016.7852647

Wicke, P., & Bolognesi, M. M. (2020). *Framing COVID-19: How we conceptualize and discuss the pandemic on Twitter*. ArXiv Preprint ArXiv:2004.06986. https:// arxiv.org/abs/2004.06986

Wukich, C. (2016). Government social media messages across disaster phases. *Journal of Contingencies and Crisis Management, 24*(4), 230–243. doi:10.1111/1468-5973.12119

Yan, X. (2018). *GitHub BTM.* https://github.com/xiaohuiyan/BTM

Yan, X., Guo, J., Lan, Y., & Cheng, X. (2013). A biterm topic model for short texts. *Proceedings of the 22nd International Conference on World Wide Web*, 1445–1456. 10.1145/2488388.2488514

Yin, F., Lv, J., Zhang, X., Xia, X., & Wu, J. (2020). COVID-19 information propagation dynamics in the Chinese Sina-microblog. *Mathematical Biosciences and Engineering, 17*(3), 2676–2692. doi:10.3934/mbe.2020146 PMID:32233560

Yu, J., Lu, Y., & Muñoz-Justicia, J. (2020). Analyzing Spanish News Frames on Twitter during COVID-19—A Network Study of El País and El Mundo. *International Journal of Environmental Research and Public Health, 17*(15), 5414. doi:10.3390/ijerph17155414 PMID:32731359

Zhang, F., Luo, J., Li, C., Wang, X., & Zhao, Z. (2014). Detecting and analyzing influenza epidemics with social media in China. In V. S. Tseng, T. B. Ho, Z.-H. Zhou, A. L. P. Chen, & H.-Y. Kao (Eds.), *Pacific-Asia Conference on Knowledge Discovery and Data Mining* (pp. 90–101). Springer. 10.1007/978-3-319-06608-0_8

Zhang, X., Fuehres, H., & Gloor, P. A. (2011). Predicting Stock Market Indicators Through Twitter "I hope it is not as bad as I fear". *Procedia - Social and Behavioral Sciences, 26*, 55–62. doi:10.1016/j.sbspro.2011.10.562

Zhao, Y., Cheng, S., Yu, X., & Xu, H. (2020). Chinese public's attention to the COVID-19 epidemic on social media: Observational descriptive study. *Journal of Medical Internet Research, 22*(5), 1–13. doi:10.2196/18825 PMID:32314976

Chapter 6
Deep Learning Approaches in Pandemic and Disaster Management

Marcello Trovati
https://orcid.org/0000-0001-6607-422X
Edge Hill University, UK

Eleana Asimakopoulou
Hellenic National Defence College, Greece

Nik Bessis
https://orcid.org/0000-0002-6013-3935
Independent Researcher, UK

ABSTRACT

A quick decision-making process in response and management of epidemics has been the most common approach, as accurate and relevant decisions have been demonstrated to have beneficial impacts on life preservation as well as on global and local economies. However, any disaster or epidemic is rarely represented by a set of single and linear parameters, as they often exhibit highly complex and chaotic behaviours, where interconnected unknowns rapidly evolve. As a consequence, any such decision-making approach must be computationally robust and able to process large amounts of data, whilst evaluating the potential outcomes based on specific decisions in real time.

DOI: 10.4018/978-1-7998-6736-4.ch006

INTRODUCTION

The occurrence of epidemics has a long-lasting impact, usually affecting a large number of individuals (UNDRR, https://www.unisdr.org/). Epidemics are often regarded as a type of disaster, similar to 'man-made' disasters but with increased impact (O'Brien, et al, 2010). In this chapter, we argue that the increasing digitalisation of the management of disasters is directly linked with epidemics, with existing and novel AI and deep learning applications having a direct impact on assessing and monitoring epidemic occurrences.

A quick decision-making process in response and management of epidemics has been the most common approach, as accurate and relevant decisions have been demonstrated to have beneficial impacts on life preservation as well as on global and local economies (Thompson, et al. 2006).

However, any disaster or epidemic is rarely represented by a set of single and linear parameters, as they often exhibit highly complex and chaotic behaviours, where interconnected unknowns rapidly evolve. As a consequence, any such decision-making approach must be computationally robust and able to process large amounts of data, whilst evaluating the potential outcomes based on specific decisions in real time. There are a variety of software products to aid practitioners during the decision-making process, including Emergency Information System (EIS), SoftRisk, EM 2000, and E-Team, which provide a range of emergency management decision support, resource management, and incident documentation functions to emergency managers (Green, et al, 2001). The emergency management and operations research literature also contains a number of examples of Decision Support Systems (DSS) designed for specific scenarios or objectives.

Table 1 depicts relevant support tools, which are widely used in disaster management scenarios. These are also applied to epidemic scenarios especially in the management of resources and infrastructures.

Table 1. Decision support tools widely used in disaster management and applicable to epidemic scenarios

Decision Support Tools	
Damage assessment	• CATS (www.saic.com/products/simulation/cats/cats.html)
Emergency logistics	• MCCADS • CALMS (www.nyc.gov/html/oem/html/response/calms/html) ARES
Evacuation	• TEDSS • CEMPS • REMS
Emergency management	• CAMEO • MIND

(Tompson, et al, 2006).

Any epidemic and disaster management approach includes four distinct components: 'mitigation'; 'preparedness'; 'response'; and 'recovery'. The aim of the mitigation component is to identify and minimise the effects of a hazardous event, while the preparedness component aims to identify the best response. Response activities follow the above phases, and they focus on plans as well as suitable emergency activities to mitigate life and economy losses. Finally, recovery identifies the best procedures to allow a return to pre-disaster levels (Yu, et al., 2018).

Figure 1. The disaster and epidemic management cycle
(Yu, et al, 2018)

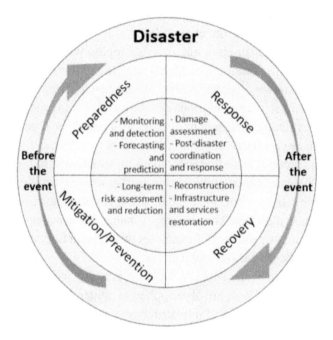

During an epidemic event, the flow of information originates from several sources, including emergency telephone calls, news, social media, and other real-time sources. However, due to the highly dynamic scenarios related to disaster events, information is likely to be incomplete, inaccurate and continually evolving.

As a consequence, technology needs to address such issues in order to support the decision-making process.

ARTIFICIAL INTELLIGENCE APPROACHES TO EPIDEMIC AND DISASTER MANAGEMENT

There are several artificial intelligence (AI) approaches utilised in epidemic and disaster management, which include supervised and unsupervised models, deep learning, reinforcement learning, and deep reinforcement learning (Sun, et al, 2020).

Supervised AI models are trained on pre-processed data by including suitable labels linking known input and output pairs. In general, supervised models infer a mapping function between input and output using different techniques such as regression and classification methods, which predict the output variable (Russell, et al, 2016). They are widely used for information extraction, pattern and speech recognition, among others.

Unsupervised AI models, on the other hand, are based on statistical techniques to identify hidden structures within unlabelled datasets without human intervention. Unsupervised models have been shown to be particularly suitable for abnormal data detection and data dimension reduction, with specific applications to data clustering and aggregation tasks.

Deep learning models belongs to artificial neural networks (ANNs), and they are defined by several interconnected layers which, following a training process, are able to identify data features. In order to design accurate deep learning models, the overall training process tends to be relatively long. Overall, deep learning algorithms have been demonstrated to produce good results in damage assessment, motion detection, and data trend prediction (Sun, et al, 2020).

Other types of models that have drawn considerable attention include reinforcement learning, which consists of punishment and reward actions associated with positive and negative signals. Reinforcement learning is particularly successful when applied to information extraction and decision-making approaches in stochastic environments (Sun, et al, 2020).

When reinforcement algorithms are combined with deep learning, also known as Deep reinforcement learning, they exhibit a considerably better performance in tasks related to computer vision, robotics, finance, stochastic modelling, etc.

Machine Learning, Neural Networks and Deep Learning

Machine learning approaches have been gathering increasing interest due to their versatility and applicability to various research areas such as pattern recognition, text mining, trend analysis, and computational learning. Most of their popularity stems from the fact that machine learning enables computers systems are capable of learning without being explicitly taught, to design algorithms directly learnt from data, whilst carrying out data-driven decision processes and predictions. Over the last few years, machine learning applications have exponentially grown, with real-time data extraction and analysis, autonomous systems, image recognition among them. However, areas remain where machine learning algorithms are still far from being comparable to information processing mechanisms, exhibiting disappointing performance in terms of accuracy, scalability and complexity.

Artificial neural networks (ANNs) have also considerably expanded over the last decade (Hou, et al, 2016), (Yang, et al, 2016), (Yu, ae al., 2016), (Yuan, et al, 2016). ANNs are defined by layers of neurons, which are mutually activated by weighted links. The corresponding parameters need to be learnt by adjusting the weights, as well as the overall topology of the network. Despite having shown significant potential in several automated tasks, the process of training an ANN may be computationally very expensive. Extensive research has focused on the training process, which has led to the introduction of the backpropagation algorithm. This is an efficient gradient descent algorithm with a high training accuracy. However, its performance is still problematic, depending on the type of training data utilised.

Deep learning has been motivated by ANNs (Hinton, et al, 2006). In Hinton (2006), the authors introduced a new training method, which initialised the birth of deep learning. The underling concept in deep learning is the *layer-wise-greedy-learning* algorithm based on the idea that unsupervised pre-learning should be carried out prior to the subsequent layer-by-layer training. This process leads to a reduction of the data dimension and a more efficient data-labelling step. The development of Big Data analytics has been one of the key factors in the increasing popularity of deep learning techniques, due to its ability to accurately and efficiently analysis large quantity of data.

In general, deep learning algorithms exhibit hierarchical architectures, whose topology is defined by several layers for a non-linear information processing capability.

Via suitably labelled training datasets, coupled with appropriate models, deep learning allows the identification, extraction and subsequent analysis of data patterns, inter-connections and relationships.

Considering the ability of deep learning to analyse and investigate large structured and unstructured datasets, it has a considerable number of applications both academic and commercial (Deng, et al., 2014), (Najafabadi, et al, 2015). Examples of applications include speech recognition, image processing and sensing scene classification (Hu, et al., 2015), as well as large-scale sentiment classification (Glorot, et al, 2011).

More specifically, the field of computer vision and pattern recognition have benefitted from deep learning, as its computational efficiency can address large datasets, otherwise complex to investigate. Feature selection is a core component of pattern classification and recognition, which tends to be challenging for traditional classification algorithms with limited generality. On the other hand, deep learning architectures, such as Convolutional NNs (CNNs), are able to automatically identify suitable features, whilst exhibiting excellent performance via GPU-based computational resources.

Deep learning methods have also achieved outstanding performance in object recognition tasks, especially compared with traditional classification algorithms (Tang, et al, 2012). Specific recent applications can be found in traffic management and prediction (Ciresan, et al, 2012), preventative and investigative medicine (Kim, et al, 2016), image labelling (Lerouge, et al, 2015), wind speed patterns classification and multi- spectral land-use classification (Hu, et al, 2016).

DATA SOURCES FOR EPIDEMIC AND DISASTER MANAGEMENT

As discussed in (Yu, et al, 2018), a comprehensive and detailed classification of the data used in epidemic and disaster management is still lacking. Currently, the main information types and sources which have been identified include spatio-temporal data, mobile-based technologies, satellite imagery, and general sensory data.

In particular, satellite remote sensing technology has been demonstrated to offer qualitative and quantitative data types which can provide tools to assess post-event damage, guidance to suitable operational assistance (Skakun, et al, 2014), as well as risk management and prediction approaches. Remote sensing is based on several methods such as higher resolution, multidimensional, and multi-technique. In particular, recent improvements in image resolution, has led to effective methods to assess geographical areas relevant to the management of resources and infrastructures (Pradhan, et al, 2016).

This type of data can be used to train suitable models and monitor the occurrence of events, which are likely to affect the appropriate response to epidemic outbursts, as well as more general disasters. In fact, the information collected via high resolution satellite imagery can identify land and urban areas structure, which might lead to an increased likelihood of the negative impacts posed by adverse events, including epidemics (Liou, et al, 2010). This has significant potential in directing rescue efforts, monitor any possible increase in disaster occurrence (Raspini, et al, 2017), adverse event reduction (Pesaresi, et al, 2015), as well as identifying and assessing the level of infrastructures relevant to the successful management of epidemics and disasters occurrences (McCallum, et al, 2016).

Other image-based data can be captured by using unmanned aerial vehicles (UAVs). UAVs can gather images with a high spatial resolution, which in turn can be processed much more efficiently compared to satellite imagery (Ofli, et al, 2016). Furthermore, UAVs are fully controllable whilst providing high resolution VHR imagery allowing the detection of fine details and detailed point clouds. UAVs can also assist health practitioners to better identify affected or isolated areas.

Wireless Sensor Network (WSN) technologies have also been shown to produce actionable data to assess disasters. They, in fact, provide reliable data transmission from different types of sensors, whilst minimising energy consumption (Chen, et al, 2013). Recently, the Inundation Monitoring and Alarm Technology in a System of Systems has been introduced to integrate smartphone data with WSN for enhanced situational awareness (Erdelj, et al, 2017). WSN technology has also been extensively applied to Internet of Things (IoT) technologies scenarios, which include BRINCO (a notification system for earthquake and tsunami warning), BRCK (communication system under low connectivity areas), and GRILLO (earthquake alarming sensor network) (Ray, et al, 2017). The most obvious advantages of IoT are its ability of managing and compensating limited infrastructure and so providing an increased data network resilience during critical situations (Sakhardande, et al, 2016).

Other data particularly relevant to disaster and epidemic management is generated by social media platforms, including Twitter, YouTube, and Facebook. Geotagged social media data can also be gathered to provide precise geolocation data.

As a consequence, social media services can significantly enhance appropriate management responses by providing a real-time communication platform (Charalabidis, et al, 2014). Furthermore, they can facilitate more efficient epidemic and disaster management response and recovery efforts (Roche, et al, 2013).

Even though social media provides implicit varieties of crowdsourced data, it is being effectively used in human dynamics modelling. In general, social media have several applications to disaster management, such as data collection, predictive analytics, information extraction, geolocation analytics, and the information sharing across social media platforms (Carley, et al, 2016).

In Bret, et al, (2019), the authors argue that Twitter has become a very effective social medium during disasters and epidemics. In fact, Twitter can be easily used with mobile devices and information can be shared with large audiences, not necessarily within one's social network (Lachlan, et al, 2014). Furthermore, despite tweets having a 280-character limit constraint, various types of information, such as URLs and images, can be easily shared. During the occurrence of several disasters including epidemics, Twitter users often shared images, geolocation and textual information. However, unfiltered messages contained irrelevant or erroneous material unsuitable for discerning useful information (O'Brien, et al, 2010).

The correct identification of geolocation information is essential is determining the spatial evolving of specific events. However, it can be challenging due to various issues, including the use of non-standard English, typographic errors and unconventional abbreviations.

In Twitter, geolocation information is captured by user location, place name, and geo-coordinates. However, some of these fields are optional and free text can be entered.

Place names are predefined within the Twitter database, with very limited granular location information. Furthermore, geolocation coordinates need to be enabled by using a GPS- enabled device. However, tweets with geo-coordinate information are uncommon. Deep learning techniques have been shown to identify location information at different granularity information levels. This has significant potential to monitor and assess the occurrence of disasters by providing location information via mobile technologies (Abhinav, et al, 2019). Table 2 depicts the main data sources phases relevant to the different disaster and epidemic management phases.

Table 2. Epidemic and disaster management phases with major data sources as discussed in (Yu, et al, 2018)

Disaster and Epidemic Management Phases	Data Source
Mitigation/Prevention	
Long-term risk assessment and reduction	• Satellite, • Crowdsourcing • Sensor web and IoT • Social mediaMobile GPS and CDR
Forecasting and Predicting	• Satellite • Social media • Sensor web and IoT
Preparedness	
Monitoring and detection	• Social Media • Sensor web and IoT • Satellite • Spatial data, • Mobile GPS and CDR • Crowdsourcing
Early warning	• Social Media • Sensor web and IoT • Crowdsourcing
Response	
Damage Assessment	• Social Media • Sensor web and IoT • UAVs • Satellite • Crowdsourcing
Post-disaster Coordination and Response	• Social Media • Sensor web and IoT • Satellite • Spatial data, • Mobile GPS and CDR • Crowdsourcing • UAVs
Recovery	
	• Satellite • Combination of various sources • Crowdsourcing

DEEP LEARNING FOR DISASTER AND EPIDEMIC MANAGEMENT

The impact of disasters and epidemics can be reduced if their occurrence can be predicted. AI-based systems have been demonstrated to predict highly volatile scenarios with usually several inter-connected parameters. As a consequence, activities and initiatives related to predicting, assessing and minimising the impact of epidemics have drawn considerable attention. Due to the high number of unknown parameters that need to be considered in any accurate model, the complexity of such tasks is likely to require large computational, storage and efficiency capabilities. The introduction and development of big data techniques and methods have enabled the analysis and utilisation of large unstructured datasets, which in turn allow more comprehensive predictive modelling capabilities.

However, the analysis of large datasets must be based on novel approaches, which are not simply related to traditional statistical investigations. Deep learning can address this issue.

As discussed above, deep learning techniques offer a robust and efficient approach to the analysis of large unstructured data, which in turn provide a set of tools to predict, assess and monitor the occurrence of epidemics and disasters. Furthermore, if any automated intelligent system is integrated with human decision into a hybrid process, this would provide a powerful way to minimise potential issues related to incomplete, inaccurate or delayed data, whilst enhancing effectiveness. Satellite imagery can be used to train deep learning system to identify infrastructure weaknesses which might impact mitigation actions (Antoniou, et al, 2020). In fact, the analysis of the main road networks, the corresponding basic infrastructure and facilities, as well as any human dynamics property related to a geographical area provides valuable information that can be used in planning any disaster response.

More importantly, deep learning can contribute to a more efficient epidemic relief management by helping experts to facilitate their decision-making process and by providing usable results in time-restricted and life-critical applications (Antoniou, et al, 2020).

Real-time analysis of classification of images shared across Twitter can provide useful information (Brett, et al, 2019). In particular, the use of deep learning can lead to high levels of accuracy, especially when ignoring text, to minimise the risk of identifying irrelevant or ambiguous information. Although deep learning may be used in this task, the existing models still exhibit a lack of accuracy (Brett, et al, 2019). It is suggested that this is due to a lack of robustness of the existing training data, which is affected by a class imbalance and limited dataset size. Potential solutions include a more comprehensive collection of training datasets, and a better pre-processing approach to filter out misinformation or incomplete data.

Figure 2. The object identification architecture as in (Antoniou, et al, 2020)

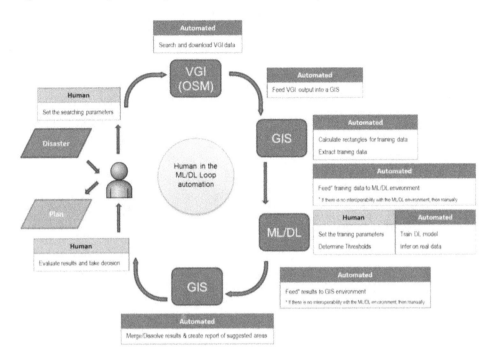

There are several deep learning applications to disaster management, which despite having different aims and targets, share a similar computation structure compared to epidemic scenarios.

An example is seismic activity monitoring and prediction. The enormous amount of seismic data which are comparable to epidemic data, has been used to train and design deep learning systems. These systems aim to predict the magnitude and patterns of earthquakes in different locations. In DeVries, et al, (2018), the authors introduce a deep learning approach to predict specific seismic events. This deep learning system was trained on a dataset containing 131,000 data points, and it was subsequently validated on a database of 30,000 similar pairs. As discussed above, Earth satellites images can be analysed to identify morphological and structural changes of natural and urban environment. Deep learning can be used to predict the risk associated with infrastructure changes or features potentially affected by epidemics and disasters in general. This would minimise damage as well as identify pre-emptive actions to minimise the overall disruption. In fact, the detection of urban structures is likely to lead to a better infrastructure and human dynamics management and modelling.

Figure 3. Diagram from Sun, et al. (2020) depicting the different applications of artificial intelligence in disaster and epidemic management.

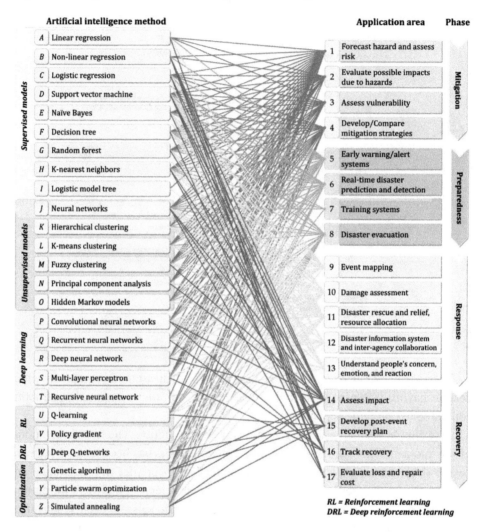

Real-time images, social media feeds and targeted messages provide a very effective approach to general warning systems. Research has focussed on AI-based systems that can be trained on historical and real-time data. Extensive experimental validation has found this type of approach to be significantly better compared to traditional systems. Furthermore, via the collection of data from social media, deep learning systems can be used to monitor and predict human behaviour and activities (Hewage, et al, 2020).

Therefore, the prediction and modelling of meteorological events is also an important factor in epidemic and disaster management activities. Satellite images and real-time information sharing (such as specialised platforms) combined with deep learning techniques provide an enhanced approach to weather prediction especially compared with the human-driven methods (Trovati, et al, 2018).

DISCUSSION

As discussed above, AI has shown significant potential in several applications and fields, its limitations have an impact in a more extensive use of the technology in real-world scenarios. Deep learning technologies, and AI in general, have demonstrated unprecedented capabilities in analysing large volumes of data at significant speed, enabling the identification of data patterns and trend. However, prediction capabilities are still lagging behind due to a number of limitations. Firstly, deep learning is over-reliant on training datasets manually annotated, which are prone to human error, leading to erroneous conclusions. secondly, the high level of skills required to adequately train deep learning is likely create an unquestioned reliance on AI is several contexts.

A major issue related to the application of AI to epidemic and disaster management is that the data is trained on prior recorded occurrences. However, prior knowledge of such disasters does not consider the continuous evolving of the relevant parameters influencing their occurrences. As a consequence, deep learning and any other AI-based approach are not able to take the surrounding environmental dynamics into consideration. And if they do, they can do so only partially. One important example is the effect of human dynamics on the management of epidemics. Since AI approaches are trained (and often validated) using historical data, these systems tend to lack predictive power when human activities are considered. Therefore, it is difficult for deep learning and AI technologies in general to provide an accurate long-term prediction of epidemics and disasters.

To mitigate these issues, financial and resource investments should be made more consistently. This would facilitate identification and hiring of experienced researchers and technology experts who are fully aware of AI limitations. In particular, a more inter-disciplinary research effort is necessary to bridge limitations in AI fields with specific mathematical and physical approaches to include the highly dynamic nature related to the occurrence of epidemics and disasters. Furthermore, training datasets need to be amended, revised and collected. This would alleviate the risks associated with incomplete or inaccurate training processes. Finally, organisations should fully embrace the potential provided by AI technologies. However, it would also imply a deeper awareness of what AI can, or cannot do at the moment. In addition to limiting the risks or over-reliance, or a 'black-box' type of utilisation, further research is needed to enhance the current state-of-the-art AI technologies and applications

It is clear that an insightful use of AI to predict, mitigate and manage disasters has significant potential in saving lives and limiting financial losses. Furthermore, AI-based systems can contribute to better planning of infrastructure in geographical areas which are likely to experience specific disasters. Therefore, a full utilisation of deep learning and AI technologies must be fully employed to take advantage of its data-drive capabilities.

Input data are likely to have different formats and types or might be partially incomplete. due to intrinsic reasons as well as legal or business issue. In particular, urban areas usually have a wider range of available data to produce accurate AI models, whereas rural areas might have limited data. It is, therefore, important to design public policies and regulations to enable efficient data gathering, pre-processing, assessment, and management procedures. Furthermore, an 'any AI fits-all' approach is unlikely to be scalable or widely applicable as different types of scenarios have different underlying parameters as well as incompatible socioeconomic requirements. However, any generalisation approach to AI-based models is typically difficult to train and implement. Finally, deep learning and general AI techniques are likely to require highly specialised knowledge and skills which limit their overall user-friendliness. Additionally, due to the computational complexity of deep learning methods, high-performance computing infrastructures might be needed. However, this might not be available for many governmental and emergency agencies in economically disadvantaged areas (Sun, et al, 2020).

As a consequence, a more focused research effort on developing more powerful, cost-effective, 'white-box' AI-based techniques are required. These would enable the implementation of better decision-making approaches to identify, assess and predict disaster occurrences with enhanced accuracy, availability and speed.

REFERENCES

Antoniou, V., & Potsiou, C. (2020). A Deep Learning Method to Accelerate the Disaster Response Process. *Remote Sensing, 12*(3), 544. doi:10.3390/rs12030544

Carley, K. M., Malik, M., Landwehr, P. M., Pfeffer, J., & Kowalchuck, M. (2016). Crowd sourcing disaster management: The complex nature of Twitter usage in Padang Indonesia. *Safety Science, 90*, 48–61. doi:10.1016/j.ssci.2016.04.002

Charalabidis, Y. N., Loukis, E., Androutsopoulou, A., Karkaletsis, V., & Triantafillou, A. (2014). Passive crowdsourcing in government using social media. *Transform. Gov. People Process Policy, 8*, 283–30. doi:10.1108/TG-09-2013-0035

Chen, D., Liu, Z., Wang, L., Dou, M., Chen, J., & Li, H. (2013). Natural disaster monitoring with wireless sensor networks: A case study of data-intensive applications upon low-cost scalable systems. *Mobile Networks and Applications, 18*(5), 651–663. doi:10.100711036-013-0456-9

Ciresan, D., Meier, U., Masci, J., & Schmidhuber, J. (2012). Multi-column deep neural network for traffic sign classification. *Neural Networks, 32*, 333–338. doi:10.1016/j.neunet.2012.02.023 PMID:22386783

Ciresan, D., Meier, U., & Schmidhuber, J. (2012). Multi-column deep neural networks for image classification. *Proceedings of IEEE Conference on Computer Vision and Pattern Recognition (CVPR)*, 3642–3649. 10.1109/CVPR.2012.6248110

Deng, L. (2014). A tutorial survey of architectures, algorithms, and applications for deep learning. *APSIPA Transactions on Signal and Information Processing, 3*, e2. doi:10.1017/atsip.2013.9

DeVries, P. M. R., Viégas, F., Wattenberg, M., & Meade, B. J. (2018). Deep learning of aftershock patterns following large earthquakes. *Nature, 560*(7720), 632–634. doi:10.103841586-018-0438-y PMID:30158606

Erdelj, M., Natalizio, E., Chowdhury, K. R., & Akyildiz, I. F. (2017). Help from the sky: Leveraging UAVs for disaster management. *IEEE Pervasive Computing, 16*(1), 24–32. doi:10.1109/MPRV.2017.11

Glorot, X., Bordes, A., & Bengio, Y. (2011). Domain adaptation for large-scale sentiment classification: A deep learning approach. *Proceedings of the 28th International Conference on Machine Learning (ICML-11)*, 513–520.

Green, W. (2001). E-emergency management in the USA: A preliminary survey of the operational state of the art. *International Journal of Emergency Management, 1*(1), 70–81. doi:10.1504/IJEM.2001.000511

Hewage, P., Behera, A., & Trovati, M. (2020). Temporal convolutional neural (TCN) network for an effective weather forecasting using time-series data from the local weather station. *Soft Computing, 24*, 16453–16482. doi:10.100700500-020-04954-0

Hinton, G. E., Osindero, S., & Teh, Y. W. (2006). A fast learning algorithm for deep belief nets. *Neural Computation, 18*(7), 1527–1554. doi:10.1162/neco.2006.18.7.1527 PMID:16764513

Hinton, G. E., & Salakhutdinov, R. R. (2006). Reducing the dimensionality of data with neural networks. *Science, 313*(5786), 504–507. doi:10.1126cience.1127647 PMID:16873662

Hou, N., Dong, H., Wang, Z., Ren, W., & Alsaadi, F. E. (2016). Non-fragile state estimation for discrete Markovian jumping neural networks. *Neurocomputing, 179*, 238–245. doi:10.1016/j.neucom.2015.11.089

Hu, F., Xia, G. S., Hu, J., & Zhang, L. (2015). Transferring deep convolutional neural networks for the scene classification of high-resolution remote sensing imagery. *Remote Sensing, 7*(11), 14680–14707. doi:10.3390/rs71114680

Hu, Q., Zhang, R., & Zhou, Y. (2016). Transfer learning for short-term wind speed prediction with deep neural networks. *Renewable Energy, 85*, 83–95. doi:10.1016/j. renene.2015.06.034

Kim, J., Calhoun, V. D., Shim, E., & Lee, J. H. (2016). Deep neural network with weight sparsity control and pre-training extracts hierarchical features and enhances classification performance: Evidence from whole-brain resting-state functional connectivity patterns of schizophrenia. *NeuroImage, 124*, 127–146. doi:10.1016/j. neuroimage.2015.05.018 PMID:25987366

Kumar & Singh. (2019). Location reference identification from tweets during emergencies: A deep learning approach. *International Journal of Disaster Risk Reduction, 33*, 365–375.

Lachlan, Spence, & Lin. (2014). Expressions of risk awareness and concern through Twitter: On the utility of using the medium as an indication of audience needs. *Computers in Human Behavior, 35*, 554–559.

Lerouge, J., Herault, R., Chatelain, C., Jardin, F., & Modzelewski, R. (2015). IODA: An input/ output deep architecture for image labeling. *Pattern Recognition, 48*(9), 2847–2858. doi:10.1016/j.patcog.2015.03.017

Liou, Y. A., Kar, S. K., & Chang, L. (2010). Use of high-resolution FORMOSAT-2 satellite images for post-earthquake disaster assessment: A study following the 12 May 2008 Wenchuan Earthquake. *International Journal of Remote Sensing, 31*(13), 3355–3368. doi:10.1080/01431161003727655

Luus, F., Salmon, B., Van Den Bergh, F., & Maharaj, B. (2015). Multiview deep learning for land-use classification. *IEEE Geoscience and Remote Sensing Letters, 12*(12), 2448–2452. doi:10.1109/LGRS.2015.2483680

McCallum, I., Liu, W., See, L., Mechler, R., Keating, A., Hochrainer-Stigler, S., Mochizuki, J., Fritz, S., Dugar, S., Arestegui, M., Szoenyi, M., Bayas, J.-C. L., Burek, P., French, A., & Moorthy, I. (2016). Technologies to support community flood disaster risk reduction. *Int. J. Disaster Risk Sci., 7*(2), 198–204. doi:10.100713753-016-0086-5

Najafabadi, M. M., Villanustre, F., Khoshgoftaar, T. M., Seliya, N., Wald, R., & Muharemagic, E. (2015). Deep learning applications and challenges in big data analytics. *Journal of Big Data*, 2(1), 1–21. doi:10.118640537-014-0007-7

O'Brien, G., O'Keefe, P., Gadema-Cooke, Z., & Swords, J. (2010). Approaching disaster management through social learning. *Disaster Prevention and Management*, *19*, 498–508. doi:10.1108/09653561011070402

Ofli, F., Meier, P., Imran, M., Castillo, C., Tuia, D., Rey, N., Briant, J., Millet, P., Reinhard, F., Parkan, M., & Joost, S. (2016). Combining human computing and machine learning to make sense of big (aerial) data for disaster response. *Big Data*, *4*(1), 47–59. doi:10.1089/big.2014.0064 PMID:27441584

Pesaresi, M., Ehrlich, D., Ferri, S., Florczyk, A., Freire, S., Haag, F., Halkia, M., Julea, A. M., Kemper, T., & Soille, P. (2015). Global human settlement analysis for disaster risk reduction. *The International Archives of the Photogrammetry, Remote Sensing and Spatial Information Sciences*, *40*(W3), 837–843. doi:10.5194/isprsarchives-XL-7-W3-837-2015

Pradhan, B., Tehrany, M. S., & Jebur, M. N. (2016). A new semiautomated detection mapping of flood extent from TerraSAR-X satellite image using rule-based classification and taguchi optimization techniques. *IEEE Transactions on Geoscience and Remote Sensing*, *54*(7), 4331–4342. doi:10.1109/TGRS.2016.2539957

Raspini, F., Bardi, F., Bianchini, S., Ciampalini, A., Del Ventisette, C., Farina, P., Ferrigno, F., Solari, L., & Casagli, N. (2017). The contribution of satellite SAR-derived displacement measurements in landslide risk management practices. *Natural Hazards*, *86*(1), 327–351. doi:10.100711069-016-2691-4

Ray, P.P., Mukherjee, M., & Shu, L. (n.d.). Internet of things for disaster management: State-of-the-art and prospects. *IEEE Access, 5*, 18818–18835.

Robertson, Johnson, Murthy, Smith, & Stephens. (2019). Using a combination of human insights and 'deep learning' for real-time disaster communication. *Progress in Disaster Science, 2*.

Roche, S., Propeck-Zimmermann, E., & Mericskay, B. (2013). GeoWeb and crisis management: Issues and perspectives of volunteered geographic information. *GeoJournal*, *78*(1), 21–40. doi:10.100710708-011-9423-9 PMID:32214617

Russell, S. J., & Norvig, P. (2016). *Learning from examples. Artificial intelligence: a modern approach* (3rd ed.). Pearson.

Sakhardande, P., Hanagal, S., & Kulkarni, S. (2016). Design of disaster management system using IoT based interconnected network with smart city monitoring. In *Proceedings of the International Conference on Internet of Things and Applications (IOTA)*. IEEE. 10.1109/IOTA.2016.7562719

Skakun, S., Kussul, N., Shelestov, A., & Kussul, O. (2014). Flood hazard and flood risk assessment using a time series of satellite images: A case study in Namibia. *Risk Analysis*, *34*(8), 1521–1537. doi:10.1111/risa.12156 PMID:24372226

Sun, W., Bocchini, P., & Davison, B. D. (2020). Applications of artificial intelligence for disaster management. *Natural Hazards*, *103*(3), 2631–2689. doi:10.100711069-020-04124-3

Tang, Y., Salakhutdinov, R., & Hinton, G. E. (2012). *Deep lambertian networks*. arXiv:1206. 6445.

Thompson, S., Altay, N., Green, W. G. III, & Lapetina, J. (2006). Improving disaster response efforts with decision support systems. *International Journal of Emergency Management*, *3*(4), 250. doi:10.1504/IJEM.2006.011295

Trovati, Asimakopoulou, & Bessis. (2018). An investigation on human dynamics in enclosed spaces. *Computers & Electrical Engineering*, *67*, 195–209. doi:10.1016/j.compeleceng.2018.03.031

Yang, F., Dong, H., Wang, Z., Ren, W., & Alsaadi, F. E. (2016). A new approach to non-fragile state estimation for continuous neural networks with time-delays. *Neurocomputing*, *197*, 205–211. doi:10.1016/j.neucom.2016.02.062

Yu, M., Yang, C., & Li, Y. (2018). Big Data in Natural Disaster Management: A Review. *Geosciences*, *8*(5), 165. doi:10.3390/geosciences8050165

Yu, Y., Dong, H., Wang, Z., Ren, W., & Alsaadi, F. E. (2016). Design of non-fragile state estimators for discrete time-delayed neural networks with parameter uncertainties. *Neurocomputing*, *182*, 18–24. doi:10.1016/j.neucom.2015.11.079

Yuan, Y., & Sun, F. (2014). Delay-dependent stability criteria for time-varying delay neural networks in the delta domain. *Neurocomputing*, *125*, 17–21. doi:10.1016/j.neucom.2012.09.040

Chapter 7
Information Extraction From Social Media for Epidemic Models

Tariq Soussan
ⓘ https://orcid.org/0000-0003-4143-756X
Edge Hill University, UK

Marcello Trovati
ⓘ https://orcid.org/0000-0001-6607-422X
Edge Hill University, UK

ABSTRACT

Social media platforms are widely used to share opinions, facts, and real-time general information on specific events. This chapter will focus on discussing and presenting data analytics approaches which combine a variety of techniques based on text mining, machine learning, network analysis, and mathematical modelling to assess real-time data extracted from social media and other suitable data related to pandemic outbreaks. The use of real-time insights regarding pandemic outbreaks provides a valuable tool to inform and validate existing modelling techniques and methods. Furthermore, this would also support the discovering process of actionable information to facilitate the decision-making process by enhancing the most informed and appropriate decision, based on the available data. The chapter will also focus on the visualisation and usability of the insight identified during the process to address a non-technical audience.

DOI: 10.4018/978-1-7998-6736-4.ch007

I. INTRODUCTION

Social Media has become popular the last decade or so. It constitutes of a group of online platforms, websites or applications that permit users to interact, interconnect, cooperate and discuss point of views and information (Doyle, 2010) (Holotescu & Grosseck, 2013) (Soussan & Trovati, 2020) (Zeng et al., 2012). It provides communication among individuals that creates a widespread volume of data (Al-garadi et al., 2016). Users create different types of content such us audiovisual, pictures, text, and geospatial data which is considered free (Schreck & Keim, 2012). Data can be utilized by diverse institutes for different grounds. Firms use it to enhance business methods, legislators utilize it to detect trends in community opinion, and public health officials need it to screen infectious disease pandemics (Schreck & Keim, 2012). Lately, online social networks have established substantial consideration as a probable tool to monitor a pandemic since they can offer a nearly real-time observation system at a less expensive rate than the old-style surveillance systems (Al-garadi et al., 2016). Social media networks such as "YouTube" and "Twitter" deliver direct reach to an extraordinary sum of content and can increase gossips and doubtful information. Considering users' preferences and attitudes, algorithms facilitate content development and thus information diffusion (Cinelli et al., 2020). In the coming sections, section 2 will discuss infodemiology and data reliability. Section 3 will give critical discussion and literature review on epidemic models. Section 4 and 5 will give discuss details about the information cake model and the SIR model. Finally, section 6 will discuss social bot detection.

II. INFODEMIOLOGY AND DATA RELIABILITY

Infodemiology (information epidemiology) is defined as the group of methods, which examine the health data on the internet for the basis of public health studies and policies (Al-garadi et al., 2016). It is also defined as a "new emerging research discipline and methodology" encompassing "the study of the determinants and distribution of health information and misinformation—which may be useful in guiding health professionals and patients to quality health information on the Internet" (Eysenbach, 2020). It is considered as a method to "identify areas where there is a knowledge translation gap between best evidence (what some experts know) and practice (what most people do or believe)" (Eysenbach, 2002).

The word infodemic has been created to highlight the threats of misinformation incidents during the managing of virus epidemics, because it could accelerate the epidemic progression by influencing and disintegrating social response (Cinelli et al., 2020). Social networks have the possibility to remove the time lag in out-of-date surveillance by allowing the mining of loads of real-time text data, which contain geographical location and data about a person's personal welfare (Al-garadi et al., 2016). The pervasiveness of social media enhances information that users share and speeds up its diffusion between them. The data diffusion method is a successive result by which users affect one another over a time duration (Woo & Chen, 2016). Another issue that affects data reliability is fakes accounts on social media often referred to as bots. These bots act like real humans and can mislead users. When a fair dataset is collected, there may be advantage in removing not wanted content incorporated by automatic bot accounts (Ferrara et al.,2016). Bots can damage community through possibly jeopardizing democracy, producing anxiety throughout crises, and influencing the stock marketplace. They can also make individuals' audience bigger, destroy the name of any business for profitable or diplomatic reasons, and penetrate group of unsuspecting people and influence them to change their views of reality, which can have an erratic outcomes (Ferrara et al.,2016). The actions of bots and their effect can incorporate the modification of analytics of social network, which may be implemented for different reasons like TV scores, specialist results, and methodical influence size (Ferrara et al.,2016). Some previous work showed that botnet can be used to uncover confidential data like phone numbers and addresses. This kind of weakness can be used to affect trust in social media and can be used in cybercrime (Ferrara et al.,2016). Some bots interfere with real individuals' identity. They create usernames which are very close to the original usernames and copy the photos and links. In addition, some bots emulate the actions of real users, through imitating the patterns of the users when publishing content and communicating with the users' acquaintances (Ferrara et al.,2016). Another example from previous work on the issue with data reliability is the data related to COVID-19 pandemic (Pennycook et al.,2020). It showed that users do not think about the precision of content before sharing it. It also showed that users who lack information about science are more prone to consider and distribute falsehoods (Pennycook et al.,2020).

III. LITERATURE REVIEW

Diffusion is defined as the procedure such that the interest (e.g., info, innovation, or disease) moves from one to another (Cliff & Haggett 2005). Because of homogeneous patterns in the outbreak of epidemics and social infection procedures, most research assumes similar theoretical ideologies for epidemics in discussing the info diffusion (Woo & Chen, 2016). The mainstream theory that clarifies the epidemic describes the disease diffusion as the outspread of memes of infection (Blackmore 2000). Thus, most epidemic models are primarily based on the contagion through the communication between people (Woo & Chen, 2016). With the development of email, internet, and social network platforms, online information diffusion has turned out to be a main topic for diffusion research and as such, epidemic models have been applicable to modeling of information diffusion on the net (Woo & Chen, 2016). (Gruhl et al. 2004) described the features of diffusing themes in the blog and suggested a technique for approximating the transmission probability for independent cascade model (ICM). The cascade generation model under the SIS framework with static transmission probability was proposed by (Leskovec et al., 2007). Another work was done by (Kubo et al. (2007) displayed the similarity between the disease propagation model, the SIR model, and web forums data posts. This work was extended including the new media effects concentrating on how new media effects can be shown in the SIR model (Woo & Chen, 2012). (Sun et al. 2009) completed the observed inspection of information diffusion using Facebook. They implemented the regression model to classify affecting features on big chain diffusion. Important pieces of information spreading in Flickr social platform were studied by (Cha et al., 2009). The work showed how popular pictures broadcasted gradually throughout the network. Another work done by (Tang et al., 2014) produced information dissemination using hashtag in Sina Weibo, micro-blogging such as Twitter by implementing the susceptible-infected (SI) model. Another model called emotion-based SIS model was proposed by (Wang et al., 2015) displayed that it outruns the SIS model in showing information diffusion with Twitter data. Moreover, another dynamic susceptible-infected-recovered (SIR) model was introduced by (Liu & Zhang, 2014) such that users can remove links and connect again with their second-order friends. Another dynamic model was also introduced by (Jalali et al., 2016) to measure the essential procedures of request diffusion including invitation, which is the contagion element, interest, consciousness, forgetting, input and reminding. Another work was done on a model known as sentiment urgency emotion detection (SUED) from previous work. This model was applied on tweets from two different periods of time, one before the start of the COVID-19 pandemic and the other after it started to show the effect of COVID-19 pandemic on the conversions of the sentiments, emotions and urgencies of the tweets (Soussan & Trovati, 2020). The work showed that the sentiments of users around the monitored brand have shifted more towards negativity over time with COVID-19 pandemic being one of the reasons for this (Soussan & Trovati, 2020).

IV. THE INFORMATION CAKE MODEL

The information Cake Model (Eysenbach, 2020) gave the initial wide roadmap on how to fight an infodemic during the COVID-19 pandemic as shown in Figure 1. The present infodemic is a crisis to extract the absolute amount of information, that

128

is happening on four levels: (1) science, (2) policy and practice, (3) news media, and (4) social media (Eysenbach, 2020). These levels are shown in Figure 1 as layers during which the bigger the size of the layer, the higher the amount information generated by this level. Science level contains the least amount of information which is why it is the smallest level in size, and this shows difficult and specific information construction cycles (Eysenbach, 2020). One issue noted was not the presence of misinformation at the science level, but the task of converting this information into actions that can be recommended, and delivering conclusions for many spectators and shareholders in other layers which is showed by the "Knowledge Translation (KT)" arrows in Figure 1.

Figure 1. The Information "Cake" Model
(Eysenbach, 2020)

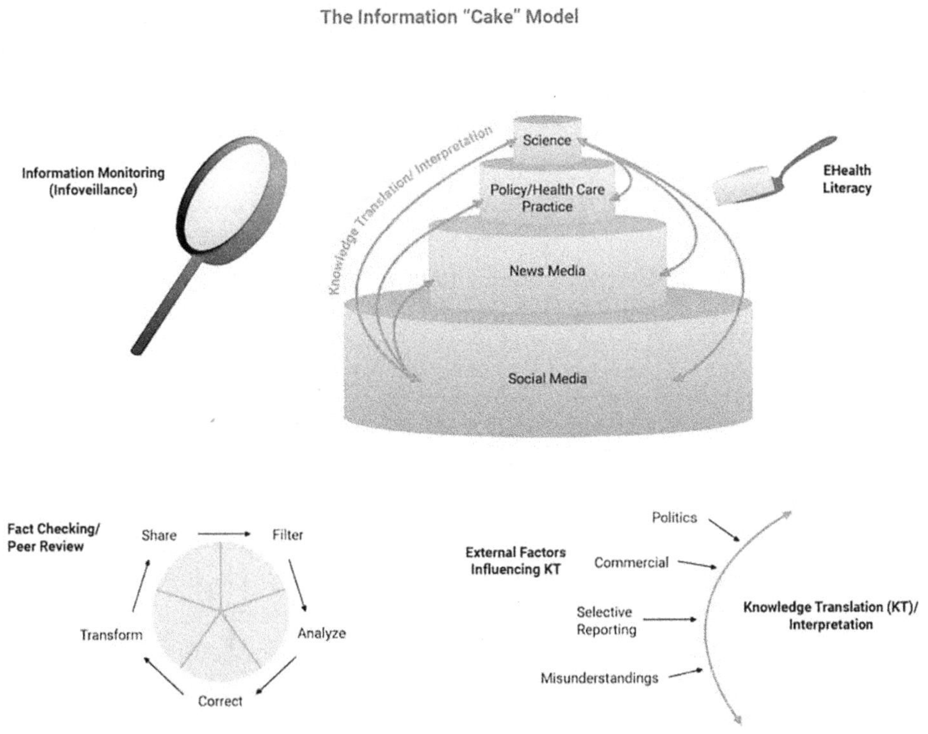

Hence, infodemic management has been summarized in four pillars.

The first pillar is referred to as: "Facilitate Accurate Knowledge Translation". When knowledge is being translated from one audience to another, the information might become misinformation due to many reasons such as policies, commercial benefits, specific reporting, and misinterpretations. Therefore, there is a need to support knowledge translation in an accurate way by minimizing the influencing factors (Eysenbach, 2020).

The second pillar for infodemic management is "Knowledge Refinement, Filtering, and Fact-Checking". These methods are required on every level, to speed up internal quality development procedures. These methods are occasionally noticeable but sometimes unseen by the user. A decent example on this is when academics peer review and publish work to filter, enhance, and expand information from previous scholars' work. Within every level, refinement of the information can be initiated on different stages showing that having information at diverse knowledge creation stages is as significant as facilitating them and speeding them up (Eysenbach, 2020).

The third pillar for infodemic management is defined as "Build eHealth Literacy" where there is an attempt to improve the ability of all participants to build eHealth literacy and to pick and evaluate health and science knowledge that are found from different levels of the information cake model from Figure 1. eHealth literacy is referred to as the capability to seek, discover, comprehend, and assess health information from e-sources and use the facts gained to deal with or solve a health problem (Eysenbach, 2020) (Norman & Skinner, 2006). With the flow of data and its easy access through the internet, information has been able to be extracted from any level and assembling eHealth literacy as a vital skill in a world network. It is the user's responsibility to refine reliable health info in this information era. There might be cases when users go through "unreviewed preprints" issued in preprint servers. Still, understanding and examining the information found needs important eHealth literacy.

The final pillar of this model is constant observation and examination the data patterns going back and forth over the internet which is referred to as "infodemiology and infoveillance "(Eysenbach, 2009). The task here is to locate occurrences of fabrication, gossip, untruthfulness, and to oppose them with truths or other involvements. Infoveillance needs producing specifications on data source on the web, such as the quality of the data, and it also needs producing specifications related to information requests such as inquiries posted on social network platforms. Infoveillance is shown in Figure 1 through patterns of information that are being communicated between different communities of the different levels of the model (Eysenbach, 2020).

The model helps to conclude that the execution of infodemic management in an imperfect and unskillful way can result in unintentional outcomes such as the suspending and repression of science due to political and business benefits. A good example of an unintentional outcome is the Twitter advertising rule that permits only specific newscast media and administrations to increase messages but does not permit this to science institutes or science editors (Eysenbach, 2020).

V. SIR MODEL FOR WEB FORUMS

To understand better how information is extracted from social media for epidemic models, the SIR model from previous work for web forums will be discussed at which the system design of this model will be based on data assembly, topic mining, time-series patterns, and model fitting (Woo & Chen, 2016).

Figure 2. System Design for the SIR Model for web forums
(Woo & Chen, 2016)

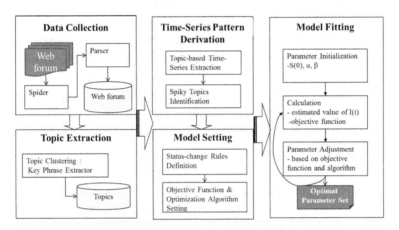

A unified and innovative system design has been showed in Figure 2 (Woo & Chen, 2016). Using the web forum, data is collected using the "forum spider and parser". The process executes when this spidorbot browses every HTML site in the forum. This spider is able go through the page to extract the data since the forum is made up of internet pages connected with one another using hyperlinks (Woo & Chen, 2016). The web crawler is made up of the page crawler which provides the URLs of the sites that have the forum's contents. The spidorbot tracks the links leading to the next page since they are connected to the current page and adjusts the cursor to the next page. This process is repeated until the final page has been reached. The crawler is also made up of the content crawler of the threads of the content as well as the responds on the content (Woo & Chen, 2016). Thread contents and their responds are linked to the web through a thread, and the threads list can be observed on every front page. Unique patterns in text are found by the parser that utilizes the regular expressions. A Distinctive tag is utilized by HTML files to show specific info. Messages in HTML files, user ID, and thread ID are all main data fields that are retrieved using the parser. (Woo & Chen, 2016)

As per Figure 2, the next step in the design for this model in topic extraction. Topic clustering is executed to extract keywords through a probabilistic topic model such as Latent Dirichlet allocation (LDA) (Blei et al., 2003). Discovering themes automatically in a large group of unorganized text is implemented through a topic modeling method (McCallum, 2002). Different themes compose a document where a theme is defined as group of words that often found together. A probability distribution over the words constitute the theme. The model attempts to discover the top group of words and to elaborate in the documents the displayed words. In order to generate new documents, a distribution over themes is selected which is followed by selecting a theme randomly depending on the distribution for every word in the document and a word can be extracted from that theme (Woo & Chen, 2016). The procedure has been reversed through statistical techniques by deducing the group of themes needed for producing a group of documents (Blei et al., 2003). Depending on the possible keywords, messages can be grouped. The theme distribution is expected to contain a Dirichlet prior in LDA which helps statistical interpretation to be basic and result in more sensible combinations of topics (Steyvers & Griffiths, 2007). Using a probability distribution, each word is allocated to a provisional theme such that it can be allocated to distinct themes in many documents. Theme allocation initiates iteratively where a word is allocated to the theme such that the word is the highly predominant and a document is allocated to a theme where the words in the document are primarily allocated (Woo & Chen, 2016). Theme modeling is completed once the iteration has been converged. Mallet has been utilized to run LDA for theme clustering (McCallum, 2002). It helps investigate the words in the topic in order to understand the meaning of the topics or themes. Words with different meaning in a theme are broad when the number of themes is low. On the other hand, a topic can have specific words that can allocate to many topics once high number of topics has been adjusted (Woo & Chen, 2016). To avoid convergence of themes, the number of themes has been changed and incremented by ten and checked to see if correct semantic clusters have been created. The topic group that contains relevant keywords, debated vigorously, and is made up of large number of posts and authors, has been assigned as the key topic (Woo & Chen, 2016). Messages are grouped in multiple classes and topic groups with significant keywords showing user needs are chosen. In addition, some keywords have helped find bigrams in order to obtain themes are relevant and having good volume.

The next step in this design is the time-series patterns stage. By combining posts that include a theme in a time period, the number of diverse authors is extracted. Topics with continuous debates, having part of the topic flow mostly decided by authors choices, is called chatter topics. The heated debates of everyday events which are related to a topic are referred to as spikey topics (Gruhl et al. 2004). High rises in posts is encouraged by the spikey theme. A spike occurs on a specific day once posts surpassed μ + 2σ (Gruhl et al., 2004). Chatter themes and chatter themes with continuous patterns have been dismissed when examining time series patterns. Topics lacking epidemic patterns were not thought to be infectious or lead to an infection between users. Spikey topics are chosen because these are the themes that attract attention (Gruhl et al., 2004).

The next step in this design is the Model fitting. An optimization algorithm called genetic algorithm (GA) was implemented to test data on the model. It is implemented for parameter approximation. Running this algorithm requires developing broad variety of methods. A linear-ranking algorithm determines a fitness function that shows how well the current population matches the objective function (Baker, 1987). The selection of the population is impacted by the fitness function. The selection method which captures chromosomes from the population must be fixed in order to create the population in every generation. Moreover, roulette wheel selection was utilized (Golberg, 1989). To create the offspring, pairs are reassembled at a given probability through the crossover process. In addition, Single-point has been applied in this work (Booker, 1987) and real value mutation has been implemented as well (Mühlenbein & Schlierkamp-Voosen, 1993).

The SIR model was analyzed concerning the righteousness of the fit using Equation 1 below that defines the "Mean Squared Error" known as (MSE) and the "R-square" (Woo & Chen, 2016).

Mean squared error (MSE) and the R-square (Woo & Chen, 2016):

$$MSE = \frac{1}{n} \sum_{i=1}^{n} \left(I_i - \hat{I}\left(t_i, \hat{\theta}\right) \right)^2$$

$$R\text{-}square = 1 - \frac{\sum_{i=1}^{n} \left(I_i - \hat{I}\left(t_i, \hat{\theta}\right) \right)^2}{\sum_{i=1}^{n} \left(I_i - \overline{I} \right)^2}$$

(1)

I_i = the number of infectives at time i

$\overline{I}$ = the average of I_i

n = the number of samples

i = time point

θ = the estimated parameter set

Experimental Results on SIR Model

The model was tested with two web forums. The first one from marketing exchange containing 10-year-old data of shareholders' opinions on different themes related to Walmart. The other forum is a political forum constituting of authors points of views on universal political subjects. In the Walmart forum, both chatter and spikey topics can be observed as shown in Figure 3 (Woo & Chen, 2016). Topic clustering was conducted using Mallet to derive themes. To minimize the convergence of keywords amongst clusters, the number of clusters is fixed. Fifty clusters have been created during which the non-peak chatter topics were removed. Main spikey topics that have vital volumes were added as well. The major topics in Walmart dataset are shown in Table 1 (Woo & Chen, 2016). The time series of picked themes are shown in Figure 4 (Woo & Chen, 2016). In addition, the Walmart web forum results for the parameter approximation is summarized ins Table 2 (Woo & Chen, 2016).

Figure 3. Spikey topic vs. chatter topic
(Woo & Chen, 2016)

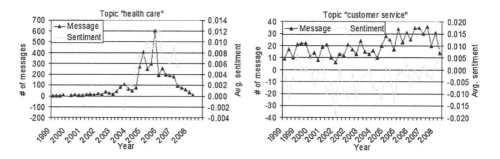

Table 1. The Walmart forum main keywords and themes

Topic group	Topic	Keywords
Investor	Stock price	Growth, share, earnings, price, stock, market
	Sales	Sales, percent, quarter, increase, fiscal, earnings, expected, results
Customer	Low price	Prices, low, economy, consumer, cost, market
	Shopping convenience	Shopping, items, manager, shoppers, service, line, door, experience
Employee	Healthcare	Healthcare, employees, insurance, medical, plan
	Labor law	Labor, illegal, federal, laws, violations, rights
	Wage	Pay, wages, benefits, employees, hour, working paid average hours, minimum, poverty, paying

(Woo & Chen, 2016)

The sales subject has a smaller number of potential original authors, a higher rate of infection, and a lesser rate of recovery than the stock price subject, suggesting that the stock price is a less spiky theme than sales. In customer-related issues, the low-price issue and in employee-related topics, the healthcare topics are less spiky than others. By solving differential equations with the ideal parameter tuned, the numbers of sensitive, infectives, and recovered at successive times are extracted (Woo & Chen, 2016).

Figure 4. Walmart selected themes' time series
(Woo & Chen, 2016)

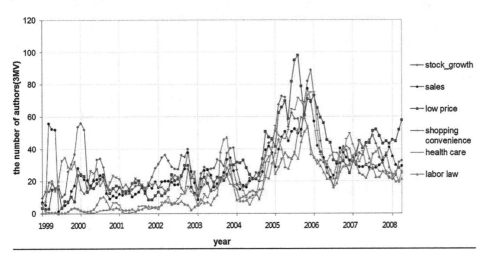

Table 2. Walmart forum parameter approximation results

Topic	MSE	R^2	S(0)	α	β	μ	K
Stock price	5.28E+03	0.6198	163	0.0045	0.6798	0.1226	1384
Sales	2.72E+03	0.6320	100	0.0081	0.7270	0.1388	997
Low price	3.64E+03	0.7262	122	0.0059	0.7506	0.1419	1401
Shopping convenience	1.98E+03	0.6433	116	0.0078	0.7914	0.1230	1000
Healthcare	3.83E+03	0.7190	116	0.0065	0.7677	0.1361	1200
Labor law	1.16E+03	0.7510	89	0.0088	0.7433	0.1324	800
Wage	6.55E+03	0.5209	100	0.0053	0.6000	0.1524	950

(Woo & Chen, 2016).

VI. SOCIAL BOT DETECTION

One of the ways to maintain data integrity in social media is detect the fake accounts or bots that might spread it. One way to detect bots is through graph based social bot detection. A competitor might manage various bots known as sybils to mimic various personalities and initiate an intrusion. This is shown in Facebook Immune System (Ferrara et al.,2016). Analyzing the composition of a social graph can help in identifying sybils. SybilRank shows that since sybil accounts need a lot of connections to look authentic, they connect mostly to other sybil accounts, with few connections to real accounts (Cao et al., 2012). It also implies that an account communicating with an authentic account is believed to be authentic (Ferrara et al.,2016). Another way to detect bots is crowdsourcing through a social Turing Test platform (Wang et al., 2013). Specialists were employed to spot bots in Renren data and Facebook data from their profile data. The decision is based on profile being detected by many people simultaneously with the majority's judgement taken (Wang et al., 2013). Another way to detect bots is based on features. By integrating machine learning methods with patterns on related to monitored behavior, users can filter out behaviors that can be regarded as bots. "Bot or Not" for example uses extremely analytical features based on a detection algorithm with 95% accuracy (Ferrara et al.,2016). In addition, user actions and scheduling data are various aspects of individual behavior which can be detected by the Renren Sybil detector (Ferrara et al.,2016).

VII. CONCLUSION

From the work of (Woo & Chen, 2016), it was noticeable that users respond to the posts of one another, confirming their communication through posts. The disease diffusion model was adopted which describes "the disease outbreak through the contact between people" (Woo & Chen, 2016). The diffusion model's purpose is to comprehend the ways of the "spread of new diseases, ideas and products", to estimate success or failure of diffusion in the early phases, and to come up with a plan to grow or decrease the probabilities of diffusion (Woo & Chen, 2016). By analyzing the early stage of the diffusion procedure, the outbreak of topics can be predicted using the general concept of the mathematical epidemic model (Woo & Chen, 2016). Overall, in modeling web forums topic diffusion, the SIR model's performance was well (Woo & Chen, 2016). From other previous work as well (Eysenbach, 2020), it can be concluded that unintentional implications, such as the suspending and repression of science for the benefit of political and commercial interests, may occur if poorly implemented infodemic management with lack of coordination has been performed (Eysenbach, 2020). This work also showed some of the ways to detect social bots which can jeopardize data integrity. Future work can involve studying more ways that helps make data for social media more reliable with less falsehoods.

REFERENCES

Al-garadi, M. A., Khan, M. S., Varathan, K. D., Mujtaba, G., & Al-Kabsi, A. M. (2016). Using online social networks to track a pandemic: A systematic review. *Journal of Biomedical Informatics*, *62*, 1–11. doi:10.1016/j.jbi.2016.05.005 PMID:27224846

Baker, J. E. (1987, July). Reducing bias and inefficiency in the selection algorithm. In *Proceedings of the second international conference on genetic algorithms (Vol. 206,* pp. 14-21). Academic Press.

Blackmore, S., & Blackmore, S. J. (2000). *The meme machine* (Vol. 25). Oxford Paperbacks.

Blei, D. M., Ng, A. Y., & Jordan, M. I. (2003). Latent dirichlet distribution. *Journal of Machine Learning Research, 3,* 993–1022.

Booker, L. (1987). Improving search in genetic algorithms. *Genetic Algorithms and Simulated Annealing,* 61-73.

Cao, Q., Sirivianos, M., Yang, X., & Pregueiro, T. (2012). Aiding the detection of fake accounts in large scale social online services. In *9th {USENIX} Symposium on Networked Systems Design and Implementation ({NSDI} 12)* (pp. 197-210). USENIX.

Cha, M., Mislove, A., & Gummadi, K. P. (2009, April). *A measurement-driven analysis of information propagation in the flickr social.* Academic Press.

Cinelli, M., Quattrociocchi, W., Galeazzi, A., Valensise, C. M., Brugnoli, E., Schmidt, A. L., . . . Scala, A. (2020). *The covid-19 social media infodemic.* arXiv preprint arXiv:2003.05004.

Cliff, A., & Haggett, P. (2005). *Modeling diffusion processes.* Academic Press.

Doyle, C. (2010). *A literature review on the topic of social media.* Academic Press.

Eysenbach, G. (2002). Infodemiology: The epidemiology of (mis) information. *The American Journal of Medicine, 113*(9), 763–765. doi:10.1016/S0002-9343(02)01473-0 PMID:12517369

Eysenbach, G. (2009). Infodemiology and infoveillance: Framework for an emerging set of public health informatics methods to analyze search, communication and publication behavior on the Internet. *Journal of Medical Internet Research, 11*(1), e11. doi:10.2196/jmir.1157 PMID:19329408

Eysenbach, G. (2020). How to fight an infodemic: The four pillars of infodemic management. *Journal of Medical Internet Research, 22*(6), e21820. doi:10.2196/21820 PMID:32589589

Ferrara, E., Varol, O., Davis, C., Menczer, F., & Flammini, A. (2016). The rise of social bots. *Communications of the ACM, 59*(7), 96–104. doi:10.1145/2818717

Golberg, D. E. (1989). *Genetic algorithms in search, optimization, and machine learning.* Addion Wesley.

Gruhl, D., Guha, R., Liben-Nowell, D., & Tomkins, A. (2004, May). Information diffusion through blogspace. In *Proceedings of the 13th international conference on World Wide Web* (pp. 491-501). 10.1145/988672.988739

Holotescu, C., & Grosseck, G. (2013). An empirical analysis of the educational effects of social media in universities and colleges. *Internet Learning*, *2*(1), 5. doi:10.18278/il.2.1.3

Jalali, M. S., Ashouri, A., Herrera-Restrepo, O., & Zhang, H. (2016). Information diffusion through social networks: The case of an online petition. *Expert Systems with Applications*, *44*, 187–197. doi:10.1016/j.eswa.2015.09.014

Kubo, M., Naruse, K., Sato, H., & Matubara, T. (2007, December). The possibility of an epidemic meme analogy for web community population analysis. In *International Conference on Intelligent Data Engineering and Automated Learning* (pp. 1073-1080). Springer. 10.1007/978-3-540-77226-2_107

Leskovec, J., Adamic, L. A., & Huberman, B. A. (2007). The dynamics of viral marketing. *ACM Transactions on the Web*, *1*(1), 5. doi:10.1145/1232722.1232727

Liu, C., & Zhang, Z. K. (2014). Information spreading on dynamic social networks. *Communications in Nonlinear Science and Numerical Simulation*, *19*(4), 896–904. doi:10.1016/j.cnsns.2013.08.028

McCallum, A. K. (2002). *Mallet: A machine learning for language toolkit.* http://mallet. cs. umass. edu

Mühlenbein, H., & Schlierkamp-Voosen, D. (1993). Predictive models for the breeder genetic algorithm i. continuous parameter optimization. *Evolutionary Computation*, *1*(1), 25–49. doi:10.1162/evco.1993.1.1.25

Norman, C. D., & Skinner, H. A. (2006). eHEALS: The eHealth literacy scale. *Journal of Medical Internet Research*, *8*(4), e27. doi:10.2196/jmir.8.4.e27 PMID:17213046

Pennycook, G., McPhetres, J., Zhang, Y., Lu, J. G., & Rand, D. G. (2020). Fighting COVID-19 misinformation on social media: Experimental evidence for a scalable accuracy-nudge intervention. *Psychological Science*, *31*(7), 770–780. doi:10.1177/0956797620939054 PMID:32603243

Schreck, T., & Keim, D. (2012). Visual analysis of social media data. *Computer*, *46*(5), 68–75. doi:10.1109/MC.2012.430

Soussan, T., & Trovati, M. (2020). Sentiment urgency emotion conversion over time for business intelligence. *International Journal of Web Information Systems*.

Steyvers, M., & Griffiths, T. (2007). *Latent semantic analysis: a road to meaning, chapter probabilistic topic models*. Laurence Erlbaum.

Sun, E., Rosenn, I., Marlow, C., & Lento, T. M. (2009, May). Gesundheit! modeling contagion through Facebook news feed. ICWSM.

Tang, M., Mao, X., Yang, S., & Zhou, H. (2014). A dynamic microblog network and information dissemination in "@" mode. *Mathematical Problems in Engineering*, *2014*, 2014. doi:10.1155/2014/492753

Wang, G., Mohanlal, M., Wilson, C., Wang, X., Metzger, M., Zheng, H., & Zhao, B. Y. (2013). Social Turing Tests: Crowdsourcing Sybil Detection. In *NDSS Symposium 2013*. Internet Society.

Wang, Q., Lin, Z., Jin, Y., Cheng, S., & Yang, T. (2015). ESIS: Emotion-based spreader–ignorant–stifler model for information diffusion. *Knowledge-Based Systems*, *81*, 46–55. doi:10.1016/j.knosys.2015.02.006

Woo, J., & Chen, H. (2012, June). An event-driven SIR model for topic diffusion in web forums. In *2012 IEEE International Conference on Intelligence and Security Informatics* (pp. 108-113). IEEE. 10.1109/ISI.2012.6284101

Woo, J., & Chen, H. (2016). Epidemic model for information diffusion in web forums: Experiments in marketing exchange and political dialog. *SpringerPlus*, *5*(1), 66. doi:10.118640064-016-1675-x PMID:26839759

Zeng, L., Hall, H., & Pitts, M. J. (2012). Cultivating a community of learners: the potential challenges of social media in higher education. In *Social Media: Usage and Impact* (pp. 111–126). Lexington Books.

Chapter 8
Towards Combating Pandemic–Related Misinformation in Social Media

Isa Inuwa-Dutse
University of St Andrews, UK

ABSTRACT

Conventional preventive measures during pandemics include social distancing and lockdown. Such measures in the time of social media brought about a new set of challenges – vulnerability to the toxic impact of online misinformation is high. A case in point is COVID-19. As the virus propagates, so does the associated misinformation and fake news about it leading to an infodemic. Since the outbreak, there has been a surge of studies investigating various aspects of the pandemic. Of interest to this chapter are studies centering on datasets from online social media platforms where the bulk of the public discourse happens. The main goal is to support the fight against negative infodemic by (1) contributing a diverse set of curated relevant datasets; (2) offering relevant areas to study using the datasets; and (3) demonstrating how relevant datasets, strategies, and state-of-the-art IT tools can be leveraged in managing the pandemic.

INTRODUCTION

Human history is intertwined with various pandemics, infectious disease on a global scale, events resulting in a dramatic high mortality rate and economic hardship. Pandemics from diseases such as smallpox, tuberculosis, and the Spanish flu resulted in a large number of lost lives (Kaur, 2020). Recently, one of the defining moments

DOI: 10.4018/978-1-7998-6736-4.ch008

of the year 2020 is the outbreak of the zoonotic Coronavirus Disease (COVID-19) that radically disrupts normal social interactions. The virus was first reported by the World Health Organisation (WHO) on December 31, 2019, in Wuhan, China. At the time of writing this chapter, the recent statistics from the WHO reported 108,153,741 confirmed cases and 2,381,295 confirmed deaths across 223 countries, areas or territories. It is easy to be oblivious of early warnings despite apparent reasons suggesting otherwise. When the prevailing pandemic was first reported, many nations were heedless in taking proactive measures to a point that the outbreak quickly overwhelmed healthcare facilities making it difficult to attend to ailing people, fatigue from health workers, distress and grieve from families of ailing and lost ones. The lacklustre attitude from some leaders and the politicisation of the pandemic further compounds the situation, resulting in confusing and conflicting narratives. As the pandemic crisis exacerbates, many forms of preventive and curative responses have been imposed to curtail the scale of spread and negative impact of the pandemic. Figure 1 shows a summary of the total number of cases globally[1].

Figure 1. A summary of the total number of COVID-19 global cases.

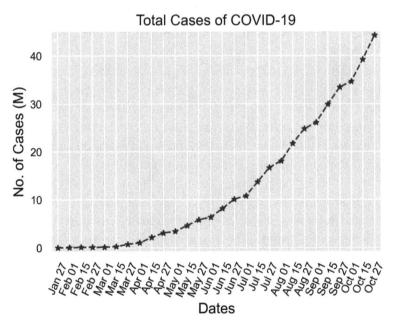

Various reactionary approaches, sometimes impulsive, have been used to flatten infection peaks to avoid overwhelming the prevailing healthcare facilities and alleviating the associated financial challenges. Typical measures to slow down the infection rate include disinfection, social distancing, contact tracing, isolation/ quarantine and some curative measures. Following the traditional approach of mitigating spread, the infamous *lockdown* measure introduced to curb the virus spread has altered many aspects of social routines in which demand for online-based services skyrocketed. While modern-day online social media networks, such as Facebook[2] and Twitter[3], facilitate the spread of information to a wide audience, making it a useful facility for instant information updates and socialisation, they also present new sets of challenges. Figure 2 shows a summary of the major events[4] since the outbreak. With a substantial proportion of the populace confined to their homes for a long period, vulnerability to the toxic impact of online misinformation is high during the COVID-19 outbreak. There is a growing body of work tackling many problems associated with the outbreak. For instance, concerning infodemic[5], coined to denote the online outburst of pandemic-related information, especially misinformation, researchers have been curating and documenting various datasets about COVID-19 pandemic. Of interest to this chapter are studies centring on online datasets, with emphasis on the online social media platforms where the bulk of the public discourse happen, regarding spurious content associated with the pandemic. Ultimately, the chapter's goal is to support the fight against online misinformation with particular emphasis on pandemic-related datasets.

Many aspects of the pandemic can be explored using such data collection – from leveraging benchmarking datasets to assess the veracity of information related to the pandemic (infodemic) to the more advanced task of modelling and tracing the propagation of the virus. Consequently, the chapter will, among other benefits, better inform how to ensure that relevant pandemic-related content dominates, and irrelevant content is suppressed, especially during critical times of the pandemic. Noting the growing vulnerability to the toxic impact of online misinformation during the pandemic, the contributions of the chapter include:

- *Datasets to neutralise negative infodemic:* the study presents a diverse set of curated relevant datasets about the pandemic to help in curtailing the proliferation of harmful information about the outbreak. The datasets will support studies investigating various aspects of the pandemic through the prism of online social media platforms.
- *How to leverage the datasets for actionable insights:* the ultimate goal is to support the fight against online misinformation on pandemic-related issues, hence, supplementing the contributed datasets with a discourse on some relevant actionable areas to focus on will be beneficial. Relevant tasks to undertake include leveraging benchmarking datasets to assess the veracity of information related to the pandemic, modelling and tracing the propagation of the virus from online signals.

Figure 2. A chronicle of some major events or topical issues related to the management of the pandemic.

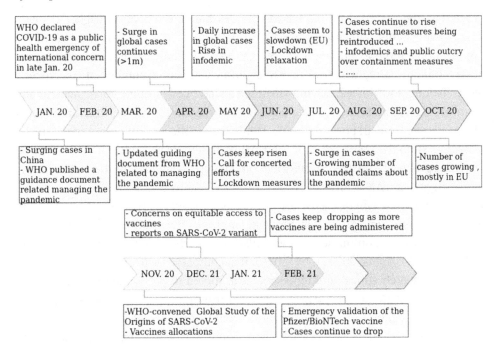

The chapter is structured as follows: Part I offers relevant background information regarding pandemics and Part II presents a detailed account of the relevant datasets, including the collection and processing steps, to use. Part III proffers some research problems worthy of investigation using the datasets. Finally, Part IV concludes the study with a closing remark.

BACKGROUND

As pointed out earlier, some of the swift measures taken to mitigate pandemics include disinfection, social distancing, contact tracing and *lockdown*. Moreover, palliatives are being provided to cushion the financial hardships brought about by the pandemic. With technological advancements, all the above-mentioned measures can be improved. Therefore, the focus in this section is on existing related work, and to highlight relevant topics that would help in achieving such goals, notably from an online social media perspective.

Pandemic in the Age of Online Connectivity

Arguably, the need for online-based services has never been in higher demand than what is being witnessed in the COVID-19-induced lockdown era. One of the implications of the lockdown is the relegation of virtually all human engagements to the online realm, which also results in an increasing number of uncensored posts. Noting how misleading information can have catastrophic consequences and hampers the fight about applying containment measures, it is pertinent to combat the pandemic from all possible fronts. While the architecture of online social media networks simplifies the spread of information to a wide audience, it also enables a breeding ground for misleading information. This opens another frontier of challenges in the fight against the virus.

Drawing from *ethnography*, a form of social research that is concerned with individual culture and group behaviour, *netnography* is a relatively new term coined to denote the use of online social media platforms to study people's interactions and behaviours (Kozinets, 2007; Pink, 2016). It encompasses aspects of data collection, analysis, research ethics, and representation, rooted in participants' observations. Because observational data can be retrieved from online communities or groups, effective aggregation of such data would yield useful insight (Kozinets, 2007). It can be argued that modern-day social interactions will be incomplete without taking online social relationships into account, where various forms of interactions among diverse users happen. This capability makes it possible to empirically quantify and evaluate social relationships among users on an unprecedented scale. Essentially, many social network theories and analytical solutions can now be tested using real social media data. Thus, a treatise on contemporary social engagements will be incomplete without reference to online social networks.

Online Social Media Ecosystem

The transformative power of technological advancements across various facets of public lives is quite enormous. Many forms of social interactions are continually evolving to support a myriad of objects to remain connected through a communication model that enables a multi-flow of information (see the influence network model of Watts and Dodds (2007)), thus contrasting it with the two-step flow model in which few users mediate communication between the media and the general public (Katz et al., 2017).

The contemporary social media ecosystem consists of numerous platforms which support various aspects of humans' social engagements and enable users to simultaneously generate and consume information (Inuwa-Dutse et al., 2020). Many forms of social interactions are continually evolving through platforms such as Twitter, Facebook, WhatsApp, TikTok, LinkedIn, Snapchat, Twitch, Pinterest, YouTube, Viber, that facilitate information diffusion and socialisation at scale. These platforms have been instrumental in socialisation, breaking news, globalisation and enabling socio-technological research (Sundaram et al. 2012). Moreover, the platforms are quite popular with the public; thus, it is worthwhile understanding the social media ecosystem in great depth and the datasets that can be retrieved.

Social Media Data

Prior to the advent of online social media, a large collection of data is exclusive to big research facilities such as weather forecast stations, astronomical stations, and scientific laboratories (Dijk van Jan 2006). Social media networks offer useful utility in understanding modern society and how it functions (Miller et al. 2015). It was estimated that 2.46 billion users will be connected in 2020, amounting to one-third of the global population.[6] Owing to the usefulness of the generated data, datafication[7], the continuous quest to turn every aspect of humans' lives into computerised data for competitive value (Cukier & Mayer-Schoenberger 2013), is being fueled by social media to supply commoditised data. Several domains have already recognised the crucial role of such data in improving productivity and gaining competitive advantages. Common use case examples include healthcare (Rojas et al. 2016, Yee et al. 2008), sport and entertainment (Davenport, 2014; Deloitte, 2014), politics (Contractor et al., 2015). The success of social media platforms has led to an increased interest in empirically testing various theories, making the platforms ideal for studying many aspects of social events. In terms of participants and data size, social media networks have profoundly transformed how various research works are being conducted, especially within the social sciences. Details about how researchers leverage theories, research constructs, and conceptual frameworks in relation to social media can be found in Ngai et al. (2015). Through *netnography*, researchers can systematically retrieve a huge amount of real-life observational data from different online social media platform's using traditional application programming interface (API) or a custom application.

Twitter and Tweets – Massive amounts of data can be easily obtained from platforms such as Twitter. Tweets, usually short text snippets, refer to the stream of posts users share on Twitter, and they enable longitudinal studies (Würschinger et al. 2016). A *tweet object* is a complex data structure, expressed in JavaScript Object-Notation (JSON) format, consisting of many extractable attributes that describe specific information about the *tweet* and the *account holder (the user)*. As a marked-up piece of text, the different fields in the tweet object define important characteristics of the tweet. The complexity of a tweet and its unstructured nature makes it difficult to process directly into a usable form, which requires a series of preprocessing before effective analysis can be conducted[8]. The stream of tweets differs from conventional stream texts in terms of posting rate, dynamism and flexibility; they are generated at a rapid rate and tend to be highly dynamic (Guille and Favre, 2015; Chakraborty et al., 2016).

Relevant Work

Since the outbreak, various stakeholders have been actively battling with the virus causing the pandemic, i.e.~SARS-Cov-2. To this end, researchers have been curating and documenting various online datasets about COVID-19, especially from social media. This endeavour is crucial towards enriching existing ground-truth data that could be used to debunk myths and misinformation around the pandemic. A collection of relevant datasets is central to tackling emerging challenges and a driving force in the various research efforts interested in combating harmful infodemic.

The following review is based on the modalities of misinformation spread, which include text, video, voice and images. It is out of the scope of the chapter to belabour or dwell on the research associated with COVID-19. There is a comprehensive catalogue of COVID-19 datasets, spanning various topics, in the work of Latif et al. (2020). The focus in this section of the chapter is on text and image modalities facilitated via social media networks, which have transformed the way sociological research is being conducted by enabling useful utility in understanding modern society and how it functions. Within a short span of the outbreak, there have been a plethora of COVID-19-related studies covering various aspects of the pandemic. Many datasets can be obtained from social media for various purposes related to the pandemic, such as in crisis management during the outbreak.

An early report about the first outbreak in China is summarised[9] in the work of Wu and McGoogan (2020). The Wikipedia projects have been maintaining comprehensive documentation about relevant articles on COVID-19. Using a large collection of diverse datasets from online social media, the *infodemics* observatory project keeps track of the digital response related to the outbreak (Valle et al., 2020). In conjunction with numerous online social media platforms, the World Health Organisation is preventing the spread of misleading information related to the pandemic[10]. Moreover, some social media platforms have put measures in place to prevent potentially inimical content from spreading. For instance, Twitter's new feature of flagging posts and the dedicated application programming interface can be used to retrieve tweets related to COVID-19[11]. A useful analysis of the impact of COVID-19 and how stakeholders can effectively act can be found in the blog post of Tomas (2020). Similarly, the focus in the work of Desvars-Larrive et. al. (2020) is on how governments have implemented nonpharmaceutical intervention strategies on tackling the outbreak. The authors present a comprehensive structured dataset of government interventions and their respective timelines of implementations. Since various intervention measures have been applied, such measures will offer additional vista to understanding the progression of the pandemic at various stages.

Social stream and evolving collection – Some useful collections of social media datasets consisting of tweets can be found in the work of Chen and Ferrara (2020), and Alqurashi et al. (2020). A preprint version of the data contributed in this chapter is given in Inuwa-Dutse and Korkontzelos (2020). The work of Zarei et al. (2020) presents a collection of multilingual COVID-19 Instagram dataset that could be used to study the propagation of misinformation related to the pandemic. Qazi et al. (2020) present a large-scale multilingual tweet on the pandemic; the collection is composed of geolocation information that could be used for location-specific analysis of COVID-19 related issues. The work of Haouari (2020) presents COVID-19 dataset from Twitter based on the Arabic language. The work of Wang et al. (2020) presents an evolving large collection of diverse datasets from multiple sources/ scientific research papers on COVID-19. Owing to its diversity, the collection is suitable for text mining and discovery systems related to the pandemic. Also, the work of Banda et al. (2020) contributes an evolving diverse dataset – biomedical, biological, and epidemiological – that captures social dynamics about the pandemic.

Datasets on misinformation – Noting the high spread of misinformation and fake health news over the Internet, there exists a plethora of studies and datasets on the topic. To help in tackling fake news and its detection in health news, Shahi and Nandini (2020) present multilingual cross-domain datasets of fact-checked news articles on COVID-19. In Dai et al. (2020), the focus is also on datasets (FakeHealth) to support fake news detection tasks. The work of Chen et al. (2020) contributes multilingual datasets suitable for tracking COVID-19-related misinformation and unverified rumours on Twitter.

The work of Memon and Carley (2020) is focused on characterising conspiracy theories and fake information to help in identifying and debunking unfounded claims. Similarly, the focus in the work of Cinelli et al. (2020) is on understanding the diffusion of information about the outbreak using datasets from various online platforms – Twitter, Instagram, YouTube, Reddit and Gab. The authors were able to track the spread of information from questionable online sources. Moreover, the following are useful websites that offer fact-checking services associated with the pandemic. *Snopes*[12] is an independent publication body that offers verification of misinformation on various topics, and *Poynter*[13] is part of the International Fact-Checking Network that provides a useful resource to help in neutralising COVID-19-related misinformation. The *Poynter* platform also initiated the hashtags *#CoronaVirusFacts* and *#DatosCoronaVirus* to gather misinformation about coronavirus.

DATASETS AND RELEVANT RESOURCES

With the growing number of pandemic-related misleading information, another frontier of challenge in the fight against the virus is open. Figure 3 shows the focused areas in the fight against the COVID-19 pandemic. The fight against the virus revolves around preventive (such as public enlightenment about the standard practice to prevent spread) and curative. The best approach is to avoid endangering the public to be exposed to the virus. Of interest to most researchers, especially within the computer science research community, is the need to neutralise the negative impacts of infodemic associated with the pandemic. Infodemic could lead to consuming misleading information that could endanger the public. One approach to achieving such goals is through a useful data collection that could be used to debunk myths and misinformation around the pandemic. Thus, it is crucial to combat the pandemic from all angles using the right set of datasets.

Figure 3. The figure shows a high-level view of focused areas in the fight against the pandemic. Infodemic could lead to consuming misleading information that could endanger the public. Thus, it is crucial to combat the pandemic from all angles.

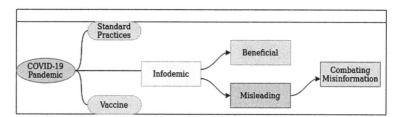

To support the fight against the spread of misinformation and rumours, the following section describes the relevant datasets about COVID-19, how to retrieve the data contributed in the chapter, and a discussion on its potential utility. The collection consists of three categories of Twitter data, information about standard practices from credible sources and a chronicle of global situation reports from WHO[14]. Regarding data from Twitter, a description of how to retrieve the hydrated version of the data and some research problems that could be addressed using the data are given.

Online Data Sources and Curation

As discussed earlier in the Background section, the advent of social media has opened a new window of obtaining a huge number of diverse research datasets across different disciplines – engineering, medicine, sociology, computer science, etc. This section is concerned with a description of how to obtain and curate relevant datasets, notably from Twitter social network. Part of Table 1 at the end of the chapter provides an overview of useful tools for retrieving data from the respective social media platforms[15]. Figure 4 shows a basic collection pipeline of the datasets.

Data Collection and Cleaning

Platforms such as Twitter offer a useful avenue to retrieve a huge amount of data on a variety of topics using relevant keywords or search terms. The use of keywords plays a central role in identifying the most useful data and relevant stakeholders as the basis for data collection. The set of datasets presented in this chapter is in response to the growing scepticism, misinformation and myths surrounding the pandemic. Thus, terms that are associated with such myths have been used to collect the data, mostly from accounts that openly dismisses COVID-19 related information as put forward by credible sources such as the WHO. For a more effective result, it will be helpful to design the collection so that the data can be classified based on whether the collection is from *specific* or *dedicated* accounts or *random* or *miscellaneous* accounts via Twitter's API. The account-based collection could be from verified or unverified accounts on Twitter and the random set from a generic collection of daily tweets on diverse topics. These are needed to provide a wider context on the prevailing topic. Because a tweet associated with a hashtag offers a high-level filter and helps in data curation, the collection can be based on some specific hashtags.

Figure 4. A schematic illustration of the data collection pipeline.

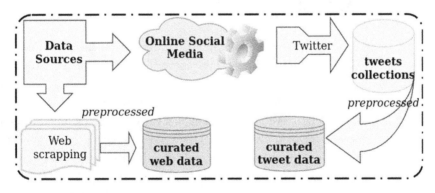

- **Tweet-based collection** - All the tweet-based collections have been collected using Twitter's API and consists of three categories from accounts that have been monitored for five weeks (March 23 to May 13, 2020). Sometimes it is better to retrieve the whole tweet-object, a complex data object composed of numerous descriptive fields, instead of selected fields using tools such as Tweepy (see Table 1) because it enables the extraction of variables that could be used for further analysis. Moreover, users on Twitter are broadly classified as *verified,* genuine users whose accounts have been authenticated by Twitter, or *unverified,* not authenticated by Twitter. The account verification helps to validate online users.

- **Non-tweet collection** - With the availability of many credible sources debunking misleading narratives about COVID-19, it will be beneficial to have a large collection of curated datasets. Consequently, the non-tweet group consists of information about standard practices from reliable sources and a chronicle of global situation reports on the pandemic. Bodies such as the World Health Organisation and nationally recognised institutions will be instrumental in providing rich and informative material for robust factual analysis. This will enable researchers to find responses to a wide range of questions related to the pandemic for a broader comparison and evaluation.

- **Data cleaning** – To support effective longitudinal and exploratory analyses of the data, some crucial preprocessing steps are required. Basic forms of which include tokenisation, stopwords removal and text formatting (involving expanding contracted terms and lemmatisation). Once the data cleaning stage is completed, data analysis proceeds with a descriptive analysis to better understand the data before delving into the detailed study. Time-series analysis is crucial in revealing interesting patterns and useful insight.

UTILITY OF PANDEMIC-RELATED DATA

The quest to turn every aspect of human life into computerised data for competitive value is rapidly growing. Depending on the interest and goal of the study, data from social media platforms can be used to conduct studies along the following dimensions: (1) Textual or multimedia data analysis: the prevalence of multimedia data (e.g., text, audio, video and graphics) enables various studies such as content and discourse analyses for many reasons (2) the second dimension is graph-based analysis, which relies on structural analysis to identify the underlying structure of relationships at various levels of granularity in social networks. Depending on which aspect or dimension is chosen, techniques or methodologies based on machine learning or deep learning can be applied to process or solve the problem at hand.

With data from online social media, there exist many useful theories, constructs, and conceptual frameworks to utilise for further investigation; the work of Ngai et al. (2015) offers more insight into the subject. Of interest to this study is to highlight areas where data from online platforms can be used to manage pandemic-related challenges in this age of hyperconnectivity. Potential problems to be addressed can be around pandemic outbreak detection and management, pandemic assessment, contingency planning, early detection or alert system for disease outbreak from online social media platforms, and modelling spread of outbreak at various levels.

Detection of Spurious and Misleading Content

One of the reasons why online social media platforms are very popular with the public has to do with the ability for users to simultaneously generate and consume content leading to various forms of information – fads, opinions, breaking news. This reason also contributes to the increasing number of uncensored posts on various social phenomena (Inuwa-Dutse et al., 2018), partly due to their short size and the speed of communication. Among the repercussions of the increasing volume of information (relevant and irrelevant) on the pandemic is the tendency to create a sense of bewilderment on the part of the public concerning what preventive measures to take, and which piece of information to believe. There exist various misinformation and conspiracy sources capable of misleading the public regarding the COVID-19 pandemic. Demand for online-based services is at its peak during the lockdown, thus exposing the populace to various vulnerabilities. Despite the measures taken by social media platforms to curtail irrelevant content, many sources of misleading information and rumours still exist. As such, it is crucial to understand how online misleading content propagate and study how to optimise methods that favour the dominance of relevant content over irrelevant ones. A comprehensive repository of both validates and spurious datasets on pandemic will facilitate the authentication of the veracity of a given piece of information on the subject.

Understanding Pockets of Outbreak

Because users can share information about virtually anything, social media platforms are ideal for conducting useful studies. For instance, the data can help in informing what action to take that will prevent the occurrence or ramp up containment measures in a given locale. For an area not hit by the pandemic, mitigation measures and scenarios can be systematically categorised as *pre-outbreak*, *in-outbreak*, and *post-outbreak* to analyse situations and answer some beneficial questions. With the right data, some of the following crucial analyses, not requiring complex modelling, can be achieved (1) determine the number of cases – susceptible, infected and death (2) analyse the impact of the estimation (3) prioritize what course of action to take based on the prevailing situation and identify the most affected areas or groups. In terms of contact tracing, it will be interesting to ask the question about how possible it would be to trace susceptible cases using social media information. A basic strategy is to utilise self-reporting information about the relevant incidence, e.g., being in contact with an infected individual. As a result, the community will be proactive in handling any eventuality related to the pandemic because the level of preparedness will be improved significantly.

Actionable Areas

The infamous pandemic-induced lockdown has its many tolls across various sectors – at individual and societal levels. Thus, it is crucial to study its impact on mental health since people have been confined indoors, usually without jobs and momentous apprehension about eventualities. With self-reporting posts, triggers for viral infection and transmission within society can be studied to understand which of the imposed measures are more effective. Insights into these aspects will inform the best strategy to adopt in reaching out to the intended audience. Moreover, the study will help mitigate the 'scarring' effect of the pandemic and possible infrastructure damages as seen during the onset of the pandemic, which has been triggered by baseless claims, e.g., that 5G causes COVID-19.

Flattening the Curves

The infection curve – COVID-19, akin to illnesses such as diabetes, seems to require prolong precautionary measures to observe in managing it. Knowledge about the impact of COVID-19 is evolving, and its long-term effect is yet to be fully established. Thus, it is pertinent to incorporate diverse information sources from social media to help in offering a useful and holistic prevention pathway that is better equipped to tackle resurgences and other related eventualities. This endeavour is crucial noting how the healthcare facilities have been overwhelmed during the peak of the pandemic. A proactive approach will help towards improving the capacity of the health care service to fight the pandemic and effectively respond in allocating relevant resources intelligently and lessen future challenges. Accordingly, the following problems will be worthy of investigation.

- COVID-19 journey via online social media platforms: By leveraging self-reporting information on pandemic-related aspects such as lockdown, contact tracing, and public perceptions will offer relevant signals about recovery pathways. To complement the existing trusted public health information sources, harnessing information from online social media to address or examine the trajectory of the journey and its consequences at various stages

– during the pandemic (pre-vaccine and post-vaccine) and after the pandemic (recovered individuals during the pandemic and post-vaccine recovery).

The infodemic curve - One of the challenges of managing pandemics during the age of online social media is the prevention of misinformation. With the prevailing situation, as the virus propagates, so is fake news or misinformation about it; hence it is equally important to simultaneously curtail propagation of the virus and its associated negative infodemic. A simple strategy that will go a long way in mitigating the harmful effect of negative infodemic will require each recipient of social media post to ascertain the veracity of seemingly problematic or controversial information before amplifying. Figure 5 shows a visual illustration from WHO where a simple verification process will prevent further spread. Abiding by this simple illustration will go a long way in curtailing the menace of misleading information, especially during the critical time of the pandemic Among other benefits, COVID-19 datasets could be used for various purposes such as the development of useful NLP-based tools for real-time digital disease surveillance from online news streams; to help identify the proliferation of spurious content, and to develop a real-time monitoring system of health-related content to inform preemptive measures.

Figure 5. A simple, albeit effective, means of filtering information is for each recipient to ascertain the veracity of the content/post
Source: ©WHO, 2020.

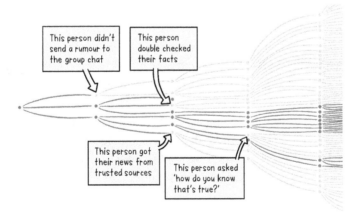

Community Detection and Sentiment Analysis

- **Community detection** - Networks are characterised by a certain degree of organisations in which groups of nodes form tightly connected units as communities. In the social science domain, sociometry is a means to measure or study social relationships between people (Wasserman & Faust 1994). Communities represent functional entities which reflect the topological relationships between elements of the underlying network (Newman 2006). Social network analysis is useful in revealing the dynamism of many forms of social relationships at various levels. Noting the level of resistance and acceptance regarding COVID-19, a high-level clustering of users could potentially unveil the distribution of users for reasons related to management, logistics, and containment of the outbreak.
- **Sentiment Analysis** – Similarly, another useful problem to tackle is understanding users' perceptions about measures taken in managing the pandemic. For instance, it will be possible to evaluate lockdown policy to understand users' willingness to comply and the attitudinal change over time.

CONCLUDING REMARK

The prevailing COVID-19 pandemic can be equated to illnesses that require prolong precautionary measures since the knowledge about its long-term impact is still evolving. Thus, it is pertinent to incorporate diverse information sources to help in tackling the pandemic crisis and offer a useful and holistic prevention pathway that is better equipped to tackle resurgences and other related eventualities. Since the outbreak, there has been a surge of studies investigating various aspects of the pandemic. Through online social media platforms, users are free to share personal information, which can be harnessed to mitigate some of the difficulties caused by the pandemic. Of interest to this chapter include studies centring on datasets from online social media platforms where the bulk of the public discourse happen. The datasets and relevant resources discussed in this chapter will play a significant role in tackling some of the pandemic-related challenges. Essentially, the following areas have been identified as crucial in the fight against the outbreak and could be studied using the datasets:

- curtailing the spread of inimical infodemic. This is needed because misleading information can have catastrophic consequences and hampers the fight about applying containment measures, which makes it pertinent to combat the pandemic from all possible fronts.

- among other benefits, the COVID-19 datasets, especially the online social stream, could be used for developing useful NLP-based tools for real-time digital disease surveillance, and to develop a real-time monitoring system of health-related content to inform preemptive measures.
- noting how the healthcare facilities have been overwhelmed during the peak of the COVID-19 pandemic, proactive strategy will help towards improving the capacity of the health care service to fight the pandemic and effectively respond in allocating relevant resources intelligently and lessening future challenges. The datasets and insights from the chapter will support studies interested in analysing the spread of fake and misleading content, evaluation of lockdown-related measures and tracking of public sentiment over time.
- the data will further enrich existing databases for debunking misinformation and fact-checking avenues, such as the International Fact-Checking Network.

Table 1. The table represents a sample of relevant tools to retrieve data from social media platforms. It is evident that Twitter dominates the list, which can be explained by the fact the data is more accessible than the rest of the platforms. Additionally, details about relevant resources for supporting studies on combating pandemic-related misinformation.

Tool	Description	URL
Brandwatch	Supported platforms include Twitter, Facebook, YouTube, Instagram, Sina Weibo, VK, QQ, Google+, Pinterest, Online blogs	https://www.brandwatch.com/
Brand24	Twitter, Facebook, Instagram, Blogs, Forums, Videp	https://brand24.com/features/#4
Audiense	Twitter	https://audiense.com/
IBM Bluemix	Twitter	https://www.ibm.com/cloud-computing/bluemix
Tweepy	Twitter	https://www.tweepy.org/
Brand24	Twitter, Facebook, Instagram, Blogs, Forums, Videp	https://brand24.com/features/#4
Covid-19 stream	A dedicated API by Twitter to retrieve Covid-19-related tweets.	https://developer.twitter.com/en/docs/labs/covid19-stream/overview
Hydrator	A tool to return the full version of tweet's objects from Twitter.	https://github.com/docnow/hydrator
Worldometer	A website for keeping track of COVID-19 global cases.	https://www.worldometers.info/coronavirus/coronavirus-cases/
	Framework for Managing Infodemics in Health Emergencies by WHO	https://www.who.int/publications/i/item/9789240010314%20/
	A joint effort between WHO and the UK in documenting online misinformation	https://www.who.int/campaigns/connecting-the-world-to-combat-coronavirus/how-to-report-misinformation-online
Fact-checking	International Fact Checking Network.	https://www.poynter.org/ifcn/
	Updates on COVID-19 diagnosis and treatment.	https://jamanetwork.com/journals/jama/pages/coronavirus-alert

Hopefully, the content of this chapter will support the computing community and policymakers in tackling present and future pandemics.

REFERENCES

Alqurashi, S., Alhindi, A., & Alanazi, E. (2020). *Large arabic twitter dataset on covid-19.* arXiv preprint arXiv:2004.04315.

Banda, J. M., Tekumalla, R., Wang, G., Yu, J., Liu, T., Ding, Y., & Chowell, G. (2020). *A large-scale COVID-19 Twitter chatter dataset for open scientific research—an international collaboration.* ArXiv preprint arXiv:2004.03688.

Chen, E., Lerman, K., & Ferrara, E. (2020). Tracking social media discourse about the covid-19 pandemic: Development of a public coronavirus twitter data set. *JMIR Public Health and Surveillance, 6*(2), e19273. doi:10.2196/19273 PMID:32427106

Chen, E., Lerman, K., & Ferrara, E. (2020). *Covid-19: The first public coronavirus twitter dataset.* arXiv preprint arXiv:2003.07372.

Cinelli, M., Quattrociocchi, W., Galeazzi, A., Valensise, C. M., Brugnoli, E., Schmidt, A. L., & Scala, A. (2020). The covid-19 social media infodemic. *Scientific Reports, 10*(1), 1–10. doi:10.103841598-020-73510-5 PMID:33024152

Dai, E., Sun, Y., & Wang, S. (2020, May). Ginger cannot cure cancer: Battling fake health news with a comprehensive data repository. In *Proceedings of the International AAAI Conference on Web and Social Media* (Vol. 14, pp. 853-862). AAAI.

Desvars-Larrive, A., Dervic, E., Haug, N., Niederkrotenthaler, T., Chen, J., Di Natale, A., Lasser, J., Gliga, D. S., Roux, A., Sorger, J., Chakraborty, A., Ten, A., Dervic, A., Pacheco, A., Jurczak, A., Cserjan, D., Lederhilger, D., Bulska, D., Berishaj, D., ... Thurner, S. (2020). A structured open dataset of government interventions in response to COVID-19. *Scientific Data, 7*(1), 1–9. doi:10.103841597-020-00609-9 PMID:32855430

Haouari, F., Hasanain, M., Suwaileh, R., & Elsayed, T. (2020). *Arcov-19: The first arabic covid-19 twitter dataset with propagation networks.* ArXiv preprint arXiv:2004.05861.

Inuwa-Dutse, I., & Korkontzelos, I. (2020). *A curated collection of COVID-19 online datasets.* arXiv preprint arXiv:2007.09703.

Inuwa-Dutse, I., Liptrott, M., & Korkontzelos, I. (2018). Detection of spam-posting accounts on Twitter. *Neurocomputing, 315,* 496–511. doi:10.1016/j.neucom.2018.07.044

John, M. L. (2001). *A dictionary of epidemiology.* Oxford University Press.

Kaur, H., Garg, S., Joshi, H., Ayaz, S., Sharma, S., & Bhandari, M. (2020). A Review: Epidemics and Pandemics in Human History. *Int J Pharma Res Health Sci, 8*(2), 3139–3142. doi:10.21276/ijprhs.2020.02.01

Kozinets, R. V. (2007). Netnography. The Blackwell Encyclopedia of Sociology, 1-2.

Latif, S., Usman, M., Manzoor, S., Iqbal, W., Qadir, J., Tyson, G., ... Crowcroft, J. (2020). *Leveraging Data Science To Combat COVID-19: A Comprehensive Review.* Academic Press.

Memon, S. A., & Carley, K. M. (2020). *Characterizing covid-19 misinformation communities using a novel twitter dataset.* ArXiv preprint arXiv:2008.00791.

Ngai, E. W., Tao, S. S., & Moon, K. K. (2015). Social media research: Theories, constructs, and conceptual frameworks. *International Journal of Information Management, 35*(1), 33–44. doi:10.1016/j.ijinfomgt.2014.09.004

Pink, S. (2016). *Digital ethnography. Innovative methods in media and communication research.* Academic Press.

Qazi, U., Imran, M., & Ofli, F. (2020). Geocov19: A dataset of hundreds of millions of multilingual covid-19 tweets with location information. *SIGSPATIAL Special, 12*(1), 6–15. doi:10.1145/3404820.3404823

Shahi, G. K., & Nandini, D. (2020). *FakeCovid—A Multilingual Cross-domain Fact Check News Dataset for COVID-19.* ArXiv preprint arXiv:2006.11343.

Tomas, P. (2020). *Coronavirus: Why You Must Act Now.* https://medium.com/@tomaspueyo/coronavirus-act-today-or-people-will-die-f4d3d9cd99ca

Valle, Sacco, Gallotti, Castaldo, & De Domenico. (2020). *Covid19 infodemics observatory.* DOI: doi:10.17605/OSF.IO/N6UPX

Wang, L. L., Lo, K., Chandrasekhar, Y., Reas, R., Yang, J., Eide, D., & Kohlmeier, S. (2020). *Cord-19: The covid-19 open research dataset.* ArXiv.

Wu, Z., & McGoogan, J. M. (2020). Characteristics of and important lessons from the coronavirus disease 2019 (COVID-19) outbreak in China: Summary of a report of 72 314 cases from the Chinese Center for Disease Control and Prevention. *Journal of the American Medical Association, 323*(13), 1239–1242. doi:10.1001/jama.2020.2648 PMID:32091533

Zarei, K., Farahbakhsh, R., Crespi, N., & Tyson, G. (2020). *A first Instagram dataset on COVID-19*. arXiv preprint arXiv:2004.12226.

ENDNOTES

[1] The data used in plotting the figure is obtained from www.worldometers.info

[2] https://www.facebook.com/

[3] https://twitter.com/

[4] For a more comprehensive information about the major events see https://www.whoint/emergencies/diseases/novel-coronavirus-2019/interactive-timeline

[5] See https://www.who.int/docs/default-source/coronaviruse/situation-reports/20200202-sitrep-13-ncov-v3.pdf?sfvrsn=195f4010_6

[6] www.statista.com/topics/1164/social-networks

[7] see https://www.foreignaffairs.com/articles/2013-04-03/rise-big-data

[8] see https://github.com/ijdutse/covid19-datasets for some relevant information about COVID-19 data preprocessing.

[9] The following blogpost also offers useful insights about the pandemic: https://medium.com/@tomaspueyo/coronavirus-act-today-or-people-will-die-f4d3d9cd99ca

[10] see https://www.who.int/publications/i/item/9789240010314%20/

[11] see https://developer.twitter.com/en/docs/labs/covid19-stream/overview

[12] See https://www.snopes.com/

[13] See https://www.poynter.org/covid-19-poynter-resources/

[14] The datasets described in the section is available on arXiv preprint at https://arxiv.org/abs/2007.09703 (Inuwa-Dutse and Korkontzelos, 2020)

[15] See https://blogs.lse.ac.uk/impactofsocialsciences/2019/06/18/using-twitter-as-a-data-source-an-overview-of-social-media-research-tools-2019/ for a more comprehensive list of relevant tools.

Section 3
Technology–Driven Challenges and Implications in Pandemic Management

Chapter 9

Ensuring Food Supply and Security During Localised Lockdowns:
An Information and Technology-Based Approach

Iman Hussain
University of Wolverhampton, UK

Lukas Jaks
University of Wolverhampton, UK

Chloë Allen-Ede
University of Wolverhampton, UK

Herbert Daly
University of Wolverhampton, UK

ABSTRACT

A pandemic crisis inevitably puts great pressure on different aspects of societal and commercial infrastructure. Paths for information and goods designed and optimised for stable conditions may fail to meet the needs of emergency situations, whether suddenly imposed or planned. This chapter discusses the effects of the 2020 pandemic on food supply chains. These issues are considered as problems of information sharing and systemic behaviour with implications for both people and technology. Based on work in Wolverhampton, UK, the effect of the 2020 lockdown period on local businesses and charities is considered. In response to these observations, the design and development of Lupe, a prototype application to support the distribution and trading of food during periods of lockdown, is described. The aim of the system is to integrate the needs of consumers, businesses, and third sector organisations. The use of blockchain technology in the Lupe system to provide appropriate functionality and security for data is explored. Initial evaluations of the prototype by stakeholders are also included.

DOI: 10.4018/978-1-7998-6736-4.ch009

INTRODUCTION

Covid-19 was first detected in the UK in the middle of January 2020 (Aspinall, 2021). The viral infection affects a patient's respiratory system and was transmitted by the vector of airborne droplets through close contact with others (Modes of transmission of virus causing COVID-19, 2021). As a result, the virus quickly spread across the country with estimates placing the rate of infection at 100,000 people a day by the time the first lockdown was initiated on the 23rd of March 2020 (Jit, 2020).

The initial lockdown meant that people were urged to stay at home and schools were shut. Workers who could work from home were encouraged to do so, whilst others were put on 'furlough' (extended period of time of paid leave). This led to a massive drive in the public 'bulk buying' goods (buying large quantities of items which are not necessary at the time of purchase) at local supermarkets and online, leaving others empty handed (Evans & Elley, 2020). Between the months of March and July, British citizens were urged to avoid contact and going outside, unless absolutely necessary. As the weeks rolled on and with no end date in sight, the availability of certain goods greatly decreased. There was major concern that the supply chains would collapse. Shops could not restock their shelves quick enough from their suppliers, as demands for certain items increased, examples include soaps, bathroom tissue and pasta.

Heightened by the limitations of imported food that Britain relies on and with more people losing their jobs or being made furloughed, foodbank usage increased by 81%. Families with children were amongst the hardest hit with over a 122% increase in food parcels delivered according to The Trussell Trust (The Trussell Trust, 2020). The Independent Food Aid Network reported 17 times greater food bank reliance than this time last year (IFAN, 2020). With more people relying on charities and fewer people being able to donate, food banks were overstretched with the availability of what they had to offer. As restrictions were lifted, the economic situation of the country was only getting worse and this led to a greater percentage of people living below the poverty line and unable to afford essential goods. Food poverty was already declared a UK health emergency in a 2019 report by Human Rights Watch despite a significant portion of the population having surplus goods.

There was an amalgamation of issues regarding food, in which such was often held in the wrong place, or hoarded beyond use, whilst others went hungry and suffered from food poverty. In many cases the problem wasn't the lack of food, it was lack of ability to get that food to where it needed to go. Examples include restaurants who, before the "Eat Out to Help Out" scheme (discussed later in this chapter), were paying to store their food, as well as hotels and offices with abundances of cleaning supplies after seeing fewer customers (Sheehan, 2020). Restaurants who were able to pivot to delivery services also had to deal with exuberant and almost predatory charges with companies such as JustEat1 and UberEats2 squeezing commissions from every sale.

It was clear that a solution was needed, it would have to be safe, efficient and accessible for people to use.

CASE STUDY

Covid-19: First Pandemic of the 21st Century

We begin with a brief examination of the Covid-19 pandemic, the main cause for the supply shocks and lockdown scenarios which form the background to the development of Lupe. The disruptive effects of infectious diseases are a well-known phenomena in human history. In the 19th Century epidemics of illnesses such as cholera, typhoid and smallpox cost millions of lives worldwide affecting many regions, nations through the rapid infection of a significant proportion of their populace. However, pandemics where an infection extends rapidly across national borders, engulfing whole regions are rarer but ultimately much more devastating. In the early 20th century, between 1918-1920, a global pandemic of influenza caused around 50 million deaths worldwide (Barro et al., 2021). Advancements in medical treatment, such as vaccination but also antibiotic and antiviral interventions resulted in the suppression of many dangerous infectious diseases such as smallpox, measles and polio (Rosenberg 1992). However, the global reservoir of pathogens occasionally throws up new candidates fast and extensive infection. Several recent examples of such, belong to the coronavirus family.

Coronaviruses commonly circulate among particular species of mammal, infecting the upper respiratory tract though many variants exist that result in mild symptoms for most humans. Three notable exceptions to this fairly limited pattern of symptoms have occurred in in the last two decades; SARS identified in 2002, MERS identified in 2012 and Covid-19 identified in December 2019. Severe Acute Respiratory Syndrome or SARS resulted in an estimated 8000 cases and around 800 deaths worldwide. The Middle East Respiratory Syndrome (MERS) outbreak infected around 2500 people resulting in around 900 deaths ("How do SARS and MERS compare with COVID-19?", 2021)

The first cases of Covid-19 also, known as SARS-CoV-2, were identified in December 2019 in Wuhan province, Peoples' Republic of China. The World Health Organisation (WHO) reported this outbreak as being due to a novel coronavirus and issued initial advice to the global health community in early January (WHO 2020). In the UK the first recorded death due to Covid-19 was on the 30th of January 2020. Following a sharp increase in the number of cases, on the 13th of March the UK government announced a ban on mass gatherings, with a national lockdown being declared on the 23rd of March 2020 which allowed people to leave their homes for only a limited range of purposes such as shopping for basic necessities. Schools and workplaces all were officially close except for certain, essential activities. There was also a ban on "all social events, including weddings, baptisms and other ceremonies, but excluding funerals" (UKGOV 2020). Pubs, bars, canteens, restaurants, public and private canteens were all effectively closed with those unable to work supported by government furlough schemes. Over the next month UK cases and deaths rose sharply as new testing regimes were considered and implemented. On the 27th of April as the UK passed 36000 deaths, the UK Prime Minister, Boris Johnson, made his first speech following hospitalisation with the virus. The first easing of Lockdown restrictions was announced on the 10th of May, with socially distanced sports and outdoor gatherings soon permitted. Limited opening of schools and outdoor markets began on the 1st of June, with high streets, retail parks, zoos and safari parks opening on June 15th. The first local lockdown was imposed in the City of Leicester on June 29th as a result of a spike in local cases. By the 30th of July special regional restrictions were applied to households in Greater Manchester, East Lancashire and West Yorkshire. By the 18th of September new restrictions were placed on households in the Midlands and parts of the North West. (Guardian 2020) (Independent 2020)

Logistical Challenges of the Lockdown

The foundations of the Covid-19 related supply crisis is found in Britain's dependence on imported food, with various factors making the standard just-in-time stocking procedures ineffective. The UK imports almost half of its food and 84% of its fresh produce, and heavily relies on other countries in doing so (Revoredo-Giha & Costa-Front, 2020). When Coronavirus forced EU countries such as Spain and Italy to lockdown, the amount of imported food decreased. Additionally, the lockdown led to less people being active within the supply chain, which increased lead times on deliveries of an already complex chain.

Even before the lockdown was announced people anticipated a shortage of food due to Britain's exit from the European Union ("Brexit: leaked papers predict food shortages and port delays", 2021), which led to panic buying of foods such as eggs, milk and bread. This started to occur as early as February and increased exponentially (Southey, 2020). It became a self-sustaining problem as other's feared they'd have no food, leading to the widespread phenomena of empty shelves. The media was plastered with imagery of vacant isles and was attributed as one of the causing factors by a Commons survey completed by MPs on the Environment, Food and Rural Affairs Select Committee in 2020.

People were also unsure of how long the lockdown was going to be; this meant that when they were 'panic buying' in which they brought goods in huge supplies. The uncertainty was further obfuscated by government orders, telling people to eat at home yet limit their purchases (Turnnidge & Chao-Fong, 2020). This compounded with adults working from home and schools being closed led to a higher demand for eating around a dining table. As a result, supermarkets reported the period of March to May 2020 as having the largest grocery sales ever recorded in the country (Jahshan, 2020). Dry goods and tinned produce topped the sales charts, whilst breads and fresh produce also remained in incredibly high demand.

Supermarkets became interaction hotspots as people would often form large queues in order to purchase bare supplies. Which created its own problem of ensuring a safe and hygienic shopping environment. A distributed platform would not have this problem.

Throughout lockdown, very limited amounts of businesses and food outlets were allowed to open. Furthermore, the government advised against all non-essential travel. This led to the hospitality industry grinding to a halt as caterers, hotels and office blocks saw less use. As mentioned above these businesses would often have large stores of goods such as cleaning supplies and food stuffs. Through their fieldwork the researchers learned that companies were still paying for the storage of their goods, despite not being able to operate as usual due to the circumstances. This proved to be particularly problematic because the lack of demand for such items meant the profit margins on the items was decreased.

As the general lockdown was lifted in the UK, the government switched to a policy of "localised lockdowns". These would allow the majority of the UK to return to normal, whilst certain areas of high transmission would be forced to adhere to stricter isolation rules. The reasoning behind the localised lockdowns was to combat the rising chance of a second wave in areas where the disease was most present, although some of the same mistakes were made in regards to stock management as shops were forced to revert back to rationing to help manage demand (Wood, 2020).

Prior Solutions and Limitations

With the fear of COVID-19 still present in the public's mind, small businesses and restaurants struggled to get the people into their establishments. As a result of the decreased footfall, the British Government introduced the 'Eat Out to Help Out' scheme in which restaurants that operated a sit-down service could offer customers 50% off of their meals between Monday and Wednesday (with various terms and conditions applying) (Slatterly, 2020). However, the researchers found that most cafes who operated this could not adequately predict the larger disparity in influx of customers from one day to the next resulting in them still having an excessive amount of food in their stores. Furthermore, not every establishment was able to offer such a discount often meaning they had fewer customers and thus less profit and more food waste. Some smaller businesses couldn't maintain adequate social distancing and as a result couldn't take advantage of the scheme.

Whilst markets and businesses in the UK remained unstable there became a heightened need for food banks, but due to the logistical factors already discussed in "Logistical Challenges of the Lockdown" section there was a shortage of food and supplies. Applications to help with food and resource distribution already exist, and are examined in depth below. The knowledge gained from such an exercise aids in forming a basis of the researcher's artefact.

The App "To Good to Go", specialising in giving away excess food, has saved over 1,000,000 meals from landfill between its use from 2016 to 2019 ("To Good To Go", 2020). Whilst this platform seems promising it's architecture wasn't able to scale quickly as seen with its limited adoption rates in the UK. Furthermore, it doesn't cater to the business to business market, instead simply providing an outlet for businesses to offload unused food to the public. Another limiting factor of the application was its inability to adapt to different scenarios and situations. The application's key selling point focuses on just restaurants and although this works well in cities with large food courts and a strong restaurant industry, the app struggles with rural areas. Currently, the application is only partnered with larger supermarket chains such as the Co-Operative and Nisa Local which aren't always available in smaller village or town communities. The app is also only available on smartphones which limits its potential users. Moreover, its focus on eateries and food products means that during the pandemic it couldn't pivot and respond quickly to the rising need for hygiene supplies.

Another platform examined was FarmDrop - this allows farmers to deliver directly to individuals. This app in particular was interesting as it catered to a niche, farmers directly selling to customers. FarmDrop itself served as a direct sales portal for farmers to utilise and proved to be successful amongst the farming community in the UK ("Farmdrop", 2020).

During Covid-19 and with Brexit related problems, migrant pickers and farm workers weren't available in the UK to assist in harvest (Morris, 2020). Although a campaign by the British government was launched to recruit fruit pickers from the UK, the program failed to meet its goals (Hymas, 2020). This meant that edible crops were not harvested which had a knock-on effect on the levels of produce available. Whilst Farmdrop was a promising application and served as an influence, due to the above factors the platform itself was unsustainable during the 2020 crop season.

Another issue is that Farmdrop was constricted to only allow industrial and career farmers to be able to sell their produce. This could serve as a problem due to the picking related factors above, but also due to an increased trend into small scale farming operations. This includes community allotments, or hobbyist gardeners. For example, an individual growing food at home would not be able to trade through the platform. The application is also limited in the areas it serves, at this time including just the South of England.

There was a clear gap in the market where an application that could connect businesses, charities and people could flourish. Although similar applications do exist, they are far too focused on specific problems and use cases, and often don't cater to the wider community or serve as accessible points of contact during a crisis.

The Lupe platform aims to rectify and plan ahead for the problems outlined above. The application's tech-stack involving the blockchain was specifically chosen to facilitate the future growth and scaling of a solution that could be used all year round for different scenarios. Additionally, the nature of the app allows for self-picking food with patrons bidding, buying and collecting the food themselves.

Charities and Their Challenges

As stated above, conventional food banks and community pantries were overwhelmed at the onset of the lockdown, with items such as milk, fresh food and baby formula running out quickly.

Food redistribution centres often found themselves left behind technologically with many using outdated systems with no official training. "Food banking doesn't have a high-tech rep and maybe that does us a disservice," states Triada Stampas, the vice president for Research and Public affairs at the Food Bank for NYC (Cosgrove, 2020). This can have a negative impact when it comes to using resources and space efficiently as well as ensuring people in need get what they require.

Feeding America, a foodbank not-for-profit, created an online platform where food banks could bid on items using virtual currency in 2015 (Lamb, 2020). The value of the currency was derived from the food bank's number of patrons as well as how urgent the supplies were required to the particular location. The result was a success with food banks given a greater amount of control as to what food they receive.

With the technological success noted; Feeding America initiated another project centred around an App that would help patrons, "Plentiful". Features included SMS updates, pick-up slot booking and tracking which supplies were available. The app was widely received and led to great acclaim and recognition.

One of the key advantages of the app was the ability to collect data on patrons, specifically what foods they were using most, and where they were collecting from. This was fed into a data model whereby Feeding America was able to create a "Hunger Heat Map" to help assist with efficient redistribution ensuring food got to where it was needed.

From 2015 to 2017, Plentiful was adopted by 235 pantries in the NYC area, enabling over a million client visits and serving 250,000 people (Fougre, 2020). Its widespread use has been accredited with helping monitor the demand and flow of food through the NYC food bank system as well as allowing data scientists to predict future demand.

Although the application was clearly a success, questions were raced on its security and privacy.

The data collection, arguably Plentiful's greatest asset could also be cause for concern as different countries and states may have different legislation as to what data a charity can collect. This could halt mass adoption or rollout of a similar system in other territories.

Some patrons were concerned about where their food had come from and the general food hygiene standards that were already strenuous in the NYC area. As all food was stored together and there was no way of tracing interactions between sources; potential for cross-contamination was high and a similar system may not be able to operate in countries with more stringent food hygiene regulations.

One of the key potential use cases of the blockchain involves the verification of logistical supply chains. In a blockchain system each stakeholder, and each owner would be able to share objects in their possession with all transactions being stored on a shared ledger. The shared ledger forms the basis of a blockchain and is a list of transactions shared between all members of the chain with consensus. This shared ledger would serve as a way of witnessing and verifying transactions which could help to ensure food safety and hygiene standards were met.

LUPE: INFORMATION SYSTEMS DESIGN

Lupe is a blockchain powered asset redistribution website for businesses, individuals and charities to offload food and supplies that would otherwise go to waste. It can be accessed from mobile devices, computers and most web browsers.

As a platform it allows businesses, charities and individuals to easily identify and signpost any such supplies that they have in excess. Nearby organisations can then bid and acquire the supplies. It serves as a distributed platform for the transfer of food and other principle household goods.

An example could be found in the hoarding of toilet paper and sanitary goods. These inedible, yet crucial items were some of the first supplies to be sold out after being brought in bulk. Lupe could be used as a means of trading inedible cleaning supplies, for edible food and vice versa. This could be done through people, or via hospitality companies such as hotels or offices who would often have an abundance of surface cleaners and detergents in the event of a lockdown.

Lupe incorporates many new and innovative cutting-edge tools such as the Blockchain and Angular to make it accessible and to help reach as many people as possible.

Blockchain

With the focus of the project being on reusable and adaptable food redistribution the group knew it was key to use new technologies and consider possible future changes in laws or scenarios. With this in mind, the developers decided to use the blockchain as a basis, using IBM's hyperledger software to help construct smart contracts to handle the transactions (buying, selling, updating) of food-based records.

One of the conclusions found in the research was that people are often apprehensive of where food has come from. One of the benefits of the blockchain is the clear transparency of the logistical journey of food. The ledger clearly states who owns the food and when the food is transferred between people.

When food or supplies are added to the system, users can define their value, amount and name as well as their "use by date", which would aid in limiting food waste. It would also help manage the auto-donate function.

The structure can be observed in Figure 1, whereby an "asset" can be seen with its attribute fields labelled.

Figure 1. Asset & Corresponding Attributes.

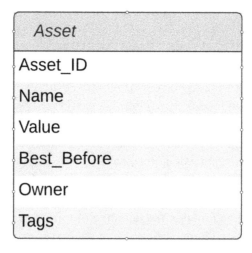

Figure 2 is a flow diagram defining the transaction of goods through Lupe.

Figure 2. Flow diagram describing the different users and clients of Lupe.

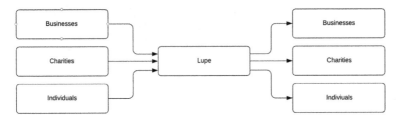

The architecture of the project would allow businesses, charities and individuals to deposit and add their items to the Lupe ledger. At this stage their items will be displayed and other businesses, charities or individuals could bid and own the items. The chaincode would have an automated method that would automatically offload any items that could potentially spoil to charities for free - the previously mentioned "auto-donate" function. Once the owners have been changed and the transaction is stored the organisations would then arrange pick up or delivery.

Figure 3. Relationship between assets and ledger via smart contract

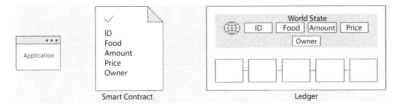

Furthermore, the blockchain offers several security benefits over traditional SQL based or document-based systems. An entire community can have consensus as to who owns what. This mutual trust and verification as well as the irrefutability that the shared ledger provides makes blockchain an attractive technology to use.

Angular

The application's front end was powered by Google's Angular platform, an open source web-application framework that had previously been used for IBM's FabCar project. Angular was chosen due to its open source nature ("Projects – Google Open Source", 2020) as well as it's integration with common testing ("Angular Testing", 2020) and development application programming language allowing for an agile development style.

Another benefit that Angular provides includes its cross-compatibility meaning a single web-app can be used on mobile, tablet and pc clients. With mobile usage at an all-time high making up 52.2% of all web traffic (BroadbandSearch, 2020) it made logical sense to develop the platform with a wide range of devices in mind as well as future-proofing support.

Cloud

Lupe is a self-contained network and offers the ability to scale to meet demands and needs. It can quickly be deployed to areas of crisis such as those locations under a localised lockdown.

Each area could have its own distinct ledger which could help prevent people traveling hundreds of miles for simple supplies that could be found locally.

Another unique feature offered by Lupe is its low processing footprint and distributed architecture. Being based off of a blockchain means it can scale rapidly as a decentralised system with instances being spun up with minimal user input and configuration. Although there is a common misconception of blockchains having absurd energy requirements, the research in this area is positive with private permissioned blockchains having minimal energy requirements compared to their crypto-currency peers (Sedlmeir, Buhl, Fridgen & Keller, 2020).

TESTING

Once the artefact was created it entered into a period of rapid testing and further development and refinement. The academics formed links in local industries and small to medium enterprises where they deployed the artefact and collected feedback.

Feedback was split into two categories, quantitative and qualitative. Quantitative feedback was made up of surveys which were given to significant stakeholders in the industry; business owners, hospitality staff and those that work in the food industry were contacted and asked for their thoughts and opinions on the crisis. These stakeholders compromise a variety of businesses based close to the urban centre of both Wolverhampton City and Redditch Town. This was done to gain a unique insight into how the industry was developing and adapting to the ever-changing conditions of the crisis.

Qualitative feedback involved constructing user stories that the initial Lupe product would serve to aid. Written feedback would then be compiled based on test subjects completing actions and scoring the application based on usability and functionality.

Quantitative

Initial Data Gathering Survey

A large survey was distributed to businesses of varying sizes in order to gain a broad understanding of how different enterprises were affected by the lockdown. The survey was sent out to different target groups: Wolverhampton business; other businesses across the UK and owners of businesses in different countries.

Justifications

When justifying whether the application would be successful or not, the academics decided to disperse a survey to businesses to get an overview of how their organisation was coping with the pandemic. The academics predicted that smaller cafes and shops catering to only instore clients would see the highest percentage of food waste and thus profit decrease.

The survey audience was limited to SMEs (small to medium enterprises) which accumulated almost half the total turnover of all UK business services. With the higher number of employment coming from Micro-companies (0-9 employees). This was the target audience as these smaller companies were usually owned and managed by locals within the community, rather than a universal investor. Thus, any economic and social impacts would be a lot more personal and hard hitting for the company.

The survey questions were based around when the UK went into lockdown. The time frame was implemented so that there was no confusion on when certain social distancing standards and other rules became compulsory. In fact, results showed that some companies were introducing increased hygiene methods and more delivery service options before this became law.

One of the immediate questions that was required was the location of the company if situated in the UK so that further analysis could be done to see the effect by region.

The style of questions had a range of quantitative and qualitative answer types. Lupe is primarily aimed at, but not limiting to, the food service industry and because of such. We allowed the option to select the type of sector that the survey's main income was from (for example, restaurant/cafe, small shop selling food items and other goods, takeaway only services and leisure facilities offering items for sale). The main reason for opening the survey up for this demographic was to see which area was most affected in line with their hypothesis, as well as seeing how other types of industry could be able to adapt Lupe's platform for their individual needs. Wolverhampton draws employees from the West Midlands region so any changes in employment contracts would directly impact the community.

Generic questions were asked about how the company adapted their business during the lockdown (e.g., use of a one-way walking system instore; increased cleaning and face coverings being compulsory). With Lupe being solely online, this reduced the strain of having to implement social distancing standards that take place in person. Social distancing limits the number of customers on the shopfloor and discourages customers from shopping completely. The economic effect was measured by the employment history and the percentage food waste made by the company during the lockdown. Questions on employment were introduced to quantify a common misconception that with the advancements of technology, there is less of a need for staff members. Because of this, it was insightful to see how the number of employees compared to what existing online services the company currently had. Modelling this with the amount of products discarded gave us an insight into what were the most profit diminishing factors for individuals and businesses.

Further questions were asked about what was done with the food waste to the company currently produced. It was important for our researchers to see how many businesses already made charitable donations or the reasons why they did not currently. One of the important features of Lupe is its ability to redirect food that is close to its use by date to charitable organisations such as food banks. The legality behind donating items can be a real hindrance for some companies and this adds to the time it takes to proceed with a donation. Many smaller companies are fearful that they will be liable for if someone was to become ill once consuming some of their products. Lupe reduces this fear by providing a clear and transparent list of owners and stakeholders in the food, as well as a list of its location history. Users could avoid certain outlets, whilst also making use of others knowing the journey that their food has taken.

Lupe's services were described in the final section of the survey, allowing those who responded a chance to trial the software and thus make further suggestions on improvement. While Lupe can be implemented in companies of different sizes, they wanted to focus on the smaller scale companies that they predicted would be the hardest hit by the pandemic. The survey was their opportunity to see how different companies responded to the pandemic and allowed us to model their Lupe solution to best fit the client.

No personal information was saved as part of the survey and information is provided totally anonymously.

Results

Food banks (and such like charities) are vital resources for the communities most vulnerable individuals. The West Midlands for example, had a recorded 168,886 food parcel deliveries during the 2019/2020 financial year. Redditch food bank operates using pen or paper systems to keep track of their stock. From their survey, they found that the majority of businesses and charities whose business were over 5yrs old were less willing to implement new technology into their daily services.

Explanations/Discussion

For the majority of their responses, the changes the companies had to make were in line with the Government guidelines, this included introducing PPE, social distancing within an enclosed space and limiting the number of customers in the establishment at any given time. These guidelines were enforced from July 2020 as the initial lockdown started to lift ("Guidance for food businesses on coronavirus (COVID-19)", 2020).

One of their respondents argued that the implementation of food delivery services saw little increase in their overall output of food. While it could be argued that there were more small food companies on the platform, the type of meals they were providing were not in line with the general public's perception of 'takeaway'. A survey from 2017 by Delieveroo showed that 28/60 of the cities surveyed in the UK would choose a burger as first choice for takeaway (with the remaining food items consisting of typical highstreet 'fast food' chains) (Hosie, 2020). To further emphasise this point, Alice's Tea Room's menu consists of single serving cakes, small food items such sandwiches and English Breakfasts. Not only are these items more difficult to package for a takeaway service but the up-price required by using existing, online takeaway services meant that the surge for the items was not worth the cost for many buyers. Owner Tony stated how it was hard to operate his cafe online knowing that there was little drive for the goods he is selling to be sent home. The experience of being in a calm, relaxing atmosphere such as the local cafe was what drove a lot of Tony's customers, he stated. This was echoed by other respondents who operate a similar facility to that of Tony's. In particular, there was a drive in the UK food industry for 'baking at home' goods and thus could be one of the reasons why smaller cafes and bakeries were unable to sell their usual foods through delivery. Grocery sales of flour were up 92% in the four weeks to 22nd March compared to the same period last year (Mathers, 2020).

Lupe understood that not every small enterprise that handled food could be considered suitable for the standard takeaway application and thus focused on the selling of whole items rather than those made for a profit purpose.

Qualitative

User Stories

The application was designed to serve as an asset redistribution platform for business, charities and individuals, as such the user stories were designed to reflect these. The current functionality was designed to be simplistic and accessible with basic create, read, update and delete abilities as well as the function to search and order entries.

Businesses, charities and individuals would be able to upload their assets which includes food or supplies. They would be able to specify amounts, and availability as well as location of the specified items. Further attributes included any allergy information as well as current state. Although food would be sold in a sealed and unused condition, entries such as chemical based cleaners could be sold if opened once identity is verified.

Other businesses, charities and individuals would then be able to bid on uploaded assets. Alternatively, they could trade assets providing that they could arrange for the transportation and collection. This would allow the transfer of resources from businesses who could open, for example Pubs or Bars, to businesses which could operate, such as take-aways. It would also allow those with ample supplies of cleaning products, such as self-employed cleaners, to trade for food.

Furthermore, businesses who couldn't offload stock to individuals or other businesses would be able to automatically handle the transfer of assets to charities in the local vicinity. These charities could include vital food banks and community pantries.

Findings and Feedback

Mount Pleasant Hotel

Through close work with various stakeholders, the researchers found the current feature set to be adequate in managing stock levels and supplies. One such organisation, the Mount Pleasant Hotel, found it simple to use across a wide range of their devices including smartphones used by staff and tablets used at reception. They found the ability to actively monitor what stocks they had as positive. Furthermore, as the hospitality industry suffered from the lockdown, Lupe allowed the owners to offload their vast supplies in toiletries and bleach-based cleaning supplies to local consumers and restaurants who were open. This allowed them to recoup an otherwise sunk cost and with the introduction of furlough, allowed them to continue operating at a reduced service rate as opposed to having to shut down.

Chick King

Another stakeholder was Chick King, a fast-food outlet in Redditch. Takeaway companies remained in service despite the lockdown and although Chick King saw fewer orders initially as the economy was uncertain they quickly grew to match pre-lockdown levels. One area that didn't grow was in the in-store service. Chick King was not able to apply the "Eat Out to Help Out" based discount due to its small dining floor, this meant eat in service was completely stopped. As imagined, this led to a lower usage of sanitary equipment and the takeaway found itself with excess stocks of cleaning fluids which were then offloaded through Lupe. Once again this gave the owner another steady source of income as he was able to offload his months' worth of cleaning supplies to local businesses and individuals that could then make use of it.

Redditch Mosque Foodbank

As previously discussed, the research many food banks still operate on pen and paper, with minimal digitalisation despite the massive use of computers and the internet in their modern lives. This creates many challenges when simplifying operations and streamlining logistical flow especially in terms of managing resources and volunteers efficiently. The Redditch Mosque Food Bank is a perfect example of this phenomenon. Although it possesses ample supply of food and toiletries, some of these stocks are lost due to inefficiencies in time and asset management.

Working closely with RMFB (Redditch Mosque Foodbank) they helped facilitate a small roll out of Lupe. Their use of Lupe allowed patrons and users within the community to remotely bid and acquire resources, this simplified the process of donating and giving food out. Furthermore, the ability to remotely arrange collections and donations cannot be understated in a period of limited contact during a pandemic.

Tony's Delicatessen

Tony's Delicatessen was the academic's insight into how small businesses struggled through the lockdown. Tony Wortley owns two neighbouring businesses in central Wolverhampton: Alice's Tea Room and Tony's Delicatessen. Prior to the lockdown, the two businesses were thriving with most of the customers coming from the nearby offices and passers-by. The store specialised in coffees and local cheeses and it was these that sought the most profit. Stock management was previously governed through use of wholesalers for generic items and local traders for the more specialised produce. A keen member of the Wolverhampton community, the store already donated leftover sandwiches to local homeless charities, with a representative collecting unused goods at the end of the working day. While these donations were easy and routine now for the company, this would not have happened without the connection made from one of the staff members; an asset that many of the other local venues do not have.

With the enforced closure of all 'sit-in' food services, Tony saw a large dip in profit. Fortunately, the company was able to make the most of what was given to them through Government schemes etc and the eatery was able to apply for a 'bounce-back' loan. This enabled the small cafe to invest in essential PPE, adjust the layout of the environment with new tables and chairs and purchase two new ovens. Naturally, this put the business in a good position for the eventual reopening of both the shop and the cafe, allowing for them to operate immediately. Common among many store owners including Tony, was the confusion that came with the regulations for reopening. Partially due to lack of communication through councils but also between businesses in how normal operations would proceed. Tony was clear from the beginning at creating new risk assessments and setting firm practices in place for the eventuality of opening during an ongoing pandemic. Food waste was a particular problem for Tony at the beginning of the non-operating period and approximately £250 of stock was wasted. Most of these compromised items such as cheese, bread and other perishables that could not otherwise have been sold or donated in such short notice. This is where Lupe could have been integrated sooner with smart contracts to donate to charity. All the staff employed are residents under the local council and thus the immediate closure resulted in the staff becoming furloughed. The closure of a small local cafe and delicatessen had a huge knock on effect on the local residence. Significant numbers of the customers are within the 50+ age demographic and many have a close relationship with the business and its owners. This demographic was both high risk and dependent on walk in eateries and supermarkets, meaning the closures of such had a great effect on them. This was because some of the older people weren't getting their food.

Marketing for the company became particularly difficult as well. As one of the few cafes serving special coffees and freshly made food, the cafe was able to operate on a contract level with some of the businesses such as the high street banks. These staff members were classed as key workers and thus would be some of the few people that were able to go to an office. Tony was able to deliver daily the amount of food ordered each day in person and thus keep the business going strong whilst not being able to open the store. Despite the deals the delicatessen had with local offices (i.e. delivering lunch for key workers), handing out physical resources was banned from many of the offices. One of the future features of Lupe is highlighting our local heroes so that companies like Tonys are able to get the recognition they deserve from serving the key workers during the pandemic without having to hand out physic assets.

With the arrival of the Governments "Eat out to help out" scheme, Tony saw a large increase in the amount of customers he had in the tea room. With more people eating in the cafe, naturally there was an increase in profit for the business; however, there was still an issue around surplus stock which they kept in their stores. The scheme was only valid from Monday to Wednesday in the month of August and being able to predict the number of customers during the whole week period proved more difficult than anticipated. The variety in numbers from the early part of the week meant that often fresh food would rot by the end of the week when fewer people were willing to visit the cafe due to having to pay full price. Balancing between having enough stock to serve while still creating profit from limiting waste was a huge strain on the business and something that individual businesses could not figure out on their own.

Owner Tony stated how previous delivery applications did not fit his business needs and that the services were too restrictive in how he wanted to use it (all whilst charging a premium). This opinion was echoed by many others in similar situations when trying to develop their existing services online. It was clear when liaising with their industry partners that even businesses struggled in setting up service-based delivery solutions such as JustEat or UberEats. What became apparent was that businesses needed a simpler solution, that would provide them with more control as to how their stock would be managed.

With the implementation of Lupe, Tony had to worry less about the risk of losing stock to waste as the majority of surplus could be uploaded online and sold to people nearby. Comparatively, Tony's eagerness to use the platform resulted in him being able to donate more food, as it was a significantly simpler process. All of his staff were able to quickly understand how to use the application and the team were able to implement it into their daily routine of running the business.

As the calendar month changed to September, "Eat Out to Help Out" scheme stopped, despite speculation and pleas from industry. A side-effect was that many restaurants and cafes offered their own special offers to retain the new footfall. Not all smaller retailers could afford to do this; even Tony stated that it was a financial strain not receiving the full amount but argued that it was worth the risk as it kept the level of customers he had previously. For the Tea Room, the first two weeks operated at a similar level but as the prices returned to normal by mid-September, the cafe saw a dip of approximately 40% in daily customers. The result of the dramatic dip in customer levels is primarily linked to the prices but also because the city of Wolverhampton entered its own 'local lockdown' from the 22nd September. While it was still possible to go out to restaurants and cafes etc, there was a greater emphasis on self-isolating and staying at home where possible as the number of confirmed cases in the city was ever rising.

Furthermore, the summer holiday period in the UK (end of July to the beginning of September for school closures) had just ended which meant that many individuals were returning to the workplace or schools. Overall this resulted in fewer people using the local cafes. The amount of stock that the company stored had to be adjusted to suit the current climate. Tony stated how it was difficult, if not impossible, to predict the level of stock that would be required for a standard week; however, he continued to shop once a week (or twice if demand called for it) for produce in an effort to reduce overall waste. The use of Lupe was fully implemented into Tony's existing infrastructure and thus leveraged some of the burden of having losing stock at full price and donating any that was close to its sell by date. Furthermore, the sharing ability of connecting business to business meant that Tony was able to connect to other local venues to trade their stock and thus support the community further.

Real World Crises

Australian Bushfires, 2019-2020

During the 2019-2020 Australian bushfire season, at least 33 people were killed (Henriques-Gomes, 2020) and more than 2100 homes were destroyed (Tiernan, 2020). Fire damage to homes and other buildings caused shortages of food and essential items in certain areas. The shortages grew as people vacated and moved around in an attempt to avoid the fires. A large amount of food, clothes and other essential items were donated by the public to support the victims of the wildfire.

More than 1 billion animals have been wiped out by the wildfires. Due to the fires destroying their natural habitats and affecting crop yields both animals and humans lacked access to food. This was partially solved by the New Wales government, who has dropped over 4,000 pounds of food to them (Wida, 2020). This meant that even more food was needed, as emergency response units had to count for those who survived wildlife as well.

In this instance Lupe could assist by helping to redistribute the donations to those who need it the most. An advantage of Lupe is that it can be split into different regions which is essential for natural disasters that affect large areas such as the bushfires. It is estimated that approximately 18.6 million hectares were burnt. Lupe could also benefit people in areas not affected by the wildfire and who had surpluses of essential items available to share with their community. This could help local food banks and emergency response units to keep track of local people willing to help and volunteer.

Sichuan Earthquake, 2008

The 7.8 magnitude 2008 Sichuan earthquake was a devastating event that occurred in the mountainous central region of Sichuan province in southwestern China. Four-fifths of structures was destroyed and approximately 90,000 people were counted as dead or missing ("Sichuan earthquake of 2008 I Overview, Damage, & Facts", 2020). On top of this, the environment suffered heavily from the impact of the tectonic shift and thus became more difficult to farm and raise livestock.

China was quick to respond to the disaster and as a result, the affected region had both phone and internet access a few days later (Phneah, 2020). With mobile networks now in place, the area could have benefited from the ability to share vital resources in a time of need. Access to nearby towns was more difficult as infrastructure was largely damaged by landslides which damaged food stores. Furthermore, the affected areas were split into smaller mountainous villages, so having the knowledge of items to trade would have been beneficial for supply management between very nearby locations. It would have also allowed for local authorities to see what reserves citizens currently have and thus manage the spread of items more easily.

It took a few days for food reserves to arrive at the centre of the Earthquake and many of the villagers were having to try and disperse food amongst themselves (Pinghui, 2020). With rescue workers deployed to the area, the ability for outsiders to track what resources people inside the villages had could have provided tremendous support. With the blockchain technology implemented in Lupe, support workers can see who has an abundance of certain items and allow those who do not to request them with embedded tracking to make sure all the resources are safe and secure. Allowing the authorities to track and make quicker decisions on what needs to be sent to the disaster zone.

Swine Flu Pandemic/Other Relevant Viral Pandemic Section

Covid-19, although the first pandemic of its kind, is not unique in its nature. Outbreaks on a smaller scale such as Swine and Avian Flu have caused problems in the past concerning food security and availability. These potential issues have been explored by others which made up a significant portion of our prior research.

In the report "supply chain disruption", Kumar and Chanda modelled scenarios and used evidence to draw conclusions on how varying levels of pandemic severity can affect the supply chains of various businesses (KUMAR, S., & CHANDRA, C. 2010). They recognised that although the administration and corporate structure remained intact and could be operated remotely; Many logistical workers (transport drivers, menial staff, general employee's) would be unwilling to work in unsafe conditions.

From this they concluded that depending on the threat level the Avian flu grew to the logistical complications would be exponential. The main industries that were affected included those that relied on a large amount of imported goods and a global supply chain as each link in that chain would be disrupted. Certain goods that originated or travelled through certain hotspots (electronics from East Asia for example) would be significantly hampered in their export and sales, potentially driving costs up.

On a local level this could mean food and supply shortages at supermarkets and smaller shops.

A significant publication published in 2015 entitled "How resilient is the United States' food system to pandemics?" tried to predict the outcome of a widespread pandemic on the U.S's food supply. The academics concluded that food shortages would start to build up over the course of 6 months, with major shortages following soon after (Huff, Beyeler, Kelley & McNitt, 2015).

The researchers then compared this to another major plague, the Spanish Flu in 1918. The Spanish Flu had far fewer cases of famine, most notably in remote settlements in the far north such as Alaskin Innuit communities. This was perhaps due to America's vast domestic farming industry.

OVERALL CONCLUSION

From the above research and the artefact's development and deployment, the academics have determined that Lupe has had a net positive impact on the local community. The ability to coordinate a neighbourhood, or city centre's resources between businesses that are open and closed was invaluable.

The feedback the researchers received from individuals, charities and businesses highlighted the need for a simple solution to the problem of excess stock, and stock management. Specific notes included praise for the ability to search in the local vicinity, especially useful during localised lockdowns. There were also considerable commendations for the accessibility features and the ease of use. Many small businesses owners cannot dedicate hours to retraining, especially in times of crisis, so the bare-bones approach was valued.

IBM's blockchain was used when verifying the transfer and exchange of goods from locations. It also provided a way of seeing where food had been and who it had been in contact with. This allowed any members of a Lupe to directly see and track where their items have come from, how long they've been stored for and their condition.

Local businesses reflected that the ability to automate the sending of food to charitable groups was simple and easy to do, meaning that they had the potential to donate a lot more and more often. This led to less food waste amongst test subjects.

There was some constructive feedback on the overall implementation involving exponential latency when transferring large items on larger blockchains. The blockchain was never designed to be an all-encompassing data storage solution, or as a replacement for traditional databases. The potential for latency to occur on a large scale would impede the experience for other users, as such the group made the design choice to stick to local Lupe systems. Smaller, localised Lupe instances would work more in agreement with the government's current advice of limiting wider travel and local lockdowns.

There are some future avenues that this research could be developed, some of which include; compartmentalisation, scoring or action based appraisals and further implementations of accessibility features. These are outlined below.

FUTURE WORK

Accessibility

With technological advancement ever growing the gap between those who have access to such resources and those who don't is becoming more prominent. The researches realised the importance of having equal access to their solution so that all can benefit from its features. Individuals marked as 'high risk' are often the least likely to be able to have access to the goods and services they need during the lockdown. High risk individuals were advised by Governments to limit as much contact with other people as possible to reduce the likelihood of contracting the virus. Relying on food delivery services was often their main source of goods; however, these services were being booked up rapidly and many were left unable to book such service (Amatulli, 2020). Therefore, it would be important to help those who need delivery services the most in particular. This would mean making the interface simple and easy to use, whilst retaining key functionality and features.

The World Health Organisation predicts there are approximately 200 million people with low vision who do not have access to assistive products for low-vision. With Lupe's mission to serve the community, the group believes that everyone should have the same access to their services and thus the implementation of a screen reader will allow those who are visually impaired to use the app. A benefit of the structure of Lupe is that the interface is not overbearing.

Text Format

Font based and filtering solutions can also be implemented for adjusting the size and format of the on-screen text. For example, this means that users with dyslexia are able to clearly understand the information presented to them.

Foreign Languages

The open-source nature of Lupe means that other countries are able to use the model and make adjustments to the on screen options in their own language as well as contribute to translations.

The new accessibility features would require more rigorous testing to make sure that the services they are providing are truly useful and helpful to those who'd need them. Further user feedback would be our key for surveying whether the changes are useful. Plans for trialling the service in certain test groups will need to take place post-lockdown.

COMMUNICATION LIMITATIONS

During a natural disaster, it may be possible that cell towers could be destroyed but unavailable. This will lead to users being unable to connect to Lupe, and leaving them unable to see, edit or add stock. This can be resolved by using the app that would use Bluetooth or Wi-Fi direct to create a peer-to-peer network and shared ledger which would then be distributed among users. With this solution, there could also be temporary receivers placed around the area of a disaster to increase the size and range of the network.

Compartmentalisation

In the future a Lupe based system being actively used in areas of natural disaster or areas of crisis. Lupe naturally serves as a central rally point when working with the safe and conscious redistribution of resources.

Through the team's user stories and ongoing work with local companies the researchers have found that excessively large ledgers lead to exponential latency in adding and updating records. This, alongside the recommendations of local lockdowns, leads us to believe that smaller more local Lupe systems are the way forward.

Currently Lupe has been set up to serve specific areas in the UK as per the local lockdown requirements, in future this feature could be used to dynamically set up Lupe instances in areas of crisis and dismay. Lupe is already a proven technology and being able to assist in the redistribution of produce and supplies after a crisis is key to restoring normality and order.

Examples include the recent explosion at Beirut's port and following fire, crippling importation of food including wheat, rice and sugar (ABC News, 2020). With Lebanon already being a net importer of food, it would be vital to ensure that all produce is redistributed intelligently. Moreover, Lupe's ability as a stock monitoring tool could be used to actively control and manage the remaining imported foods from Lebanon's other ports more effectively.

The ability to actively respond and scale based on natural disasters and current events is one of Lupe's key abilities. The more data that goes through a Lupe system, the better it can adapt and supply its surrounding areas.

Scoring for Consumers and Distributors

A point system in which businesses can gain virtual credits is a useful tool to encourage those with surplus goods to distribute as much as they can through the application. It also allows for the customers to appreciate the good deeds that various enterprises are doing. Additionally, this will work in the distributors favour as customers are more likely to support the services that have done more for their local community.

An example of where this has had previous effect was during the tragic Manchester Bombings of 2017. Uber had a surge in the price as it saw an increase in traffic from the amount of people trying to use the service. Naturally this brought anger and frustration on a national scale towards the service and as a result saw a decrease in Ubers stock price. Consequently, Uber offered refunds to those affected by the price increase but the popularity of the service in comparison to local black cabs never fully recovered (Marinova, 2020). The local black cabs did the opposite of their competitors and it was recorded that many taxi drivers went significantly out of their way to serve their local community (Bursa, 2020), As a result, they were hailed as some of the unsung heroes of the tragic situation and thus prevail in the city centre to this day over companies such as Uber and Lyft.

In a recent survey, 35% of people said they were more likely to buy from businesses that did support their local communities (Klaviyo, 2020). Lupe can be a catalyst for driving a charitable change as well as an economic drive in both smaller businesses and those on a larger scale. With the ability to see which companies are making a conscious effort to support their local community so easily available on the app, this is sure to drive economic success for those who are serving their local area. Furthermore, larger companies with multiple stores across the country would be able to broadcast their achievements to their relevant local audiences.

CRITICAL ANALYSIS

This project suffered from limitations in the scope of testing and development. Some of these factors were determined by external measures, whilst others were due to design constraints.

COVID-19, and the effects of food disparity are found globally, but due to the pandemic and limitations on international travel the researchers were only able to test their Lupe system in the UK. Their results are positive and Lupe remain confident that the technology will be versatile and adaptable to other situations and locations, they didn't have the opportunity to collect user data from other areas.

With the lockdown coming into place they were also constricted with their local testing. Due to limitations on non-essential travel their initial testing and feedback process was limited to communities based around Wolverhampton City centre and Redditch Town centre. This relatively small sample of test subjects could lead to anomalous results that would need a process or period of larger more wide scale testing to eliminate. The problem that this creates is that it could go against government legislation on essential travel and may have to wait until restrictions are sufficiently loosened.

Factors that could affect Lupe's usage in other countries include changes in food safety laws which could limit what products are available through Lupe. Furthermore, changes in climate would limit sell-by-dates and may force a faster cycle of food products through the system. Whilst factors such as accessibility to the internet could limit potential users.

The application will require an installer before being released to the public. Due to the closed nature of current deployments this has yet to be implemented. A proper onboarding process would need to be developed, that would be usable by any end user regardless of prior technological knowledge. It could be based on a single master Lupe website, with individual Lupe communities; or as a simple, self-hosted distributed web-app.

REFERENCES

Allen-Kinross, P. (2020). *When did lockdown begin in the UK? Full Fact.* Retrieved 12 September 2020, from https://fullfact.org/health/coronavirus-lockdown-hancock-claim/

Amatulli, J. (2020). *HuffPost is now a part of Verizon Media.* Retrieved 4 October 2020, from https://www.huffingtonpost.co.uk/entry/grocery-delivery-coronavirus-online_l_5e7be548c5b6cb08a92766f

Angular Testing. Angular.io. (2020). Retrieved 3 September 2020, from https://angular.io/guide/testing

Aspinall, E. (2021). *COVID-19 Timeline - British Foreign Policy Group.* Retrieved 4 February 2021, from https://bfpg.co.uk/2020/04/covid-19-timeline/

Barro. (2020). *The Coronavirus and the Great Influenza Pandemic: Lessons from the "Spanish Flu" for the Coronavirus's Potential Effects on Mortality and Economic Activity*. National Bureau of Economic Research Working Paper 2020.

Brexit: leaked papers predict food shortages and port delays. (2021). *The Guardian*. Retrieved 11 February 2021, from https://www.theguardian.com/politics/2019/aug/18/brexit-leaked-papers-predict-food-shortages-and-port-delays-operation-yellowhammer

Bursa, M. (2020). Northern taxi drivers hailed as heroes after offering free rides for stranded Manchester Arena terror victims. *Professional Driver Magazine*. Retrieved 5 October 2020, from https://www.prodrivermags.com/news/northern-taxi-drivers-hailed-as-heroes-after-offering-free-rides-for-stranded-manchester-arena-terror-victims/

Coronavirus consumer trends poll insights from April 21, 2020. (2020). *Klaviyo*. Retrieved 5 October 2020, from https://www.klaviyo.com/covid-19-daily-ecommerce-insights/marketing-consumer-insights-04212020

Cosgrove, E. (2020). How Emergency Food Providers Are Developing Tech to Help Them Give More. *AgFunderNews*. Retrieved 4 September 2020, from https://agfundernews.com/emergency-food-providers-tech.html

Evans, J., & Elley, J. (2020). *UK food suppliers battle to fill the empty shelves*. Ft.com. Retrieved 3 September 2020, from https://www.ft.com/content/fe10b7e0-69f8-11ea-800d-da70cff6e4d3

Farmdrop - Mind-blowing groceries, delivered. (2020). *Farmdrop*. Retrieved 4 August 2020, from https://www.farmdrop.com/shop

Fougre, D. (2020). *App Connects People in Need of Food with Nearby Pantries and Soup Kitchens*. Retrieved 11 August 2020, from https://www.ny1.com/nyc/all-boroughs/coronavirus/2020/03/26/app-connects-people-in-need-of-food-with-nearby-pantries-and-soup-kitchens

Guardian. (2020). *Covid chaos: how the UK handled the coronavirus crisis*. Retrieved 11 February 2021 https://www.theguardian.com/world/ng-interactive/2020/dec/16/covid-chaos-a-timeline-of-the-uks-handling-of-the-coronavirus-crisis

Guidance for food businesses on coronavirus (COVID-19). (2020). Retrieved 1 January 2021, from https://www.gov.uk/government/publications/covid-19-guidance-for-food-businesses/guidance-for-food-businesses-on-coronavirus-covid-19

Health Organisation. (2020). *Modes of transmission of virus causing COVID-19: implications for IPC precaution recommendations.* Retrieved 9 February 2021, from https://www.who.int/news-room/commentaries/detail/modes-of-transmission-of-virus-causing-covid-19-implications-for-ipc-precaution-recommendations

Henriques-Gomes, L. (2020). Bushfires death toll rises to 33 after body found in burnt out house near Moruya. *The Guardian.* Retrieved 5 September 2020, from https://www.theguardian.com/australia-news/2020/jan/24/bushfires-death-toll-rises-to-33-after-body-found-in-burnt-out-house-near-moruya

Hosie, R. (2020). *This is the most popular takeaway in your UK town or city.* Independent.co.uk. Retrieved 1 August 2020, from https://www.independent.co.uk/life-style/food-and-drink/deliveroo-takeaway-food-most-popular-a7573141.html

How do SARS and MERS compare with COVID-19? (2021). Medicalnewstoday.com. Retrieved 12 February 2021, from https://www.medicalnewstoday.com/articles/how-do-sars-and-mers-compare-with-covid-19

Huff, A., Beyeler, W., Kelley, N., & McNitt, J. (2015). How resilient is the United States' food system to pandemics? *Journal of Environmental Studies and Sciences, 5*(3), 337–347. doi:10.100713412-015-0275-3 PMID:32226708

Huge fire breaks out at Beirut port, a month after crippling explosion. (2020). Abc.net.au. Retrieved 17 September 2020, from https://www.abc.net.au/news/2020-09-10/lebanon-beirut-port-huge-fire-month-after-explosion/12652664

Hymas, C. (2020). Only 112 of 50,000 UK applicants for fruit pickers take jobs amid farmers' fears over skills and application. *The Telegraph.* Retrieved 4 August 2020, from https://www.telegraph.co.uk/news/2020/04/27/112-50000-uk-applicants-fruit-pickers-take-jobs-amid-farmers/

IFAN data since COVID-19 - Independent Food Aid Network UK. Independent Food Aid Network UK. (2020). Retrieved 14 September 2020, from https://www.foodaidnetwork.org.uk/ifan-data-since-covid-19

Independent. (2020). Coronavirus: Timeline of key events since UK was put into lockdown six months ago. *The Independent.*

Jahshan, E. (2020). *UK grocery enjoys biggest sales jump in 26 years - Retail Gazette.* Retrieved 4 February 2021, from https://www.retailgazette.co.uk/blog/2020/05/uk-grocery-enjoys-biggest-sales-jump-in-26-years/

Jit, M. (2020). *100,000 infections every day – why the UK lockdown came just in time | LSHTM*. Retrieved 7 February 2021, from https://www.lshtm.ac.uk/newsevents/expert-opinion/100000-infections-every-day-why-uk-lockdown-came-just-time

Kumar, S., & Chandra, C. (2010). Supply Chain Disruption by Avian flu Pandemic for U.S. Companies: A Case Study. *Transportation Journal, 49*(4), 61-73. Retrieved February 11, 2021, from http://www.jstor.org/stable/40904915

Lamb, C. (2020). *Plentiful is a Free, SMS-Based Reservation System for Food Pantry Visitors*. Retrieved 4 September 2020, from https://thespoon.tech/plentiful-is-a-free-sms-based-reservation-system-for-food-pantry-visitors/

Local restrictions: areas with an outbreak of coronavirus (COVID-19). GOV.UK. (2020). Retrieved 4 October 2020, from https://www.gov.uk/government/collections/local-restrictions-areas-with-an-outbreak-of-coronavirus-covid-19

Marinova, P. (2020). Here's What Uber Is Doing to Raise Money for Manchester Bombing Victims. *Fortune*. Retrieved 5 May 2020, from https://fortune.com/2017/06/01/uber-ariana-grande-concert-manchester-bombing/

Mathers, M. (2020). *Explained: Why it's so hard to find flour in the shops right now*. Independent.co.uk. Retrieved 7 September 2020, from https://www.independent.co.uk/life-style/coronavirus-lockdown-flour-shops-shortages-explained-a9457351.html

Morris, S. (2020). Quarantine measures may lead to shortage of fruit pickers in Britain. *The Guardian*. Retrieved 4 October 2020, from https://www.theguardian.com/business/2020/may/19/quarantine-shortage-fruit-pickers-immigration-bill-coronavirus-britain

MPs on the Environment, Food and Rural Affairs Select Committee. (2020). *What effect did the coronavirus pandemic have on our food supply?* London: House of Commons.

New report reveals how coronavirus has affected food bank use - The Trussell Trust. The Trussell Trust. (2020). Retrieved 4 October 2020, from https://www.trusselltrust.org/2020/09/14/new-report-reveals-how-coronavirus-has-affected-food-bank-use/

Nothing Left in the Cupboards. Human Rights Watch. (2020). Retrieved 2 March 2020, from https://www.hrw.org/report/2019/05/20/nothing-left-cupboards/austerity-welfare-cuts-and-right-food-uk

Online Marketplace | Feeding America. Feedingamerica.org. (2020). Retrieved 4 June 2020, from https://www.feedingamerica.org/about-us/partners/become-a-product-partner/online-marketplace

Phneah, E. (2020). *China telcos, Internet firms restore services after Sichuan quake | ZDNet.* ZDNet. Retrieved 1 October 2020, from https://www.zdnet.com/article/china-telcos-internet-firms-restore-services-after-sichuan-quake/

Pinghui, Z. (2020). Sichuan quake: Food supplies finally arrived, but still it wasn't enough. *South China Morning Post.* Retrieved 1 October 2020, from https://www.scmp.com/comment/blogs/article/1222212/sichuan-quake-food-supplies-finally-arrived-still-it-wasnt-enough

Projects – Google Open Source. Angular. (2020). Retrieved 13 September 2020, from https://opensource.google/projects/angular

Revoredo-Giha, C., & Costa-Front, M. (2020). The UK's fresh produce supply under COVID-19 and a no-deal Brexit. *LSE Business Review.* Retrieved 4 July 2020, from https://blogs.lse.ac.uk/businessreview/2020/06/22/the-uks-fresh-produce-supply-under-covid-19-and-a-no-deal-brexit/

Rosenberg. (1992). *Charles E Rosenberg Explaining Epidemics and other studies in the history of medicine.* Cambridge University Press.

Sedlmeir, J., Buhl, H., Fridgen, G., & Keller, R. (2020). The Energy Consumption of Blockchain Technology: Beyond Myth. *Business & Information Systems Engineering, 62*(6), 599–608. doi:10.100712599-020-00656-x

Sheehan, D. (2020). *COVID-19 the biggest threat to the hotel industry.* Hospitalityandcateringnews.com. Retrieved 8 July 2020, from https://www.hospitalityandcateringnews.com/2020/03/covid-19-unwanted-solution-hospitalitys-people-skills-shortages/

Sichuan earthquake of 2008 | Overview, Damage, & Facts. Encyclopedia Britannica. (2020). Retrieved 1 October 2020, from https://www.britannica.com/event/Sichuan-earthquake-of-2008

Slatterly, L. (2020). Eat Out to Help Out: Diners claim 100 million meals. *BBC News.* Retrieved 4 October 2020, from https://www.bbc.co.uk/news/business-54015221

Southey, F. (2020). *Panic buying amid coronavirus fears: How much are we spending… and why is it a problem?* foodnavigator.com. Retrieved 4 September 2020, from https://www.foodnavigator.com/Article/2020/03/27/Panic-buying-amid-coronavirus-fears-How-much-are-we-spending-and-why-is-it-a-problem

Tiernan, F. (2020). Australia's 2019-20 bushfire season. *The Canberra Times.* Retrieved 6 September 2020, from https://www.canberratimes.com.au/story/6574563/australias-2019-20-bushfire-season/

To Good To Go. (2020). Retrieved 10 July 2020, from https://toogoodtogo.co.uk/en-gb

Turnnidge, S., & Chao-Fong, L. (2020). *People Shielding From Coronavirus Question 'Confusing And Contradictory' Government Message.* Huffingtonpost. co.uk. Retrieved 4 August 2020, from https://www.huffingtonpost.co.uk/entry/shielding-coronavirus-lockdown-vulnerable_uk_5ed3c182c5b61691ddb5d11c

UKGOV. (2020). *Prime Minister's statement on coronavirus (COVID-19).* Retrieved 10 February 2021 https://www.gov.uk/government/speeches/pm-address-to-the-nation-on-coronavirus-23-march-2020

WHO. (2020). *Listings of WHO's response to COVID-19.* Retrieved 3 February 2021 https://www.who.int/news/item/29-06-2020-covidtimeline

Wida, E. (2020). *Australian government airdrops more than 4K pounds of food to hungry animals.* TODAY.com. Retrieved 6 September 2020, from https://www.today.com/food/australian-government-airdrops-food-animals-amid-fires-t171683

Wood, Z. (2020). *Morrisons becomes first large supermarket to reinstate Covid rationing.* Retrieved 3 October 2020, from https://www.theguardian.com/business/2020/sep/24/morrisons-becomes-first-large-supermarket-to-reinstate-covid-rationing-purchase-limit-toilet-roll-empty-shelves

ENDNOTES

[1]   UK food/restaurant delivery service UK based food delivery service: https://www.just-eat.co.uk/

[2]   Food based delivery service as part of Uber: https://www.ubereats.com/gb

APPENDIX A

Figure 4.

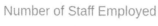
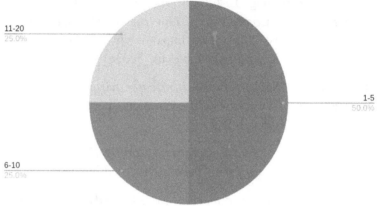

Number of Staff Employed

11-20
25.0%

1-5
50.0%

6-10
25.0%

Figure 5.

What sector is your business in?

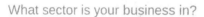
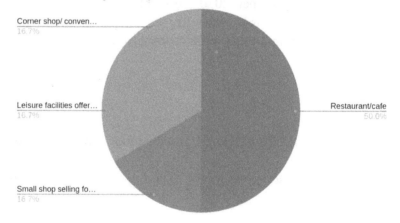

Corner shop/ conven…
16.7%

Leisure facilities offer…
16.7%

Restaurant/cafe
50.0%

Small shop selling fo…
16.7%

Figure 6.

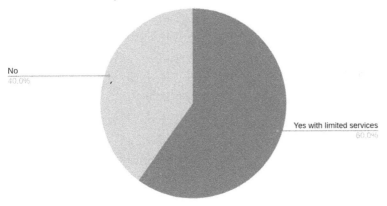

In the initial stages of lockdown (first 3 weeks) was your business able to operate?

No
40.0%

Yes with limited services
60.0%

APPENDIX B

Figure 7.

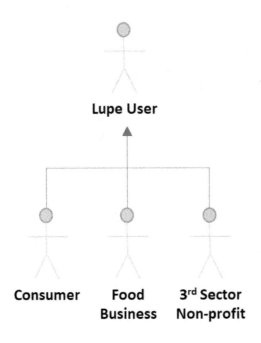

Lupe User

Consumer   Food   3rd Sector
Business Non-profit

Figure 8.

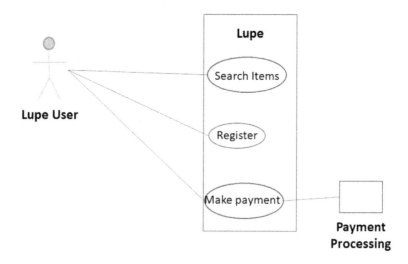

Figure 9.

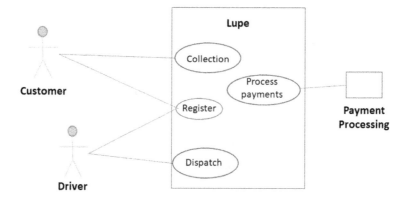

Figure 10.

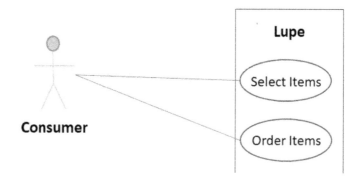

Figure 11.

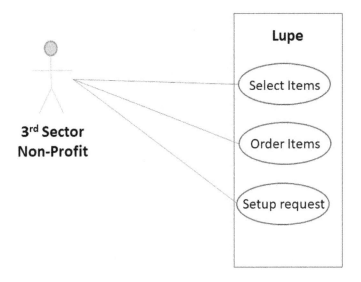

APPENDIX C

Lupe Architectural Diagram

Figure 12.

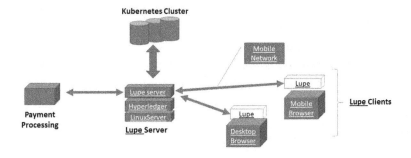

Chapter 10
Privacy–Preserving Pandemic Monitoring

Thu Yein Win
University of Gloucestershire, UK

Hugo Tianfield
Glasgow Caledonian University, UK

ABSTRACT

The recent COVID-19 pandemic has presented a significant challenge for health organisations around the world in providing treatment and ensuring public health safety. While this has highlighted the importance of data sharing amongst them, it has also highlighted the importance of ensuring patient data privacy in doing so. This chapter explores the different techniques which facilitate this, along with their overall implementations. It first provides an overview of pandemic monitoring and the privacy implications associated with it. It then explores the different privacy-preserving approaches that have been used in existing research. It also explores the strengths as well as their limitations, along with possible areas for future research.

INTRODUCTION

The recent COVID-19 pandemic has posed a significant challenge for health organisations around the world in providing treatment and ensuring public health safety. While healthcare professionals have risen up to this challenge, it has also highlighted the limitations amongst the health organisations in being able to detect it in a timely and accurate manner.

DOI: 10.4018/978-1-7998-6736-4.ch010

Due to the global nature of this pandemic, health organisations have obtained a growing amount of both unstructured and structured patient data which could potentially be leveraged to obtain insights to improve treatment as well as well control its spread. Due to increasing concerns over user data privacy, however, they are not allowed to be shared and stored in a centralised repository to ensure compliance with different data protection regulations (e.g., GDPR). This makes it an obstacle for traditional machine learning framework which requires the use of a centrally-stored data for both training and prediction. Privacy-preserving paradigms are essentially required.

Approaches in Existing Research

The different approaches which have been developed to implement privacy-preserving pandemic monitoring can be categorised in terms of four techniques, which are namely:

1. Differential privacy
2. Federated Learning
3. Social media-based approaches
4. Data Sharing and Access Control

Differential Privacy

The primary premise of differential privacy involves making sure a data subject is not affected (e.g., not harmed) by their entry or participation in a database, while maximizing utility/data accuracy (as opposed to random/empty outputs) for the queries.

Differential privacy guarantees that: (i) The raw data will not be viewed (and does not need to be modified); (ii) Maintaining the subject's privacy will be valued over mining insights from data; (iii) Resilience to post-processing; post-processing the output of a differentially private algorithm will not affect the differential privacy of the algorithm. In other words, a data analyst that does not have additional knowledge about the database cannot simply increase the privacy loss by thinking about the output of the differential privacy algorithm (Dwork & Roth, 2014).

The workflow of differential privacy can be described as follows (as shown in Figure 1):

1. Analyst sends a query to an intermediate piece of software, the differential privacy guard.
2. The guard assesses the privacy impact of the query using a special algorithm.

Figure 1. Differential Privacy overview
(Microsoft, 2012)

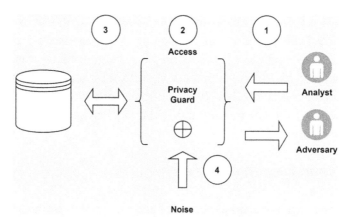

3.   The guard sends the query to the database, and gets back a clean answer based on data that has not been distorted in any way.
4.   The guard then adds the appropriate amount of "noise," scaled to the privacy impact, thus making the answer (hopefully slightly) imprecise in order to protect the confidentiality of the individuals whose information is in the database, and sends the modified response back to the analyst.

Aktay, et al. (2020) used differential privacy to obtain insights of user behaviour in response to the lockdown measures imposed in response to the pandemic. This involves using the data obtained from Google products, and applying ε-differential privacy prior to performing analytics on them. This enabled the researchers to obtain insights into user work patterns and the impact working from home has had on them.

Federated Learning

Data science has received broadest attentions both in academia and industry and has generated profound impacts in a wide range of applications.

In a traditionally assumed paradigm, data is available in a centralised point, to which a desired model can thus be applied and trained. In such a paradigm, the effectiveness of the solution lies at the model. However, the assumption of data being available at a centralised point does not necessarily stand. In fact, in most of the real-would problems, data is intrinsically located in distributed sources.

Moving data from distributed sources to a centralised point is practically impossible because it is either technically inviable, formidably costly, or would bring forth fundamental privacy risks. Federated Learning aims to be technically viable, cost-effective and most importantly privacy preserving data analysis framework over distributed datasets. The basic procedure of Federated Learning can be stated as follows:

1. Firstly, the distributed nodes each train their local models based on their local data;
2. Secondly, distributed nodes send their locally trained models to the aggregator node;
3. Thirdly, the aggregator node applies a proper mechanism to synchronise the local models so as to coordinate an ensemble model, which represents the global knowledge;
4. Fourthly, the latest ensemble model is deployed to all the distributed nodes to replace their local models;
5. Iterate the above cycle until the system converges.

Assuming that the datasets at the distributed nodes are statistically i.i.d. (independent and identically distributed), then Federated Learning would converge.

Federated learning is used together with deep learning in detecting COVID-19 infections from Chest X-ray images (Liu, et al., 2020). It involves using four different COVID-19 specific deep learning frameworks namely Covid-Net (Wang, et al., 2020), ResNeXt (Sharma & Muttoo, 2018), MobileNet-v2 (Sandler, et al., 2018) and ResNet (Ayyachamy, et al., 2019) on the publicly available COVIDx dataset containing penumonia images. Implemented using PyTorch, it achieved an average accuracy of approximately 90.34%.

Social Media Based Approaches

Traditional means of pandemic monitoring involves the use of patient data in training a machine learning model. While the use of patient data in model training allows for a granular analysis of symptoms and thereby improved prediction accuracy, accquiring them in real-time tends to be a significant time lag between proper patient diagnosis and eventual storage on the hospital systems. This is further exacerbated by the time taken to anonymised the patient data collected due to user data privacy concerns.

By contrast online social media data provides a real-time view of the public concerns over the pandemic. In addition the posts made online usually contains a geographical-related information which allows for pandemic monitoring and prediction in a given geographical location.

Two types of online data are usually used in current pandemic monitoring solutions, i.e.,

1.   Online search data;
2.   Twitter tweets.

2. 1 Online Search Data

During a pandemic outbreak, there tends to be an increase in online search on the pandemic as the public look for information on it as well as possible cure. This is also exacerbated by people who are suffering from it, as they look online for symptoms as well as measures for addressing them. These search queries usually are attached with timestamps, if properly anonymised, making them a useful data source to be used in real-time pandemic monitoring.

Lampos, et al. (2020) used patient surveys of COVID-19 symptoms together with online search data to track the outbreak of pandemic across eight different countries. This involves first using the Google Health Trends API to extract searches containing specific terms related to the pandemic in a given country and then filtering the relevant ones using the patient symptoms survey obtained from the National Healthcare Service (NHS). To further ensure that the search results obtained are indicative of the actual infections, the proportion of the pandemic coverage in the local media is used as a normalisation measurement. The search data obtained for one country is then used to build a time-series prediction model, before using the model to predict the pandemic status in other countries using transfer learning. Trained using the data obtained from Italy, it was able to forecast pandemic spread in eight countries with high pandemic occurrences over a two week period.

Keane and Neal (2021) adopted a similar approach to model consumer panic using online search data across 54 countries. Designed to understand the impact of government policies on panic buying, the proposed approach first collects user Google search data over a four month period using specific keywords. Factor analysis is then applied on the collected data to combine the ten search terms from each of the countries, before using Weighed Least Squares (WLS) method to build country-specific prediction models. Evaluation results from the proposed approach demonstrated that panic buying tends to be more affected by restriction policies in foreign countries, rather than internal restrictions.

Lu and Reis (2020) used a similar approach, and found that there is a correlation between an increase in COVID-related online searches and an increase in infection cases. It involves first collecting patient statistics from 32 different countries, before collecting anonymised search results. A correlation model is then developed using the data obtained. It is found that certain COVID-19-specific terms (e.g., "fever") can be used to predict increases in pandemic cases up to 22.16 days in advance.

Kogan, et al. (2020) also explored the near real-time prediction of COVID-19 outbreaks, similar to Lu & Reis (2020). However it features the use of six different data sources ranging from search data to metapopulation models, in addition to patient statistics. This involves first building a time-series model for case prediction using the Incidence Decay and Exponential Adjustment (IDEA) model (Fisman, et al., 2013), before using Least Square Regression (LSR) to build another time-series model using the data from the Centre for Disease Control. The two models are then combined together using Baysian-based model. Evaluation results indicate that the combined model is able to predict outbreaks with a maximum delay of 2 days.

A similar approach is used by Yom-Tov, et al. (2020) to predict regional pandemic outbreaks based on Bing search results. This involves collecting searches on Influenza-Like Illnesses (ILI) for each Upper Tier Local Authority (UTLA). Time-series analysis is then done on each UTLA as well as other UTLAs within a 50 km distance to predict regional pandemic spread. Used together with the demographic statistics obtained from the UK Office of National Statistics (ONS), it achieved an Area Under Curve (AUC) accuracy of 63%.

To monitor outbreaks of influenza-like illnesses (ILI) in different countries, Zou, et al. (2019) built a machine learning model using regularised regression together with transfer learning. Using the influenza outbreak data in the United States, a "source" supervised regularised machine learning model is trained. The model is then transferred to other countries in which limited ground truth training data exists, to monitor outbreaks in those countries. Evaluated against three different countries, the proposed approach is able to monitor ILI outbreaks with an accuracy of 91.6%.

2.2 Use of Twitter

In addition to anonymised online search queries, another key source for information for pandemic monitoring is social media data, more specifically, micro-blogging services such as Twitter. Due to its ability to post condensed messages and its ability to reach a wide audience, social media enables people to provide latest updates on the status of pandemic spread within a given region. Tweets usually are companied with timestamps and geographical locations, making them a valuable resource in temporal-based regional pandemic monitoring.

Gencoglu and Gruber (2020) modelled the causality between the user sentiment on Twitter and the characteristics of the pandemic as a means of pandemic monitoring. This involves first extracting daily tweets containing keywords related to the pandemic and then representing them as feature vectors. They are then passed along with different pandemic characteristics (e.g., mortality statistics, infection statistics, etc.) into a Bayesian Network which learns their conditional probabilities for pandemic monitoring. Implemented using publicly-available pandemic datasets, the proposed approach is able to achieve an average accuracy of 83.3%.

Dewhurst et al (2020) also used the Twitter dataset to conduct an exploratory analysis on pandemic outbreaks, but combined clustering with time-series model in doing so. Using one percent of the COVID19-related tweets across multiple languages, the proposed approach creates two clusters, one of which monitors discussions on treatments and the other monitoring the collective attention towards the pandemic.

In studying the user attention towards the pandemic spread, Cui and Kertesz (2021) applied a similar approach focusing on the Chinese social media Sina Weibo. This involves first collecting COVID-19 related posts from randomly sampled users, using the service's Hot Search List (HSL). A time-series model is the built which monitors how long a given hashtag word trends on the site. Evaluation results show that the life of a given COVID-related hashtag tends to decrease in direct proportion with the amount of government measures against it.

Zhang et al (2016) used pervasive social network (PSN) together with blockchain to securely share health data in wireless body area networks (WBAN). It first uses an improved version of the IEEE 802.15.6 protocol to establish secure connections between the sensor nodes. It then uses a separate data sharing protocol to exchange healthcare and adding their encrypted versions to the dedicated healthcare blockchain. While the experiment results indicate the proposed approach is able to exchange data securely between the nodes, it did not provide the implementation details of the data sharing protocol.

While social media provides a real-time updates on the pandemic spread and user sentiment in a given area, it can be difficult to discern accurate information from misinformation. This is due to relative lack of fact-checking on social media on a given topic, as well as the speed with which misinformation tends to spread amongst the users on a given platform (Wang, et al., 2019). In addition, privacy breaches in recent times such as the Cambridge Analytic scandal (Isaak & Hanna, 2018) has also created user concerns over their data privacy thereby have become less open to sharing certain aspects of their data. In certain situations, they might be tempted to provide inaccurate data in an attempt to protect their data privacy. All of these present a challenge to solely rely on social media to discern the spread of pandemic such as COVID-19.

Data Access and Sharing

Multi-Authority ABE (MA-ABE)

Originally proposed by Chase (2007), multi-authority attribute based encryption enables data to be encrypted using a specific set of attributes for each authority to which data is to be sent. It involves the use of a central authority that is responsible for the key management as well as regulating access control amongst different

Figure 2. Multi-authority Attibute-Based Encryption overview

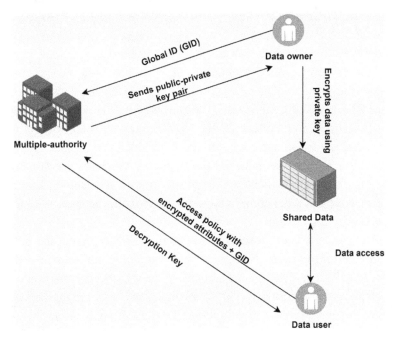

parties which need access to an object. Figure 2 illustrates how Multi-Authority Attribute-Based Encryption works.

When a data owner (**DO**) wishes to make data available for multiple authorities, he/she first registers with them using his/her Global ID (**GID**) such as NI number. Upon receiving the public-private key-pair which are specific to each authority, he/she then uses it along with the required access control policy attributes to encrypt data before storing it in a shared data server. When a data user (DU) wishes to access the encrypted data, he/she first sends his/her GID along with the access policy attributes which are encrypted using the public key of the Data Owner. Each of the participating authorities then verifies the policy attributes based on their pre-defined policies. If the access policy contains t out of n required attributes, the decryption key is then sent to the Data User who can then access the encrypted data.

Yu et al (2020) incorporated multi-authority ABE together with blockchain in implementing a tamper-resistant verification scheme. Designed to support access revocation, the proposed approach features the use of two separate blockchains one of which is used to maintain data and the other used for regulating access control.

Qian et al (2015) used multi-authority ABE in protecting the privacy of personal health records (PHR) in cloud environments using a protocol which generates secret user keys anonymously. It features the use of an access tree for the encrypting user to define fine-grained access policies for different authorities which he/she wants to share data with. To prevent the authorities from collusion, it features the use of an anonymous secret key generation algorithm by running a 2-party secure computation protocol between the user and each participating authority.

While the aforementioned techniques involve the in-device encryption of ciphertext, Policy-Hidden Outsourced ABE (PHOABE) involves outsourcing it to an external party (Belguith, et al., 2018). Designed to be used in Internet of Things (IoT) environments, it features the use of a Semi-Trusted Computing Server (STCS) to offload the intensive computation workload. To protect the privacy of user information, it hides the values of the attributes which are used to encrypt the ciphertext together with the access control structure. It is tested on five resource-constrained devices, and the computational costs remains the same with increasing number of encryption attributes.

A similar approach is proposed by Tian et al (2019) to protect the privacy and integrity in auditing user data in fog-to-cloud computing environments. Designed for Internet of Things (IoT) environments, it uses homomorphic encryption to generate data tags at each mobile sink which then sends them to the fog nodes. The fog nodes then generates the corresponding fog tags before sending the encrypted data to the cloud for processing. The third-party auditor (TPA) at the cloud end then performs auditing on the encrypted tags. The experimental results show that it is able to provide privacy preserving data auditing with minimal performance overhead.

The use of distributed authorities for data encryption and data access helps to address the issues associated with one centralised authority. However it is possible for participating authorities as well as parties to collude in obtaining the decryption keys as Meamari et al (2020) discussed.

Smart Contracts and Blockchain

Azaria *et.al* (2016) proposed the use of blockchain for secure electronic medical record sharing with access control in their implementation of *MedRec*. Designed to be used by patients as well as researchers, it involves the use of three smart contracts using Etherum to associate patient health records with different healthcare providers. Upon registration the registrator contracts associate the patient identities with their Ethereum addresses. Throughout their time within the system, the patient-provider contract is responsible for the access management of patient data with the summary contract maintaining a record of access by other parties within the system.

To provide an added protection layer for the secret keys Guo et al (2019) proposed the use of smart contracts along with multi-authority attribute-based access control. This involves the data owner first encrypting the data using his secret key together with AES (Advanced Encryption System) encryption. Smart contracts are used in this set-up to obtain the different attributes which are provided to the user by different authorities. They are then used to create an access control structure and the user is granted access if the number of correct attributes is beyond a pre-defined threshold.

Blockchain is also used together with ABE to provide anonymous user authentication and multi-party healthcare data access (Guo et al, 2020). It first uses an attribute-based multi-signature (ABMS) scheme to encrypt the patient attributes using the keys provided by the attribute authority, before storing the resulting signature on a blockchain. The patient data is encrypted in a similar manner, however it features the use of a user-defined access control policy in doing so. The healthcare providers in the network then uses the aforementioned key to access the patient attributes before using them to access the encrypted data. Implemented on the Hyperledger Fabric and Hyperledger Ursa plaform for the multi-party signature and multi-party ABE respectively, the performance of the approach is found to increase with the increase in patient attributes.

DISCUSSION

In response to the challenges posed by the COVID-19 pandemic, a number of different privacy-preserving data sharing techniques have been proposed to facilitate the sharing and analysis of patient health data. While they have proven to be effective in addressing different aspects of data sharing, a number of issues need further exploration to facilitate widespread adoption.

One of the key aspects of existing approaches is the performance overhead associated with their operations. Federated learning-based approaches reduce the need for a centralised data server by allowing model training to take place at each local node, before sharing the model parameters to create a shared global model. While this allows the use of local data at each node, the communication overhead tends to increase with increase in the number of participating nodes. By the same token, blockchain-based approaches also suffer from the same issue in generating the Proof-of-Work (PoW) amongst the participating nodes. Given the heterogeneous nature of participating nodes (e.g., mobile and IoT devices) as well as its reliance on the underlying network infrastructure, the need for a low-latency and efficient network communication protocol is an open research problem which is worth exploring.

The second aspect of existing approaches is the guarantee provided by existing techniques in ensuring user data privacy. MA-ABE-based approaches allow for a means of exchanging patient data amongst different participating authorities in a privacy-preserving manner. Similar to federated learning-based approaches, this reduces the need for a central authority which regulates access control by distributing the responsibility amongst the authorities. However the possibility of collusion attacks exists in which either participating authorities or parties can collude to obtain the access control attributes needed to decrypt patient data.

CONCLUSION

The global nature of the current pandemic has increased the need for international collaboration in their efforts to addressing it. To ensure compliance with different international patient and user data privacy regulations (e.g., HIPPAA, GDPR), a number of techniques have been proposed and used in addressing different aspects of addressing the pandemic from outbreak prediction to monitoring user sentiments towards topics associated with it. This chapter presents these techniques by first providing a technical overview of each, before discussing the different approaches in existing research which feature its application. It is then followed by a critical evaluation of the existing approaches, highlighing both their strengths as well as their limitations.

While the different techniques in existing research address different aspects of ensuring user data privacy, they have not seen a widespread adoption due to different reasons ranging from high computational requirements to user concerns over their privacy. As government and healthcare organisations strive to find a cure against COVID-19, it is of critical importance to explore the combined use of these aforementioned techniques. This will not only be able to complement the limitations of each techniques, but will also help provide a holistic perspective on the pandemic while ensuring user privacy is maintained.

REFERENCES

Aktay, A. (2020). *Google COVID-19 community mobility reports: Anonymization process description (version 1.0).* arXiv preprint arXiv:2004.04145.

Ayyachamy, S., Alex, V., Khened, M. & Krishnamurthi, G. (2019). *Medical image retrieval using Resnet-18.* Academic Press.

Azaria, A. E. A. V. T. L. A. (2016). *Medrec: Using blockchain for medical data access and permission management.* IEEE.

Belguith, S. (2018). Phoabe: Securely outsourcing multi-authority attribute based encryption with policy hidden for cloud assisted iot. Computer Networks, 133, 141-156.

Chase, M. (2007). Multi-authority attribute based encryption. In Theory of cryptography conference. Springer. doi:10.1007/978-3-540-70936-7_28

Cui, H., & Kertesz, J. (2021). Attention dynamics on the Chinese social media Sina Weibo during the COVID-19 pandemic. *EPJ Data Science, 10*(1), 8. doi:10.1140/epjds13688-021-00263-0 PMID:33552838

Dewhurst, D. R. (2020). *Divergent modes of online collective attention to the COVID-19 pandemic are associated with future caseload variance.* arXiv preprint arXiv:2004.03516.

Dodds, P. S. (2020). *Long-term word frequency dynamics derived from Twitter are corrupted: A bespoke approach to detecting and removing pathologies in ensembles of time series.* arXiv preprint arXiv:2008.11305.

Dwork, C. & Roth, A. (2014). The algorithmic foundations of differential privacy. *Foundations and Trends in Theoretical Computer Science, 9*(3-4), 211-407.

Fisman, D. N., Hauck, T. S., Tuite, A. R., & Greer, A. L. (2013). An IDEA for short term outbreak projection: Nearcasting using the basic reproduction number. *PLoS One, 8*(12), e83622. doi:10.1371/journal.pone.0083622 PMID:24391797

Gencoglu, O., & Gruber, M. (2020). *Causal Modeling of Twitter Activity During COVID-19.* arXiv preprint arXiv:2005.07952.

Guo, H., Meamari, E. & Shen, C.-C. (2019). *Multi-authority attribute-based access control with smart contract.* Academic Press.

Isaak, J. & Hanna, M. J. (2018). User data privacy: Facebook, Cambridge Analytica, and privacy protection. *Computer, 51*(8), 56-59.

Keane, M. & Neal, T. (2021). Consumer panic in the COVID-19 pandemic. *Journal of Econometrics, 220*(1), 86-105.

Kogan, N. E. (2020). *An early warning approach to monitor COVID-19 activity with multiple digital traces in near real-time.* arXiv preprint arXiv:2007.00756.

Kumar, R. (2020). *Blockchain-federated-learning and deep learning models for covid-19 detection using ct imaging.* arXiv preprint arXiv:2007.06537.

Lampos, V. (2020). *Tracking COVID-19 using online search.* arXiv preprint arXiv:2003.08086.

Liu, B. (2020). *Experiments of federated learning for covid-19 chest x-ray images.* arXiv preprint arXiv:2007.05592.

Meamari, E., Guo, H., Shen, C.-C., & Hur, J. (2020). *Collusion Attacks on Decentralized Attributed-Based Encryption: Analyses and a Solution.* arXiv preprint arXiv:2002.07811.

Microsoft. (2012). *Differential Privacy for Everyone.* Available at: http://download.microsoft.com/download/D/1/F/D1F0DFF5-8BA9-4BDF-8924-7816932F6825/Differential_Privacy_for_Everyone.pdf

Qian, H., Li, J., Zhang, Y., & Han, J. (2015). Privacy-preserving personal health record using multi-authority attribute-based encryption with revocation. *International Journal of Information Security*, 487–497.

Sandler, M. (2018). *Mobilenetv2: Inverted residuals and linear bottlenecks.* Academic Press.

Sharma, A., & Muttoo, S. K. (2018). Spatial image steganalysis based on resnext. In *2018 IEEE 18th International Conference on Communication Technology (ICCT).* IEEE.

Tian, H. (2019). Privacy-preserving public auditing for secure data storage in fog-to-cloud computing. *Journal of Network and Computer Applications*, *127*, 59–69.

Wang, L., Lin, Z. Q., & Wong, A. (2020). Covid-net: A tailored deep convolutional neural network design for detection of covid-19 cases from chest x-ray images. *Scientific Reports*, *10*, 1–12.

Wang, Y., McKee, M., Torbica, A., & Stuckler, D. (2019). Systematic literature review on the spread of health-related misinformation on social media. *Social Science & Medicine*, 240.

Yom-Tov, E., Lampos, V., Cox, I. J., & Edelstein, M. (2020). *Providing early indication of regional anomalies in COVID19 case counts in England using search engine queries.* arXiv preprint arXiv:2007.11821.

Yu, G. (2020). Enabling Attribute Revocation for Fine-Grained Access Control in Blockchain-IoT Systems. *IEEE Transactions on Engineering Management.*

Zhang, J., Xue, N., & Huang, X. (2016). A secure system for pervasive social network-based healthcare. *IEEE Access : Practical Innovations, Open Solutions*, *4*, 9239–9250.

Chapter 11
Strategies for Upskilling in Data Science After the COVID 19 Pandemic

Guru K.

https://orcid.org/0000-0003-4563-6398
SRM Valliammai Engineering College, India

Umadevi A.
SRM Valliammai Engineering College, India

ABSTRACT

The World Health Organization (WHO) declared COVID-19, an infectious disease caused by the virus SARS-CoV-2, as a pandemic in March 2020. More than 2.8 million people tested positive at the time of publication. Infections are exponentially increasing, and immense attempts are being made to tackle the epidemic. In this chapter, the authors aim to systematize data science works and evaluate the fast-growing community of recent studies. They also analyze public datasets and repositories that can be used to map COVID-19 dissemination and mitigation strategies. As part of that, they suggest a library review of the papers produced in this short period of time. Finally, they emphasize typical issues and pitfalls found in the surveyed works on the basis of these observations. Data science, narrowly established, will play a critical role in the global COVID-19 pandemic response. This chapter addresses the implications of data science for policymakers and strategists and allows them to resolve the threats, possibilities, and pitfalls inherent in using data science for tackling the COVID-19 pandemic.

DOI: 10.4018/978-1-7998-6736-4.ch011

INTRODUCTION

The SARS COV-2 virus was first detected in Wuhan City (China) in December 2019 and related disease was first announced to exist in the World Health Organization (WHO on 11 March 2020). More than 24,000 academic papers related to pandemic have been published in peer-reviewed journals and available online since December 2019. It is particularly difficult to comprehend the fast moving scientific environment as much of this literature has not yet been peer reviewed. This Chapter aims to address this problem with a detailed description and survey of COVID-19 data science studies. It is intended as a shared resource to make the vast number of data and publications released in recent months available. We use the word 'data science' as a primary concept for learning from organised and unstructured data using all approaches that use mathematical processes, algorithms and programs. We understand the significance of related viewpoints in the fields of social sciences, ethics, history and other humanities.

STRATEGIES FOR UPSKILLING IN DATA SCIENCE

The Covid-19 crisis has improved organizational infrastructure and continuity. As data and analytics progress, organizations will use data to assess the expertise and approaches needed to educate and hire employees and provide them with new skills available for what lies ahead. Data scientists are important to market development and creativity and must be equipped to respond to an ever-changing digital world. Career growth includes the development and diversification of skills and experience required for future success and work. And as an information scientist, it is important to be competitive and excellent, and to help organizations continue to succeed on a future that will continue to leverage modern IT architectures and remote infrastructure. Leadership should take action to implement new skills plans to allow its workers to continue being an asset throughout the continuing global disruption of the pandemic.

Predict Future Talent Needs

Business executives must take a selective approach to change and in order to do so, predict a reliable understanding of how capabilities will become and how many workers will be expected to drive future business targets. Think about the company's general needs and the latest talents to address current talent holes and possible potential investment in new technology and instruments that need new skills and abilities, such as artificial intelligence (AI).

Talent Analysis to Guide Skill Priorities

It is easier to develop existing employee skills than to recruit new talent, especially in light of the current shortage of data scientists. Consider undertaking an analyses of the worker talent to determine the company's specific job needs, allowing the enterprise to create staff profiles that can guide advanced decision-making. In an increasing work climate, talent growth is vital to improving efficiencies, and companies need to pursue the correct approach internally.

Encourage Strategic Skill Procurement

As a market executive, you need to put your workers in modern job environments and circumstances to thrive and innovate. Continuous preparation and advancement of expertise and immersive training in some areas of data science direct career development and improvements towards unique priorities such as collaborating successfully with emerging technology such as machine learning (ML) and cloud computing. It will be highly acceptable to facilitate new skills procurement in an ML programming language like Python or Julia, or risk management.

Help Employees Navigate New Dynamics

Your workforce must be diverse in expertise, education and community and be able to proceed with the complexities of continual and evolving job – a reality in any work situation. Accept the importance of a current employee, such as a market analyst, with specialized business experience. The employee is well worth the additional commitment in experience in data science, such as SQL, Tensorflow or Tableau. This approach blends challenging industry experience with data science guiding quantitative and statistical expertise, and returns your initial commitment many times to talent that supports your particular business in countless ways.

KEY FOCUS AREAS IN DATA SCIENCE

The epidemic of coronaviruses has prompted businesses to transform their corporate continuity plans. With the rising need for digital adoption, employment for AI, ML and data science practitioners will increase. Professionals in data science need to reorient their work plans to find jobs. When automation becomes more popular, some data science skills for businesses are becoming redundant. Data science has become a large field; it is crucial for a profession to narrow down on main target fields. The outbreak of the COVID-19 pandemic urged businesses to transform their policies to ensure economic stability in the post-lockdown environment. In exchange, this offered data scientists the ability to update their expertise with appropriate skills to retain their usefulness. Thus, data science experts have been imperative to reconsider their career strategy. In addition to the automation revolution, numerous data science capabilities are outdated for market performance. As a result, firms are currently trying to employ experts with specialized experience that will be important to businesses in the world post-COVID-19. In reality, in the tough times, data science practitioners are cautiously hopeful about work prospects, according to a recent LinkedIn survey. However, 63 per cent of those polled who are successful career seekers, 65 percent of full-time workers and 61 per cent of the self-employed said that their reliance on skills to sustain this recession would be increased. Zairus Master (2017), CEO of Shine Learning, an online training program, also told media outlets that the number of learners who want to develop their qualifications in courses such as data science, blockchain and software education has risen dramatically. "With remote work becoming the norm increasingly, we can see more demand for certain talents in this area," Master said. To thrive in the post-COVID world, data science experts must learn specialized skills to make them available for hire after this pandemic:

Natural Language Processing (NLP)

Businesses aim to gather as much data from multiple sources as possible in order to enhance customer experience. For businesses focused on new-age customer relationship management software, the NLP may be an advantage. In the near future, data science experts with NLP expertise will see great demand. With companies today seeking to gather as much data as possible for a better consumer experience in the middle of the recession, NLP may be an opportunity for enterprises. Many businesses still use self-service software, such as bots with NLP embedded with several languages to help solve consumer concerns. In order for organizations to render artificial alternatives for a better post-COVID world result, data scientists must grasp and learn NLP. In reality, Mercedes-Benz, a multinational car manufacturer in Germany, reported in recent media that the company is developing technology for profound learning (DL) and natural languages processing (NLP) to enhance driving experience. "The smart technology of the company enables a unique driving experience by automating responses by measuring the driver's needs and moods," the media reported.

Computer Vision

In the post-covid age, the technology would gain massive momentum. The ability to recognize trends and anticipate outcomes in a vast volume of photographs is a tremendous use in medical practice. In urban areas, machine vision technology is now being used to monitor people through video monitoring, contactless driving, scanning and personnel tracking. Doctors may use machine vision software to detect x-ray images in the healthcare industry. Companies constantly employ automation to develop their workflows. Computer vision would become another invention which would gain tremendous traction from COVID world because of its ability to recognize trends in a large amount of images. The use of technologies for facial recognition will become the standard after the pandemic. In the present state, computer vision technology is heavily used to preserve social isolation and to track individuals who wear masks. To do this the technology has been deployed in urban environments to monitor people through video surveillance, contactless monitoring and monitoring of employee behaviours in organizations. In recent news, a start-up of Chennai-based AI, RayReach Technologies, uses this technology to create intelligent CCTVs for its clients to detect social distance breaches. The knowledge gained in computer vision technologies would also make data scientists more accessible in the post-COVID world where social distance can be the rule. This technology has immense promise in the healthcare field as well and helps doctors to detect abnormalities in chest x-ray images by profound learning. Through leveraging this technology aggressively to develop their workflows, it is important that data scientists master this branch of artificial intelligence in order to support the after-pandemic market.

Geospatial Technology

In the Covid-19 pandemic geospatial technology was proved useful. Companies and policymakers do this to globally map the outbreak of diseases and chart the country's affected regions. With more people working on data-driven decision-making systems, geospatial information is being useful in improved system planning and processing. Geospatial technology has proved useful during the COVID-19 pandemic for businesses and governments around the world, using geographical data to map outbreaks and identify affected areas in the region. Geospatial data also helped to further prepare and process the system, with more staff working on data-driven decision-making processes. The technology will also help industrial and retail sectors recognize the disease's density areas during this lockout. In reality, Transerve Technologies has recently announced that Transerve Online Stack is providing geospatial data for the COVID-19 density zones. In keeping with the market, this technology has allowed SMBs, major dealers and supply chain practitioners to improve and revive their business in the post-COVID environment the company says. And hence businesses are looking to recruit specialists with experience in geospatial data analysis. A geospatial data scientist will need to study comprehensive geospatial data sets, including images from satellite, google maps, population data, social data and topography to help firms make money.

Data Visualisation

The visualisation of data has always been demanding. With analytics being the prime concern for businesses in all sectors, data visualisation would be needed. Powerful storytelling lets corporate executives make the best choices. This also increases the likelihood of being more sustainable in the post-covid world. With data analytics becoming a big concern for businesses across sectors, the need for effective data storage has increased. Such a skill would make a data scientist more useful to market executives as persuasive storytelling would make it easy for customers and leaders to grasp abstract numbers and statistics. Data scientists would quickly provide their audiences with complex business knowledge, which in turn can help them differentiate themselves from other practitioners on the market.

SKILLS REQUIRED FOR DATA SCIENTISTS

This also increases the ability to be more sustainable in the post-COVID world. "We can remember information up to 22 times more accurately when they are part of the narrative than when viewed as separate data points, according to researchers. Any knowledge provided as a tale also allows to improve our interpretation and decrypt trends in complicated data sets". As data storytelling helps business leaders with strong perspectives, it can help business leaders in turn leverage consumer prospects in the field of the post-pandemic. Pavan Kumar Thatha, an emerging technology pioneer at Unisys, said at his interview that without mastering storytelling ability you could not become a computer scientist.

Artificial Intelligence (AI)

With AI penetrating almost every area of human life, companies have become imperative to have faith in these devices and their decisions. Companies currently aim to incorporate AI models that can forecast reliable insight and offer explanations. Data scientists who know very well about explainable AI then become a safer choice for companies. The emphasis for many years has been on the precision and efficiency of AI models, but the recent unwillingness of many businesses to embrace AI has meant transparency in the AI models' forecast. In reality, 82 percent of market leaders decided to be well clarified in order to trust artificial intelligence. In joining the initiative, Microsoft announced in recent reports that it is actively focused on designing resources to create more accountable and fairer AI frameworks. In addition, Pegasystems App Development Company has revealed its solutions to help businesses recognize and remove the secret preconditions of their AI models. According to the company's venturer — As AI falls within almost every aspect of customer commitment, some highly prominent incidents have made companies more aware of the risk of unintentional prejudice and its painful effect on customers as a result, businesses in the post COVID world are trying to recruit experts who can handle their AI systems services.

SKILLS RELATED TO HEALTHCARE DOMAIN

Post-COVID, there will be a massive interest worldwide of healthcare technology and thus there was a huge quest for data analytics experts with experience in the area of healthcare. Data science has proven highly helpful to treating COVID patients by exploiting the data from patients, but these projections may be unreliable and also have a detrimental impact on the production of drugs and medicines without fundamental domain expertise. Healthcare will continue to be a primary concern for states, corporations and people long after the pandemic. As a result, the market for data experts will grow exponentially who can use real-time medical data to produce information and allow doctors to make better decisions. Indeed, in the aftermath of the pandemic epidemic, China's tech giant Baidu launched its Linearfold algorithm to help medical investigators combat the virus. Similarly, several other organizations have since built devices to help physicians tackle this problem. Data scientists with specialized technical expertise and experience in the healthcare field will also be more important for post-COVID enterprises.

CONCLUSION

Data scientists have been interested in solving the current COVID-19 problems. This chapter was written to make a review of the continued work for the broader community accessible easily. We tried to make five broad contributions. We introduced for the first time important applications of data science that can assist with the pandemic. This is by no means a complete list and in the coming months we plan to extend. We then worked on summarizing publicly accessible study datasets. Again this is meant to shorten the time required to uncover the necessary knowledge as a shared resource. After that, we reviewed some of the continuing research in this area. As the chapter is primarily meant for a computer science and engineering public, we have once again analyzed the various types of usable data sets. We then expanded our research and in recent months we have published a bibliometric review with thousands of publications. Finally, we outlined some of the common issues that we encountered in our comprehensive analysis, such as data access and privacy concerns. We note also that many of the systems discussed here are not yet operational. In this light, we plan to update the chapter again and again with new details. In future the workplace of executive development company may be found with some new AI staff. In 2019, it was rose by 18 percent. The study of Paul Petrone (2019) was also proposed that in 2031, 80% of new jobs requires AI-literate employees and businesses would face with the lack of such workers. To hire and attract skilled people with the requisite skills prosper in an AI environment, many organizations recognize that they must develop the talent they will use to retrain and strengthen their current skills in workforce to leverage the ability of AI. This update benefits employees also. In a world where a "lifespan" ability has deteriorated on average from 30 to 5 years. It is a challenging task to staff to keep up to date, appropriate, employable where the job market is changing rapidly.

REFERENCES

Bullock, J., Pham, K. H., Lam, C. S. N., & Luengo-Oroz, M. (2020). *COVID-19 Artificial Intelligence Landscape*. arXiv preprint arXiv:2003.11336.

Dave, J., Dubey, V. N., Doubey, J., & Coppini, D. (2019). The prediction of risk levels of diabetic neuropathy using artificial neural networks based on diabetes subject clinical characteristics. *Diabetic Medicine*, 144–144.

Floto, Gimson, Scholtes, Wood, McKinney, Jarrett, & Lio. (2020). *How artificial intelligence can assist health systems in responding to COVID-19*. Academic Press.

Guru, K. (2019). Application of Data Science and Research Trends in Marketing through Big Data. Think India Journal, 22, 118-125.

Huang, Wang, Li, Ren, Zhao, Hu, Zhang, Fan, Xu, & Gu. (2020). Wuhan 2019 novel coronavirus infected patients, clinical features. *The Lancet, 395*(10223), 497–506.

Khorana. (2018). Artificial TRI evaluation—response. *Lancet Haematology, A*, e391-e392.

Marr. (n.d.). *8 Job Skills to Succeed In A Post-Coronavirus World*. https:// www.forbes. com/sites/bernardmarr/2020/04/17/8-job-skills-to-succeed-in-apost-coronavirus-world/#1459257d2096

Petrone. (n.d.). *The Skills Companies Need Most in 2019 – And How to Learn Them.* LinkedIn.com. https://learning.linkedin.com/blog/ top-skills/the-skills-companies-need-most-in-2019--and-how-to-learn-them

Rick. (2020). *Over 24,000 papers on Coronavirus Research published on 16-March-2020, are now available at one place.* https:/tinyurl.com/MITTECHREV24000papers

Wu, Leung, & Leung. (2020). Potential for domestic and foreign spreading the epidemic of 2019-ncov originating in Wuhan, China: a modelling analysis. The Lancet, 395(10225), 689-697.

Zhu, N., Zhang, D., Wang, W., Li, X., Yang, B., Sing, J., Zhao, X., Huang, B., Shi, W., Lu, R., & ... . (2020). *A novel coronavirus from pneumonia patients in China, 2019. New England Medicine Journal.* doi:10.1056/NEJMoa2001017

Compilation of References

Abd-Alrazaq, A., Alhuwail, D., Househ, M., Hai, M., & Shah, Z. (2020). Top concerns of tweeters during the COVID-19 pandemic: A surveillance study. *Journal of Medical Internet Research*, *22*(4), 1–9. doi:10.2196/19016 PMID:32287039

Afriyie, D. K., Asare, G. A., Amponsah, S. K., & Godman, B. (2020). COVID-19 pandemic in resource-poor countries: Challenges, experiences and opportunities in Ghana. *Journal of Infection in Developing Countries*, *14*(08), 838–843. doi:10.3855/jidc.12909 PMID:32903226

Ahuja, V., & Shakeel, M. (2017). Twitter Presence of Jet Airways-Deriving Customer Insights Using Netnography and Wordclouds. *Procedia Computer Science*, *122*, 17–24. doi:10.1016/j.procs.2017.11.336

Aktay, A. (2020). *Google COVID-19 community mobility reports: Anonymization process description (version 1.0)*. arXiv preprint arXiv:2004.04145.

Al-garadi, M. A., Khan, M. S., Varathan, K. D., Mujtaba, G., & Al-Kabsi, A. M. (2016). Using online social networks to track a pandemic: A systematic review. *Journal of Biomedical Informatics*, *62*, 1–11. doi:10.1016/j.jbi.2016.05.005 PMID:27224846

Alkouz, B., Al Aghbari, Z., & Abawajy, J. H. (2019). Tweetluenza: Predicting flu trends from twitter data. *Big Data Mining and Analytics*, *2*(4), 273–287. doi:10.26599/BDMA.2019.9020012

Allen-Kinross, P. (2020). *When did lockdown begin in the UK? Full Fact*. Retrieved 12 September 2020, from https://fullfact.org/health/coronavirus-lockdown-hancock-claim/

Alqurashi, S., Alhindi, A., & Alanazi, E. (2020). *Large arabic twitter dataset on covid-19*. arXiv preprint arXiv:2004.04315.

Alsafi, Z., Abbas, A. R., Hassan, A., & Ali, M. A. (2020). The coronavirus pandemic: adaptations in medical education. International Journal of Surgery.

Altay, N., & Green, W. G. III. (2006). OR/MS research in disaster operations management. *European Journal of Operational Research*, *175*(1), 475–493. doi:10.1016/j.ejor.2005.05.016

Amatulli, J. (2020). *HuffPost is now a part of Verizon Media*. Retrieved 4 October 2020, from https://www.huffingtonpost.co.uk/entry/grocery-delivery-coronavirus-online_l_5e7be548c5b6cb08a92766f

Compilation of References

Anderson M R. (n.d.). Data is King for Government Crisis Response. *Informatica*.

ANDS. (n.d.). *Geospatial data and metadata*. Retrieved from https://www.ands.org.au/working-with-data/metadata/geospatial-data-and-metadata

Angled, L. (2020). *GitHub Stanford Corenlp*. https://github.com/stanfordnlp/python-stanford-corenlp

Angular Testing. Angular.io. (2020). Retrieved 3 September 2020, from https://angular.io/guide/testing

Antoniou, V., & Potsiou, C. (2020). A Deep Learning Method to Accelerate the Disaster Response Process. *Remote Sensing*, *12*(3), 544. doi:10.3390/rs12030544

Anuta, D., Churchin, J., & Luo, J. (2017). *Election bias: Comparing polls and twitter in the 2016 us election*. ArXiv Preprint ArXiv:1701.06232.

Apolloni, A., Poletto, C., Ramasco, J. J., Jensen, P., & Colizza, V. (2014). Metapopulation epidemic models with heterogeneous mixing and travel behaviour. *Theoretical Biology & Medical Modelling*, *11*(1), 3. doi:10.1186/1742-4682-11-3 PMID:24418011

Arshadi, A. K., Webb, J., Salem, M., Cruz, E., Calad-Thomson, S., Ghadirian, N., ... Yuan, J. S. (2020). Artificial Intelligence for COVID-19 Drug Discovery and Vaccine Development. *Front. Artif. Intell*, *3*, 65. doi:10.3389/frai.2020.00065

Aspinall, E. (2021). *COVID-19 Timeline - British Foreign Policy Group*. Retrieved 4 February 2021, from https://bfpg.co.uk/2020/04/covid-19-timeline/

Attigeri, G. V., Manohara Pai, M. M., Pai, R. M., & Nayak, A. (2016). Stock market prediction: A big data approach. *IEEE Region 10 Annual International Conference, Proceedings/TENCON*. 10.1109/TENCON.2015.7373006

Awais, M., Raza, M., Singh, N., Bashir, K., Manzoor, U., ul Islam, S., & Rodrigues, J. J. (2020). LSTM based Emotion Detection using Physiological Signals: IoT framework for Healthcare and Distance Learning in COVID-19. *IEEE Internet of Things Journal*.

Awais, M., Chiari, L., Ihlen, E. A. F., Helbostad, J. L., & Palmerini, L. (2018). Physical activity classification for elderly people in free-living conditions. *IEEE Journal of Biomedical and Health Informatics*, *23*(1), 197–207. doi:10.1109/JBHI.2018.2820179 PMID:29994291

Awais, M., Palmerini, L., Bourke, A. K., Ihlen, E. A., Helbostad, J. L., & Chiari, L. (2016). Performance evaluation of state of the art systems for physical activity classification of older subjects using inertial sensors in a real life scenario: A benchmark study. *Sensors (Basel)*, *16*(12), 2105. doi:10.339016122105 PMID:27773434

Awais, M., Raza, M., Ali, K., Ali, Z., Irfan, M., Chughtai, O., Khan, I., Kim, S., & Ur Rehman, M. (2019). An Internet of Things based bed-egress alerting paradigm using wearable sensors in elderly care environment. *Sensors (Basel)*, *19*(11), 2498. doi:10.339019112498 PMID:31159252

Aylien Ltd. (2020a). *The News Intelligence Platform - AYLIEN News API.* https://aylien.com/

Aylien Ltd. (2020b). *Using Entity-level Sentiment Analysis to understand News Content - AYLIEN News API.* https://aylien.com/blog/using-entity-level-sentiment-analysis-to-understand-news-content

Ayyachamy, S., Alex, V., Khened, M. & Krishnamurthi, G. (2019). *Medical image retrieval using Resnet-18.* Academic Press.

Azaria, A. E. A. V. T. L. A. (2016). *Medrec: Using blockchain for medical data access and permission management.* IEEE.

Baccianella, S., Esuli, A., & Sebastiani, F. (2010). SENTIWORDNET 3.0: An enhanced lexical resource for sentiment analysis and opinion mining. *Proceedings of the 7th International Conference on Language Resources and Evaluation, LREC 2010*, 2200–2204.

Bag, D. (2016). Business Analytics. In *Business Analytics* (2nd ed.). Routledge. doi:10.4324/9781315464695

Baker, J. E. (1987, July). Reducing bias and inefficiency in the selection algorithm. In *Proceedings of the second international conference on genetic algorithms* (*Vol. 206*, pp. 14-21). Academic Press.

Baker, S. B., Xiang, W., & Atkinson, I. (2017). Internet of things for smart healthcare: Technologies, challenges, and opportunities. *IEEE Access: Practical Innovations, Open Solutions*, *5*, 26521–26544. doi:10.1109/ACCESS.2017.2775180

Bakharia, A. (2019). On the Equivalence of Inductive Content Analysis and Topic Modeling. In Advances in Quantitative Ethnography (pp. 291–298). doi:10.1007/978-3-030-33232-7_25

Banda, J. M., Tekumalla, R., Wang, G., Yu, J., Liu, T., Ding, Y., & Chowell, G. (2020). *A large-scale COVID-19 Twitter chatter dataset for open scientific research—an international collaboration.* ArXiv preprint arXiv:2004.03688.

Bansal, B., & Srivastava, S. (2018). On predicting elections with hybrid topic based sentiment analysis of tweets. *Procedia Computer Science*, *135*, 346–353. doi:10.1016/j.procs.2018.08.183

Bansal, B., & Srivastava, S. (2019). Lexicon-based Twitter sentiment analysis for vote share prediction using emoji and N-gram features. *International Journal of Web Based Communities*, *15*(1), 85–99. doi:10.1504/IJWBC.2019.098693

Barro. (2020). *The Coronavirus and the Great Influenza Pandemic: Lessons from the "Spanish Flu" for the Coronavirus's Potential Effects on Mortality and Economic Activity.* National Bureau of Economic Research Working Paper 2020.

Bastian, M., Heymann, S., & Jacomy, M. (2009). Gephi: An open source software for exploring and manipulating networks. *BT - International AAAI Conference on Weblogs and Social. International AAAI Conference on Weblogs and Social Media*, 361–362.

Batini, Rula, A., Scannapieco, M., & Viscusi, G. (2015, January). From Data Quality to Big Data Quality. *Journal of Database Management, 26*(1), 60–82. doi:10.4018/JDM.2015010103

Belguith, S. (2018). Phoabe: Securely outsourcing multi-authority attribute based encryption with policy hidden for cloud assisted iot. Computer Networks, 133, 141-156.

Benson, T. (2020), *Twitter Bots Are Spreading Massive Amounts of COVID-19 Misinformation.* URL: https://spectrum.ieee.org/tech-talk/telecom/internet/twitter-bots-are-spreading-massive-amounts-of-covid-19-misinformation

Birjali, M., Beni-Hssane, A., & Erritali, M. (2017). Analyzing Social Media through Big Data using InfoSphere BigInsights and Apache Flume. *Procedia Computer Science, 113*, 280–285. doi:10.1016/j.procs.2017.08.299

Blackmore, S., & Blackmore, S. J. (2000). *The meme machine* (Vol. 25). Oxford Paperbacks.

Blei, D. M., Ng, A. Y., & Jordan, M. I. (2003). Latent dirichlet distribution. *Journal of Machine Learning Research, 3*, 993–1022.

Boatwright, A., & Wynne, W. A. (2020), *Record Global GDP Contraction Indicative of COVID-19's Cross-Country Effect.* https://www.dallasfed.org/research/economics/2020/1006

Bodas, M., & Peleg, K. (2020). Self-Isolation Compliance In The COVID-19 Era Influenced By Compensation: Findings from a recent survey in Israel: public attitudes toward the COVID-19 outbreak and self-isolation: a cross sectional study of the adult population of Israel. *Health Affairs, 39*(6), 936–941. doi:10.1377/hlthaff.2020.00382 PMID:32271627

Boersma, F. K., Passenier, D. F., Mollee, J. S., & van der Wal, C. N. (Eds.). (2012). *Proceedings of the 26th European Conference on Modelling and Simulation, ECMS2012.* Koblenz: ECMS.

Boersma, K., & Fonio, C. (2019). *Big data, surveillance and crisis management.* Routledge.

Booker, L. (1987). Improving search in genetic algorithms. *Genetic Algorithms and Simulated Annealing*, 61-73.

Borshchev, A., & Filippov, A. (2004, July). From system dynamics and discrete event to practical agent based modeling: reasons, techniques, tools. In *Proceedings of the 22nd international conference of the system dynamics society (Vol. 22).* Academic Press.

Boulos, K. M. N., Resch, B., & Crowley, D. N. (2011). Crowdsourcing, citizen sensing and sensor web technologies for public and environmental health surveillance and crisis management: Trends, OGC standards and application examples. *International Journal of Health Geographics, 10*(1), 67. doi:10.1186/1476-072X-10-67 PMID:22188675

Brexit: leaked papers predict food shortages and port delays. (2021). *The Guardian.* Retrieved 11 February 2021, from https://www.theguardian.com/politics/2019/aug/18/brexit-leaked-papers-predict-food-shortages-and-port-delays-operation-yellowhammer

Buckee, C. (n.d.). Improving epidemic surveillance and response: big data is dead, long live big data. *The Lancet Open Access*. doi:10.1016/S2589-7500(20)30059-5

Budiharto, W., & Meiliana, M. (2018). Prediction and analysis of Indonesia Presidential election from Twitter using sentiment analysis. *Journal of Big Data*, 5(1), 51. doi:10.118640537-018-0164-1

Bullock, J., Pham, K. H., Lam, C. S. N., & Luengo-Oroz, M. (2020). *COVID-19 Artificial Intelligence Landscape*. arXiv preprint arXiv:2003.11336.

Bullock, J., Luccioni, A., Pham, K. H., Lam, C. S. N., & Luengo-Oroz, M. (2020). Mapping the landscape of artificial intelligence applications against COVID-19. *Journal of Artificial Intelligence Research*, 69, 807–845. doi:10.1613/jair.1.12162

Burnap, P., Gibson, R., Sloan, L., Southern, R., & Williams, M. (2016). 140 characters to victory?: Using Twitter to predict the UK 2015 General Election. *Electoral Studies*, 41, 230–233. Advance online publication. doi:10.1016/j.electstud.2015.11.017

Bursa, M. (2020). Northern taxi drivers hailed as heroes after offering free rides for stranded Manchester Arena terror victims. *Professional Driver Magazine*. Retrieved 5 October 2020, from https://www.prodrivermags.com/news/northern-taxi-drivers-hailed-as-heroes-after-offering-free-rides-for-stranded-manchester-arena-terror-victims/

Cao, Q., Sirivianos, M., Yang, X., & Pregueiro, T. (2012). Aiding the detection of fake accounts in large scale social online services. In *9th {USENIX} Symposium on Networked Systems Design and Implementation ({NSDI} 12)* (pp. 197-210). USENIX.

Carley, K. M., Malik, M., Landwehr, P. M., Pfeffer, J., & Kowalchuck, M. (2016). Crowd sourcing disaster management: The complex nature of Twitter usage in Padang Indonesia. *Safety Science*, 90, 48–61. doi:10.1016/j.ssci.2016.04.002

Car, Z., Baressi Šegota, S., Anđelić, N., Lorencin, I., & Mrzljak, V. (2020). Modeling the spread of COVID-19 infection using a multilayer perceptron. *Computational and Mathematical Methods in Medicine*, 2020, 2020. doi:10.1155/2020/5714714 PMID:32565882

Castro, R., Kuffó, L., & Vaca, C. (2017). Back to #6D: Predicting Venezuelan states political election results through Twitter. *2017 4th International Conference on EDemocracy and EGovernment, ICEDEG 2017*. 10.1109/ICEDEG.2017.7962525

Centers for Disease Control and Prevention (CDC). National Center for Immunization and Respiratory Diseases (NCIRD). (2019a) *Pandemic (H3N2 virus) 1968*. Available: https://www.cdc.gov/flu/pandemic-resources/1968-pandemic.html

Centers for Disease Control and Prevention. National Center for Immunization and Respiratory Diseases (NCIRD). (2019b) *Pandemic (H2N2 virus) 1957-1958*. https://www.cdc.gov/flu/pandemic-resources/1957-1958-pandemic.html

Cerchiello, P., & Giudici, P. (2016). Big data analysis for financial risk management. *Journal of Big Data*, 3(1), 18. doi:10.118640537-016-0053-4

Cha, M., Mislove, A., & Gummadi, K. P. (2009, April). *A measurement-driven analysis of information propagation in the flickr social.* Academic Press.

Chakraborty, G., Pagolu, M., & Garla, S. (2014). *Text mining and analysis: practical methods, examples, and case studies using SAS.* SAS Institute.

Chang, Y.-C., Ku, C.-H., & Chen, C.-H. (2017). Social media analytics: Extracting and visualizing Hilton hotel ratings and reviews from TripAdvisor. *International Journal of Information Management.*

Chan, H. S., Shan, H., Dahoun, T., Vogel, H., & Yuan, S. (2019). Advancing drug discovery via artificial intelligence. *Trends in Pharmacological Sciences, 40*(8), 592–604. doi:10.1016/j.tips.2019.06.004 PMID:31320117

Charalabidis, Y. N., Loukis, E., Androutsopoulou, A., Karkaletsis, V., & Triantafillou, A. (2014). Passive crowdsourcing in government using social media. *Transform. Gov. People Process Policy, 8*, 283–30. doi:10.1108/TG-09-2013-0035

Chase, M. (2007). Multi-authority attribute based encryption. In Theory of cryptography conference. Springer. doi:10.1007/978-3-540-70936-7_28

Chatterjee, S., & Krystyanczuk, M. (2017). *Python Social Media Analytics.* Packt Publishing Ltd.

Chauhan, P., Sharma, N., & Sikka, G. (2020). The emergence of social media data and sentiment analysis in election prediction. *Journal of Ambient Intelligence and Humanized Computing*, 1–27. doi:10.100712652-020-02423-y

Chen, E., Lerman, K., & Ferrara, E. (2020). *Covid-19: The first public coronavirus twitter dataset.* arXiv preprint arXiv:2003.07372.

Chen, D., Liu, Z., Wang, L., Dou, M., Chen, J., & Li, H. (2013). Natural disaster monitoring with wireless sensor networks: A case study of data-intensive applications upon low-cost scalable systems. *Mobile Networks and Applications, 18*(5), 651–663. doi:10.100711036-013-0456-9

Chen, E., Lerman, K., & Ferrara, E. (2020). Tracking social media discourse about the covid-19 pandemic: Development of a public coronavirus twitter data set. *JMIR Public Health and Surveillance, 6*(2), e19273. doi:10.2196/19273 PMID:32427106

Choy, M., Cheong, M. L. F., Ma, N. L., & Koo, P. S. (2012). US Presidential Election 2012 Prediction using Census Corrected Twitter Model. *Research Collection School Of Information Systems*, 1–12. https://arxiv.org/abs/1211.0938

Cinelli, M., Quattrociocchi, W., Galeazzi, A., Valensise, C. M., Brugnoli, E., Schmidt, A. L., . . . Scala, A. (2020). *The covid-19 social media infodemic.* arXiv preprint arXiv:2003.05004.

Cinelli, M., Quattrociocchi, W., Galeazzi, A., Valensise, C. M., Brugnoli, E., Schmidt, A. L., . . . Scala, A. (2020). *The COVID-19 Social Media Infodemic.* https://arxiv.org/abs/2003.05004

Cinelli, M., Quattrociocchi, W., Galeazzi, A., Valensise, C. M., Brugnoli, E., Schmidt, A. L., & Scala, A. (2020). The covid-19 social media infodemic. *Scientific Reports*, *10*(1), 1–10. doi:10.103841598-020-73510-5 PMID:33024152

Ciresan, D., Meier, U., Masci, J., & Schmidhuber, J. (2012). Multi-column deep neural network for traffic sign classification. *Neural Networks*, *32*, 333–338. doi:10.1016/j.neunet.2012.02.023 PMID:22386783

Ciresan, D., Meier, U., & Schmidhuber, J. (2012). Multi-column deep neural networks for image classification. *Proceedings of IEEE Conference on Computer Vision and Pattern Recognition (CVPR)*, 3642–3649. 10.1109/CVPR.2012.6248110

Cliff, A., & Haggett, P. (2005). *Modeling diffusion processes*. Academic Press.

Coronavirus consumer trends poll insights from April 21, 2020. (2020). *Klaviyo*. Retrieved 5 October 2020, from https://www.klaviyo.com/covid-19-daily-ecommerce-insights/marketing-consumer-insights-04212020

Cosgrove, E. (2020). How Emergency Food Providers Are Developing Tech to Help Them Give More. *AgFunderNews*. Retrieved 4 September 2020, from https://agfundernews.com/emergency-food-providers-tech.html

Cui, H., & Kertesz, J. (2021). Attention dynamics on the Chinese social media Sina Weibo during the COVID-19 pandemic. *EPJ Data Science*, *10*(1), 8. doi:10.1140/epjds13688-021-00263-0 PMID:33552838

Culotta, A. (2010). Towards detecting influenza epidemics by analyzing Twitter messages. *SOMA 2010 - Proceedings of the 1st Workshop on Social Media Analytics*, 115–122. 10.1145/1964858.1964874

Culotta, A., & Cutler, J. (2016). Mining Brand Perceptions from Twitter Social Networks. *Marketing Science*, *35*(3), 343–362. doi:10.1287/mksc.2015.0968

Currie, C. S., Fowler, J. W., Kotiadis, K., Monks, T., Onggo, B. S., Robertson, D. A., & Tako, A. A. (2020). How simulation modelling can help reduce the impact of COVID-19. *Journal of Simulation*, *14*(2), 1–15. doi:10.1080/17477778.2020.1751570

Dai, E., Sun, Y., & Wang, S. (2020, May). Ginger cannot cure cancer: Battling fake health news with a comprehensive data repository. In *Proceedings of the International AAAI Conference on Web and Social Media* (Vol. 14, pp. 853-862). AAAI.

Das, T. K., Savachkin, A. A., & Zhu, Y. (2008). A large-scale simulation model of pandemic influenza outbreaks for development of dynamic mitigation strategies. *IIE Transactions*, *40*(9), 893–905. doi:10.1080/07408170802165856

Dave, J., Dubey, V. N., Doubey, J., & Coppini, D. (2019). The prediction of risk levels of diabetic neuropathy using artificial neural networks based on diabetes subject clinical characteristics. *Diabetic Medicine*, 144–144.

Davenport, T., & Kalakota, R. (2019). The potential for artificial intelligence in healthcare. *Future Healthcare Journal*, 6(2), 94–98. doi:10.7861/futurehosp.6-2-94 PMID:31363513

De Santis, E., Martino, A., & Rizzi, A. (2020). An Infoveillance System for Detecting and Tracking Relevant Topics from Italian Tweets during the COVID-19 Event. *IEEE Access: Practical Innovations, Open Solutions*, 8, 132527–132538. doi:10.1109/ACCESS.2020.3010033

Deng, L. (2014). A tutorial survey of architectures, algorithms, and applications for deep learning. *APSIPA Transactions on Signal and Information Processing*, 3, e2. doi:10.1017/atsip.2013.9

Depoux, A., Martin, S., Karafillakis, E., Preet, R., Wilder-Smith, A., & Larson, H. (2020). The pandemic of social media panic travels faster than the COVID-19 outbreak. *Journal of Travel Medicine*, 27(3), 1–2. doi:10.1093/jtm/taaa031 PMID:32125413

Desvars-Larrive, A., Dervic, E., Haug, N., Niederkrotenthaler, T., Chen, J., Di Natale, A., Lasser, J., Gliga, D. S., Roux, A., Sorger, J., Chakraborty, A., Ten, A., Dervic, A., Pacheco, A., Jurczak, A., Cserjan, D., Lederhilger, D., Bulska, D., Berishaj, D., ... Thurner, S. (2020). A structured open dataset of government interventions in response to COVID-19. *Scientific Data*, 7(1), 1–9. doi:10.103841597-020-00609-9 PMID:32855430

Devlin, J. (2020). *GitHub Bert*. https://github.com/google-research/bert

Devlin, J., Chang, M. W., Lee, K., & Toutanova, K. (2019). BERT: Pre-training of deep bidirectional transformers for language understanding. *NAACL HLT 2019 - 2019 Conference of the North American Chapter of the Association for Computational Linguistics: Human Language Technologies - Proceedings of the Conference*, 1(Mlm), 4171–4186.

DeVries, P. M. R., Viégas, F., Wattenberg, M., & Meade, B. J. (2018). Deep learning of aftershock patterns following large earthquakes. *Nature*, 560(7720), 632–634. doi:10.103841586-018-0438-y PMID:30158606

Dewhurst, D. R. (2020). *Divergent modes of online collective attention to the COVID-19 pandemic are associated with future caseload variance*. arXiv preprint arXiv:2004.03516.

Di Maio, P. (2008). *Ontology for ER: An open ontology for open source emergency response system abstract*. Retrieved from http://citeseerx.ist.psu.edu/viewdoc/summary?doi=10.1.1.93.1829

Dodds, P. S. (2020). *Long-term word frequency dynamics derived from Twitter are corrupted: A bespoke approach to detecting and removing pathologies in ensembles of time series*. arXiv preprint arXiv:2008.11305.

Doogan, C., Buntine, W., Linger, H., & Brunt, S. (2020). Public Perceptions and Attitudes Towards COVID-19 Non-Pharmaceutical Interventions Across Six Countries: A Topic Modeling Analysis of Twitter Data (Preprint). *Journal of Medical Internet Research*, 22(9), e21419. Advance online publication. doi:10.2196/21419 PMID:32784190

Doyle, C. (2010). *A literature review on the topic of social media*. Academic Press.

DuCharme, B. (n.d.). What Do RDF and SPARQL bring to Big Data Projects? *Big Data, 1*(1). doi:10.1089/big.2012.0004

Dwork, C. & Roth, A. (2014). The algorithmic foundations of differential privacy. *Foundations and Trends in Theoretical Computer Science, 9*(3-4), 211-407.

Erdelj, M., Natalizio, E., Chowdhury, K. R., & Akyildiz, I. F. (2017). Help from the sky: Leveraging UAVs for disaster management. *IEEE Pervasive Computing, 16*(1), 24–32. doi:10.1109/MPRV.2017.11

Ereth, J. (2017). If Data is the New Oil, Metadata is the New Gold. *Cutting-Edge Analytics.* Retrieved from https://www.eckerson.com/articles/if-data-is-the-new-oil-metadata-is-the-new-gold

Esuli, A. (2019). *GitHub SentiWordNet.* https://github.com/aesuli/SentiWordNet

Evans, J. R. (2017). Business analytics (2nd ed.). Pearson Education Limited.

Evans, J., & Elley, J. (2020). *UK food suppliers battle to fill the empty shelves.* Ft.com. Retrieved 3 September 2020, from https://www.ft.com/content/fe10b7e0-69f8-11ea-800d-da70cff6e4d3

Eysenbach, G. (2002). Infodemiology: The epidemiology of (mis) information. *The American Journal of Medicine, 113*(9), 763–765. doi:10.1016/S0002-9343(02)01473-0 PMID:12517369

Eysenbach, G. (2009). Infodemiology and infoveillance: Framework for an emerging set of public health informatics methods to analyze search, communication and publication behavior on the Internet. *Journal of Medical Internet Research, 11*(1), e11. doi:10.2196/jmir.1157 PMID:19329408

Eysenbach, G. (2020). How to fight an infodemic: The four pillars of infodemic management. *Journal of Medical Internet Research, 22*(6), e21820. doi:10.2196/21820 PMID:32589589

Fang, Y., Nie, Y., & Penny, M. (2020). Transmission dynamics of the COVID-19 outbreak and effectiveness of government interventions: A data-driven analysis. *Journal of Medical Virology, 92*(6), 645–659. doi:10.1002/jmv.25750 PMID:32141624

Farmdrop - Mind-blowing groceries, delivered. (2020). *Farmdrop.* Retrieved 4 August 2020, from https://www.farmdrop.com/shop

Ferrara, E., Varol, O., Davis, C., Menczer, F., & Flammini, A. (2016). The rise of social bots. *Communications of the ACM, 59*(7), 96–104. doi:10.1145/2818717

Fisman, D. N., Hauck, T. S., Tuite, A. R., & Greer, A. L. (2013). An IDEA for short term outbreak projection: Nearcasting using the basic reproduction number. *PLoS One, 8*(12), e83622. doi:10.1371/journal.pone.0083622 PMID:24391797

Floto, Gimson, Scholtes, Wood, McKinney, Jarrett, & Lio. (2020). *How artificial intelligence can assist health systems in responding to COVID-19.* Academic Press.

Fougre, D. (2020). *App Connects People in Need of Food with Nearby Pantries and Soup Kitchens.* Retrieved 11 August 2020, from https://www.ny1.com/nyc/all-boroughs/coronavirus/2020/03/26/app-connects-people-in-need-of-food-with-nearby-pantries-and-soup-kitchens

Funk, S., Salathé, M., & Jansen, V. A. (2010). Modelling the influence of human behaviour on the spread of infectious diseases: A review. *Journal of the Royal Society, Interface*, 7(50), 1247–1256. doi:10.1098/rsif.2010.0142 PMID:20504800

Fusco, A., Dicuonzo, G., Dell'Atti, V., & Tatullo, M. (2020). Blockchain in healthcare: Insights on COVID-19. *International Journal of Environmental Research and Public Health*, 17(19), 7167. doi:10.3390/ijerph17197167 PMID:33007951

Gatherer, D. (2009). The 2009 H1N1 influenza outbreak in its historical context. *Journal of Clinical Virology*, 45(3), 174–178. doi:10.1016/j.jcv.2009.06.004 PMID:19540156

Gencoglu, O., & Gruber, M. (2020). *Causal Modeling of Twitter Activity During COVID-19.* arXiv preprint arXiv:2005.07952.

Gephi. (2020). *Gephi - The Open Graph Viz Platform.* https://gephi.org/

Ghosh, I., & Chakraborty, T (2020). *An integrated deterministic-stochastic approach for forecasting the long-term trajectories of COVID-19.* Academic Press.

Gilbert, C. H. E., & Hutto, E. (2014). Vader: A parsimonious rule-based model for sentiment analysis of social media text. *Eighth International Conference on Weblogs and Social Media (ICWSM-14).* http://comp. social. gatech. edu/papers/icwsm14

Giordano, G., Blanchini, F., Bruno, R., Colaneri, P., Di Filippo, A., Di Matteo, A., & Colaneri, M. (2020). Modelling the COVID-19 epidemic and implementation of population-wide interventions in Italy. *Nature Medicine*, 26(6), 855–860. doi:10.103841591-020-0883-7 PMID:32322102

Glorot, X., Bordes, A., & Bengio, Y. (2011). Domain adaptation for large-scale sentiment classification: A deep learning approach. *Proceedings of the 28th International Conference on Machine Learning (ICML-11)*, 513–520.

Glowacki, E. M., Wilcox, G. B., & Glowacki, J. B. (2020). Identifying #addiction concerns on twitter during the COVID-19 pandemic: A text mining analysis. *Substance Abuse*, 0(0), 1–8. doi:10.1080/08897077.2020.1822489 PMID:32970973

Goel, A., & Mittal, A. (2012). *Stock prediction using twitter sentiment analysis.* Stanford University.

Golberg, D. E. (1989). *Genetic algorithms in search, optimization, and machine learning.* Addion Wesley.

Google. (2020). *Get an API Key | Maps Embed API | Google Developers.* https://developers.google.com/maps/documentation/embed/get-api-key

Gostic, K., & Ana, C. R. (2020). Estimated effectiveness of symptom and risk screening to prevent the spread of COVID-19. *eLife*, 9, e55570. doi:10.7554/eLife.55570 PMID:32091395

GOV.uk. (2020a). *Guidance: The R number and growth rate in the UK.* Online available at: https://www.gov.uk/guidance/the-r-number-in-the-uk

GOV.uk. (2020b). *Guidance New National Restrictions from 5 November.* Online available at: https://www.gov.uk/guidance/new-national-restrictions-from-5-november

Grandjean, M. (2016). A social network analysis of Twitter: Mapping the digital humanities community. *Cogent Arts & Humanities, 3*(1), 1–14. doi:10.1080/23311983.2016.1171458

Green, W. (2001). E-emergency management in the USA: A preliminary survey of the operational state of the art. *International Journal of Emergency Management, 1*(1), 70–81. doi:10.1504/IJEM.2001.000511

Grimaldi, D., Diaz, J., & Arboleda, H. (2020). *Inferring the votes in a new political landscape. The case of the 2019 Spanish Presidential elections.* Research Square; doi:10.21203/rs.3.rs-16463/v1

Grover, P., Kar, A. K., Dwivedi, Y. K., & Janssen, M. (2018). Polarization and acculturation in US Election 2016 outcomes – Can twitter analytics predict changes in voting preferences. *Technological Forecasting and Social Change,* (September), 1–23. doi:10.1016/j.techfore.2018.09.009

Gruhl, D., Guha, R., Liben-Nowell, D., & Tomkins, A. (2004, May). Information diffusion through blogspace. In *Proceedings of the 13th international conference on World Wide Web* (pp. 491-501). 10.1145/988672.988739

Guardian. (2020). *Covid chaos: how the UK handled the coronavirus crisis.* Retrieved 11 February 2021 https://www.theguardian.com/world/ng-interactive/2020/dec/16/covid-chaos-a-timeline-of-the-uks-handling-of-the-coronavirus-crisis

Guidance for food businesses on coronavirus (COVID-19). (2020). Retrieved 1 January 2021, from https://www.gov.uk/government/publications/covid-19-guidance-for-food-businesses/guidance-for-food-businesses-on-coronavirus-covid-19

Guo, H., Meamari, E. & Shen, C.-C. (2019). *Multi-authority attribute-based access control with smart contract.* Academic Press.

Guru, K. (2019). Application of Data Science and Research Trends in Marketing through Big Data. Think India Journal, 22, 118-125.

Haleem, A., Javaid, M., & Khan, I. H. (2020). Internet of things (IoT) applications in orthopaedics. *Journal of Clinical Orthopaedics and Trauma, 11,* S105–S106. doi:10.1016/j.jcot.2019.07.003 PMID:31992928

Haleem, A., Vaishya, R., Javaid, M., & Khan, I. H. (2020). Artificial Intelligence (AI) applications in orthopaedics: An innovative technology to embrace. *Journal of Clinical Orthopaedics and Trauma, 11,* S80–S81. doi:10.1016/j.jcot.2019.06.012 PMID:31992923

Han, X., Wang, J., Zhang, M., & Wang, X. (2020). Using social media to mine and analyze public opinion related to COVID-19 in China. *International Journal of Environmental Research and Public Health, 17*(8), 2788. Advance online publication. doi:10.3390/ijerph17082788 PMID:32316647

Haouari, F., Hasanain, M., Suwaileh, R., & Elsayed, T. (2020). *Arcov-19: The first arabic covid-19 twitter dataset with propagation networks.* ArXiv preprint arXiv:2004.05861.

Health Organisation. (2020). *Modes of transmission of virus causing COVID-19: implications for IPC precaution recommendations.* Retrieved 9 February 2021, from https://www.who.int/news-room/commentaries/detail/modes-of-transmission-of-virus-causing-covid-19-implications-for-ipc-precaution-recommendations

Heaven, W. D. (2020). *Israel is using AI to flag high-risk covid-19 patients.* https://www.technologyreview.com/2020/04/24/1000543/israel-ai-prediction-medical-testing-data-high-risk-covid-19-patients/

Hellewell, J., Abbott, S., Gimma, A., Bosse, N. I., Jarvis, C. I., Russell, T. W., ... Flasche, S. (2020). Feasibility of controlling COVID-19 outbreaks by isolation of cases and contacts. *The Lancet. Global Health, 8*(4), e488–e496. doi:10.1016/S2214-109X(20)30074-7 PMID:32119825

Henriques-Gomes, L. (2020). Bushfires death toll rises to 33 after body found in burnt out house near Moruya. *The Guardian.* Retrieved 5 September 2020, from https://www.theguardian.com/australia-news/2020/jan/24/bushfires-death-toll-rises-to-33-after-body-found-in-burnt-out-house-near-moruya

Hewage, P., Behera, A., & Trovati, M. (2020). Temporal convolutional neural (TCN) network for an effective weather forecasting using time-series data from the local weather station. *Soft Computing, 24,* 16453–16482. doi:10.100700500-020-04954-0

Hiltz, S. R., & Plotnick, L. (2013). *Dealing with information overload when using social media for emergency management: Emerging solutions.* ISCRAM.

Hinton, G. E., Osindero, S., & Teh, Y. W. (2006). A fast learning algorithm for deep belief nets. *Neural Computation, 18*(7), 1527–1554. doi:10.1162/neco.2006.18.7.1527 PMID:16764513

Hinton, G. E., & Salakhutdinov, R. R. (2006). Reducing the dimensionality of data with neural networks. *Science, 313*(5786), 504–507. doi:10.1126cience.1127647 PMID:16873662

Hiscott, J., Alexandridi, M., Muscolini, M., Tassone, E., Palermo, E., Soultsioti, M., & Zevini, A. (2020). The global impact of the coronavirus pandemic. *Cytokine & Growth Factor Reviews, 53,* 1–9. doi:10.1016/j.cytogfr.2020.05.010 PMID:32487439

Hollander, J. E., & Carr, B. G. (2020). Virtually perfect? Telemedicine for COVID-19. *The New England Journal of Medicine, 382*(18), 1679–1681. doi:10.1056/NEJMp2003539 PMID:32160451

Holotescu, C., & Grosseck, G. (2013). An empirical analysis of the educational effects of social media in universities and colleges. *Internet Learning, 2*(1), 5. doi:10.18278/il.2.1.3

Hosie, R. (2020). *This is the most popular takeaway in your UK town or city.* Independent.co.uk. Retrieved 1 August 2020, from https://www.independent.co.uk/life-style/food-and-drink/deliveroo-takeaway-food-most-popular-a7573141.html

Hou, N., Dong, H., Wang, Z., Ren, W., & Alsaadi, F. E. (2016). Non-fragile state estimation for discrete Markovian jumping neural networks. *Neurocomputing, 179,* 238–245. doi:10.1016/j.neucom.2015.11.089

How do SARS and MERS compare with COVID-19? (2021). Medicalnewstoday.com. Retrieved 12 February 2021, from https://www.medicalnewstoday.com/articles/how-do-sars-and-mers-compare-with-covid-19

Huang, Wang, Li, Ren, Zhao, Hu, Zhang, Fan, Xu, & Gu. (2020). Wuhan 2019 novel coronavirus infected patients, clinical features. *The Lancet, 395*(10223), 497–506.

Hu, F., Xia, G. S., Hu, J., & Zhang, L. (2015). Transferring deep convolutional neural networks for the scene classification of high-resolution remote sensing imagery. *Remote Sensing, 7*(11), 14680–14707. doi:10.3390/rs71114680

Huff, A., Beyeler, W., Kelley, N., & McNitt, J. (2015). How resilient is the United States' food system to pandemics? *Journal of Environmental Studies and Sciences, 5*(3), 337–347. doi:10.100713412-015-0275-3 PMID:32226708

Huge fire breaks out at Beirut port, a month after crippling explosion. (2020). Abc.net.au. Retrieved 17 September 2020, from https://www.abc.net.au/news/2020-09-10/lebanon-beirut-port-huge-fire-month-after-explosion/12652664

Hu, M., & Liu, B. (2004). Mining and summarizing customer reviews. *Proceedings of the 2004 ACM SIGKDD International Conference on Knowledge Discovery and Data Mining - KDD '04,* 168. 10.1145/1014052.1014073

Hu, Q., Zhang, R., & Zhou, Y. (2016). Transfer learning for short-term wind speed prediction with deep neural networks. *Renewable Energy, 85,* 83–95. doi:10.1016/j.renene.2015.06.034

Hutto, C. J. (2020). *GitHub Vader Sentiment.* https://github.com/cjhutto/vaderSentiment

Hymas, C. (2020). Only 112 of 50,000 UK applicants for fruit pickers take jobs amid farmers' fears over skills and application. *The Telegraph.* Retrieved 4 August 2020, from https://www.telegraph.co.uk/news/2020/04/27/112-50000-uk-applicants-fruit-pickers-take-jobs-amid-farmers/

IDC. (2011). *Leveraging Metadata Framework Technology to Take Control of the Information Explosion.* IDC Report.

IDC. (n.d.). The Digital Universe in 2020: Big Data, Bigger Digital Shadows, and Biggest Growth in the Far East. In *Big Data Governance and Metadata Management. Big data governance and Metadata management: Standards roadmap.* IEEE. Available from https://standards.ieee.org/industry-connections/BDGMM-index.html

IFAN data since COVID-19 - Independent Food Aid Network UK. Independent Food Aid Network UK. (2020). Retrieved 14 September 2020, from https://www.foodaidnetwork.org.uk/ifan-data-since-covid-19

Independent. (2020). Coronavirus: Timeline of key events since UK was put into lockdown six months ago. *The Independent.*

Inuwa-Dutse, I., & Korkontzelos, I. (2020). *A curated collection of COVID-19 online datasets.* arXiv preprint arXiv:2007.09703.

Inuwa-Dutse, I., Liptrott, M., & Korkontzelos, I. (2018). Detection of spam-posting accounts on Twitter. *Neurocomputing*, *315*, 496–511. doi:10.1016/j.neucom.2018.07.044

Isaak, J. & Hanna, M. J. (2018). User data privacy: Facebook, Cambridge Analytica, and privacy protection. *Computer, 51*(8), 56-59.

ISO/IEC 11179-1:2015 Information technology — Metadata registries (MDR) — Part 1: Framework.

Jahanbin, K., & Rahmanian, V. (2020). Using twitter and web news mining to predict COVID-19 outbreak. *Asian Pacific Journal of Tropical Medicine*, *13*(8), 378–380. doi:10.4103/1995-7645.279651

Jahshan, E. (2020). *UK grocery enjoys biggest sales jump in 26 years - Retail Gazette*. Retrieved 4 February 2021, from https://www.retailgazette.co.uk/blog/2020/05/uk-grocery-enjoys-biggest-sales-jump-in-26-years/

Jalali, M. S., Ashouri, A., Herrera-Restrepo, O., & Zhang, H. (2016). Information diffusion through social networks: The case of an online petition. *Expert Systems with Applications*, *44*, 187–197. doi:10.1016/j.eswa.2015.09.014

Jit, M. (2020). *100,000 infections every day – why the UK lockdown came just in time | LSHTM*. Retrieved 7 February 2021, from https://www.lshtm.ac.uk/newsevents/expert-opinion/100000-infections-every-day-why-uk-lockdown-came-just-time

Jockers, M. (2017a). *Introduction to the Syuzhet Package*. https://cran.r-project.org/web/packages/syuzhet/vignettes/syuzhet-vignette.html

JockersM. (2017b). *Package 'syuzhet'*. https://github.com/mjockers/syuzhet

John, M. L. (2001). *A dictionary of epidemiology*. Oxford university press.

Jones, K. H., Daniels, H., Heys, S., & Ford, D. V. (2018, July). Challenges and Potential Opportunities of Mobile Phone Call Detail Records in Health Research [Review]. *JMIR mHealth and uHealth*, *6*(7), e161. doi:10.2196/mhealth.9974 PMID:30026176

Kale, G. Ö. (2016). Marka İletişiminde Instagram Kullanımı. *The Turkish Online Journal of Design. Art and Communication*, *6*(2), 119–127. doi:10.7456/10602100/006

Karalis, T., (2020). Planning and evaluation during educational disruption: Lessons learned from COVID-19 pandemic for treatment of emergencies in education. *European Journal of Education Studies*.

Kaur, H., Garg, S., Joshi, H., Ayaz, S., Sharma, S., & Bhandari, M. (2020). A Review: Epidemics and Pandemics in Human History. *Int J Pharma Res Health Sci*, *8*(2), 3139–3142. doi:10.21276/ijprhs.2020.02.01

Keane, M. & Neal, T. (2021). Consumer panic in the COVID-19 pandemic. *Journal of Econometrics, 220*(1), 86-105.

Kermack, W. O., & McKendrick, A. G. (1927). A contribution to the mathematical theory of epidemics. *Proceedings of the Royal Society of London. Series A, Containing Papers of a Mathematical and Physical Character, 115*(772), 700–721. doi:10.1098/rspa.1927.0118

Ketter, E. (2016). Destination image restoration on facebook: The case study of Nepal's Gurkha Earthquake. *Journal of Hospitality and Tourism Management, 28*, 66–72. doi:10.1016/j.jhtm.2016.02.003

Khalid, M., Awais, M., Singh, N., Khan, S., Raza, M., Malik, Q. B., & Imran, M. (2021). *Autonomous Transportation in Emergency Healthcare Services: Framework, Challenges and Future Work. IEEE Internet of Things Magazine.*

Khorana. (2018). Artificial TRI evaluation—response. *Lancet Haematology, A*, e391-e392.

Kim, E., Sung, Y., & Kang, H. (2014). Brand followers' retweeting behavior on Twitter: How brand relationships influence brand electronic word-of-mouth. *Computers in Human Behavior, 37*, 18–25. doi:10.1016/j.chb.2014.04.020

Kim, J., Calhoun, V. D., Shim, E., & Lee, J. H. (2016). Deep neural network with weight sparsity control and pre-training extracts hierarchical features and enhances classification performance: Evidence from whole-brain resting-state functional connectivity patterns of schizophrenia. *NeuroImage, 124*, 127–146. doi:10.1016/j.neuroimage.2015.05.018 PMID:25987366

Kirsal, Y., Ever, Y. K., Mapp, G. E., & Raza, M. (2021). *3D Analytical Modelling and Iterative Solution for High Performance Computing Clusters. IEEE Transactions on Cloud Computing.*

Kogan, N. E. (2020). *An early warning approach to monitor COVID-19 activity with multiple digital traces in near real-time.* arXiv preprint arXiv:2007.00756.

Kozinets, R. V. (2007). Netnography. The Blackwell Encyclopedia of Sociology, 1-2.

Kubo, M., Naruse, K., Sato, H., & Matubara, T. (2007, December). The possibility of an epidemic meme analogy for web community population analysis. In *International Conference on Intelligent Data Engineering and Automated Learning* (pp. 1073-1080). Springer. 10.1007/978-3-540-77226-2_107

Kumar & Singh. (2019). Location reference identification from tweets during emergencies: A deep learning approach. *International Journal of Disaster Risk Reduction, 33*, 365–375.

Kumar, R. (2020). *Blockchain-federated-learning and deep learning models for covid-19 detection using ct imaging.* arXiv preprint arXiv:2007.06537.

Kumar, S., & Chandra, C. (2010). Supply Chain Disruption by Avian flu Pandemic for U.S. Companies: A Case Study. *Transportation Journal, 49*(4), 61-73. Retrieved February 11, 2021, from http://www.jstor.org/stable/40904915

Lachlan, Spence, & Lin. (2014). Expressions of risk awareness and concern through Twitter: On the utility of using the medium as an indication of audience needs. *Computers in Human Behavior, 35*, 554–559.

Lamb, C. (2020). *Plentiful is a Free, SMS-Based Reservation System for Food Pantry Visitors.* Retrieved 4 September 2020, from https://thespoon.tech/plentiful-is-a-free-sms-based-reservation-system-for-food-pantry-visitors/

Lampos, V. (2020). *Tracking COVID-19 using online search.* arXiv preprint arXiv:2003.08086.

Lanfranchi, V. (2017). Machine learning and social media in crisis management: agility vs ethics WiPe/CoRe Paper – T4 – Ethics Legal and Social Issues. *Proceedings of the 14th ISCRAM Conference.*

Latif, S., Usman, M., Manzoor, S., Iqbal, W., Qadir, J., Tyson, G., ... Crowcroft, J. (2020). *Leveraging Data Science To Combat COVID-19: A Comprehensive Review.* Academic Press.

Lda Project. (2020). *GitHub LDA.* https://github.com/lda-project/lda

Lepan, N. (2020). *Visualizing the History of Pandemics.* URL: https://www.visualcapitalist.com/history-of-pandemics-deadliest/

Lerouge, J., Herault, R., Chatelain, C., Jardin, F., & Modzelewski, R. (2015). IODA: An input/output deep architecture for image labeling. *Pattern Recognition, 48*(9), 2847–2858. doi:10.1016/j.patcog.2015.03.017

Leskovec, J., Adamic, L. A., & Huberman, B. A. (2007). The dynamics of viral marketing. *ACM Transactions on the Web, 1*(1), 5. doi:10.1145/1232722.1232727

Li, J., & Guo, X. (2020). *Covid-19 contact-tracing apps: A survey on the global deployment and challenges.* arXiv preprint arXiv:2005.03599.

Li, C., Chen, L. J., Chen, X., Zhang, M., Pang, C. P., & Chen, H. (2020). Retrospective analysis of the possibility of predicting the COVID-19 outbreak from Internet searches and social media data, China, 2020. *Eurosurveillance, 25*(10), 1–5. doi:10.2807/1560-7917.ES.2020.25.10.2000199 PMID:32183935

Li, L., Zhang, Q., Wang, X., Zhang, J., Wang, T., Gao, T. L., Duan, W., Tsoi, K. K. F., & Wang, F. Y. (2020). Characterizing the Propagation of Situational Information in Social Media during COVID-19 Epidemic: A Case Study on Weibo. *IEEE Transactions on Computational Social Systems, 7*(2), 556–562. doi:10.1109/TCSS.2020.2980007

Li, M. Y., Smith, H. L., & Wang, L. (2001). Global dynamics of an SEIR epidemic model with vertical transmission. *SIAM Journal on Applied Mathematics, 62*(1), 58–69. doi:10.1137/S0036139999359860

Lin, Q., Zhao, S., Gao, D., Lou, Y., Yang, S., Musa, S. S. & He, D. (2020). A conceptual model for the outbreak of Coronavirus disease 2019 (COVID-19) in Wuhan, China with individual reaction and governmental action. *International Journal of Infectious Diseases.*

Liou, Y. A., Kar, S. K., & Chang, L. (2010). Use of high-resolution FORMOSAT-2 satellite images for post-earthquake disaster assessment: A study following the 12 May 2008 Wenchuan Earthquake. *International Journal of Remote Sensing, 31*(13), 3355–3368. doi:10.1080/01431161003727655

Li, R., Wang, W., & Di, Z. (2017). Effects of human dynamics on epidemic spreading in Côte d'Ivoire. *Physica A, 467*, 30–40. doi:10.1016/j.physa.2016.09.059

Liu, B. (2020). *Experiments of federated learning for covid-19 chest x-ray images.* arXiv preprint arXiv:2007.05592.

Liu, C., & Zhang, Z. K. (2014). Information spreading on dynamic social networks. *Communications in Nonlinear Science and Numerical Simulation, 19*(4), 896–904. doi:10.1016/j.cnsns.2013.08.028

Local restrictions: areas with an outbreak of coronavirus (COVID-19). GOV.UK. (2020). Retrieved 4 October 2020, from https://www.gov.uk/government/collections/local-restrictions-areas-with-an-outbreak-of-coronavirus-covid-19

Luna, S., & Pennock, M. J. (2018). Social media applications and emergency management: A literature review and research agenda. *International Journal of Disaster Risk Reduction, 28*, 565–577. doi:10.1016/j.ijdrr.2018.01.006

Luus, F., Salmon, B., Van Den Bergh, F., & Maharaj, B. (2015). Multiview deep learning for land-use classification. *IEEE Geoscience and Remote Sensing Letters, 12*(12), 2448–2452. doi:10.1109/LGRS.2015.2483680

Mahrouf, M., Lotfi, E. M., Maziane, M., Hattaf, K., & Yousfi, N. (2017). Stability Analysis for Stochastic Differential Equations in Virology. *Journal of Advances in Mathematics and Computer Science*, 1-12.

Makazhanov, A., Rafiei, D., & Waqar, M. (2014). Predicting political preference of Twitter users. *Social Network Analysis and Mining, 4*(1), 193. Advance online publication. doi:10.100713278-014-0193-5

Maliszewska, M., Mattoo, A., & Van Der Mensbrugghe, D. (2020). *The potential impact of COVID-19 on GDP and trade: A preliminary assessment.* Academic Press.

Mangoni, L., & Pistilli, M. (2020). *Epidemic analysis of Covid-19 in Italy by dynamical modelling.* Academic Press.

Manning, C. D., Bauer, J., Finkel, J. R., Bethard, S. J., Surdeanu, M., Bauer, J., Finkel, J. R., Bethard, S. J., & McClosky, D. (2014). The Stanford CoreNLP natural language processing toolkit. *Proceedings of 52nd Annual Meeting of the Association for Computational Linguistics: System Demonstrations*, 55–60. http://macopolo.cn/mkpl/products.asp

Marbouh, D., Abbasi, T., Maasmi, F., Omar, I. A., Debe, M. S., Salah, K., Jayaraman, R., & Ellahham, S. (2020). Blockchain for COVID-19: Review, Opportunities, and a Trusted Tracking System. *Arabian Journal for Science and Engineering, 45*(12), 1–17. doi:10.100713369-020-04950-4 PMID:33072472

Marinova, P. (2020). Here's What Uber Is Doing to Raise Money for Manchester Bombing Victims. *Fortune.* Retrieved 5 May 2020, from https://fortune.com/2017/06/01/uber-ariana-grande-concert-manchester-bombing/

Marr. (n.d.). *8 Job Skills to Succeed In A Post-Coronavirus World*. https:// www.forbes.com/sites/ bernardmarr/2020/04/17/8-job-skills-to-succeed-in-apost-coronavirus-world/#1459257d2096

Mata, A. (2021). An overview of epidemic models with phase transitions to absorbing states running on top of complex networks. *Chaos (Woodbury, N.Y.), 31*(1), 1. doi:10.1063/5.0033130

Mathers, M. (2020). *Explained: Why it's so hard to find flour in the shops right now*. Independent. co.uk. Retrieved 7 September 2020, from https://www.independent.co.uk/life-style/coronavirus-lockdown-flour-shops-shortages-explained-a9457351.html

McAfee, A., Brynjolfsson, E., Davenport, T., Patil, D. J., & Barton, D. (2012). Big data: The management revolution. *Harvard Business Review, 90*, 61–67. PMID:23074865

McCallum, A. K. (2002). *Mallet: A machine learning for language toolkit*. http://mallet. cs. umass. edu

McCallum, I., Liu, W., See, L., Mechler, R., Keating, A., Hochrainer-Stigler, S., Mochizuki, J., Fritz, S., Dugar, S., Arestegui, M., Szoenyi, M., Bayas, J.-C. L., Burek, P., French, A., & Moorthy, I. (2016). Technologies to support community flood disaster risk reduction. *Int. J. Disaster Risk Sci., 7*(2), 198–204. doi:10.100713753-016-0086-5

McNeill, W. H., & McNeill, W. (1998). *Plagues and peoples*. Anchor.

Meamari, E., Guo, H., Shen, C.-C., & Hur, J. (2020). *Collusion Attacks on Decentralized Attributed-Based Encryption: Analyses and a Solution*. arXiv preprint arXiv:2002.07811.

MeaningCloud LLC. (2020). *Sentiment Analysis API | MeaningCloud*. https://www.meaningcloud. com/developer/sentiment-analysis

Medford, R. J., Saleh, S. N., Sumarsono, A., Perl, T. M., & Lehmann, C. U. (2020). An "Infodemic": Leveraging High-Volume Twitter Data to Understand Early Public Sentiment for the Coronavirus Disease 2019 Outbreak. *Open Forum Infectious Diseases, 7*(7), ofaa258. Advance online publication. doi:10.1093/ofid/ofaa258 PMID:33117854

Meloni, S., Perra, N., Arenas, A., Gómez, S., Moreno, Y., & Vespignani, A. (2011). Modeling human mobility responses to the large-scale spreading of infectious diseases. *Scientific Reports, 1*(1), 62. doi:10.1038rep00062 PMID:22355581

Memon, S. A., & Carley, K. M. (2020). *Characterizing covid-19 misinformation communities using a novel twitter dataset*. ArXiv preprint arXiv:2008.00791.

Mettler, M. (2016, September). Blockchain technology in healthcare: The revolution starts here. In *2016 IEEE 18th international conference on e-health networking, applications, and services (Healthcom)* (pp. 1-3). IEEE.

Microsoft. (2012). *Differential Privacy for Everyone*. Available at: http://download.microsoft. com/download/D/1/F/D1F0DFF5-8BA9-4BDF-8924-7816932F6825/Differential_Privacy_for_Everyone.pdf

Misirlis, N., & Vlachopoulou, M. (2018). Social media metrics and analytics in marketing – S3M: A mapping literature review. *International Journal of Information Management*, *38*(1), 270–276. doi:10.1016/j.ijinfomgt.2017.10.005

Mohammad, S. M. (2020). *NRC Emotion Lexicon*. http://saifmohammad.com/WebPages/NRC-Emotion-Lexicon.htm

Mohammad, S. M., & Turney, P. D. (2013). Crowdsourcing a word-emotion association lexicon. *Computational Intelligence*, *29*(3), 436–465. doi:10.1111/j.1467-8640.2012.00460.x

Mooney, S. J., Westreich, D. J., & El-Sayed, A. M. (2015, May). Commentary. *Epidemiology in the Era of Big Data Epidemiology.*, *26*(3), 390–394. doi:10.1097/EDE.0000000000000274 PMID:25756221

Morris, S. (2020). Quarantine measures may lead to shortage of fruit pickers in Britain. *The Guardian.* Retrieved 4 October 2020, from https://www.theguardian.com/business/2020/may/19/quarantine-shortage-fruit-pickers-immigration-bill-coronavirus-britain

Moschou, K., Theodouli, A., Terzi, S., Votis, K., Tzovaras, D., Karamitros, D., & Diamantopoulos, S. (2020). Performance Evaluation of different Hyperledger Sawtooth transaction processors for Blockchain log storage with varying workloads. In *2020 IEEE International Conference on Blockchain (Blockchain)* (pp. 476-481). 10.1109/Blockchain50366.2020.00069

MPs on the Environment, Food and Rural Affairs Select Committee. (2020). *What effect did the coronavirus pandemic have on our food supply?* London: House of Commons.

Mühlenbein, H., & Schlierkamp-Voosen, D. (1993). Predictive models for the breeder genetic algorithm i. continuous parameter optimization. *Evolutionary Computation*, *1*(1), 25–49. doi:10.1162/evco.1993.1.1.25

Najafabadi, M. M., Villanustre, F., Khoshgoftaar, T. M., Seliya, N., Wald, R., & Muharemagic, E. (2015). Deep learning applications and challenges in big data analytics. *Journal of Big Data*, *2*(1), 1–21. doi:10.118640537-014-0007-7

New report reveals how coronavirus has affected food bank use - The Trussell Trust. The Trussell Trust. (2020). Retrieved 4 October 2020, from https://www.trusselltrust.org/2020/09/14/new-report-reveals-how-coronavirus-has-affected-food-bank-use/

Ngai, E. W., Tao, S. S., & Moon, K. K. (2015). Social media research: Theories, constructs, and conceptual frameworks. *International Journal of Information Management*, *35*(1), 33–44. doi:10.1016/j.ijinfomgt.2014.09.004

Nielsen, F. Å. (2011). *AFINN sentiment analysis in Python: Wordlist-based approach for sentiment analysis*. Technical University of Denmark. https://github.com/fnielsen/afinn

Nielsen, F. Å. (2019). *GitHub Afinn*. https://github.com/fnielsen/afinn

Norman, C. D., & Skinner, H. A. (2006). eHEALS: The eHealth literacy scale. *Journal of Medical Internet Research*, *8*(4), e27. doi:10.2196/jmir.8.4.e27 PMID:17213046

North, M. (2012). *Data mining for the masses* (Vol. 615684378). Global Text Project Athens.

Nothing Left in the Cupboards. Human Rights Watch. (2020). Retrieved 2 March 2020, from https://www.hrw.org/report/2019/05/20/nothing-left-cupboards/austerity-welfare-cuts-and-right-food-uk

O'Brien, G., O'Keefe, P., Gadema-Cooke, Z., & Swords, J. (2010). Approaching disaster management through social learning. *Disaster Prevention and Management*, *19*, 498–508. doi:10.1108/09653561011070402

O'Neill, P. D. (2002). A tutorial introduction to Bayesian inference for stochastic epidemic models using Markov chain Monte Carlo methods. *Mathematical Biosciences*, *180*(1-2), 103–114. doi:10.1016/S0025-5564(02)00109-8 PMID:12387918

Odlum, M., Cho, H., Broadwell, P., Davis, N., Patrao, M., Schauer, D., Bales, M. E., Alcantara, C., & Yoon, S. (2020). Application of topic modeling to tweets as the foundation for health disparity research for COVID-19. In Studies in Health Technology and Informatics (Vol. 272). doi:10.3233/SHTI200484

Ofli, F., Meier, P., Imran, M., Castillo, C., Tuia, D., Rey, N., Briant, J., Millet, P., Reinhard, F., Parkan, M., & Joost, S. (2016). Combining human computing and machine learning to make sense of big (aerial) data for disaster response. *Big Data*, *4*(1), 47–59. doi:10.1089/big.2014.0064 PMID:27441584

Omitola, T., & Wills, G. (2019). Emergency Response Ontology Informatics: Using Ontologies to Improve Emergency and Hazard Management. *International Journal of Intelligent Computing Research*, *10*(3).

Online Marketplace | Feeding America. Feedingamerica.org. (2020). Retrieved 4 June 2020, from https://www.feedingamerica.org/about-us/partners/become-a-product-partner/online-marketplace

Open, A. I. (2019). *Better Language Models and Their Implications*. https://openai.com/blog/better-language-models/

Ordun, C., Purushotham, S., & Raff, E. (2020). *Exploratory analysis of covid-19 tweets using topic modeling, umap, and digraphs*. https://arxiv.org/abs/2005.03082

Otte, E., & Rousseau, R. (2002). Social network analysis: A powerful strategy, also for the information sciences. *Journal of Information Science*, *28*(6), 441–453. doi:10.1177/016555150202800601

Öztürk, N., & Ayvaz, S. (2018). Sentiment analysis on Twitter: A text mining approach to the Syrian refugee crisis. *Telematics and Informatics*, *35*(1), 136–147. doi:10.1016/j.tele.2017.10.006

Palen, L., Vieweg, S., Sutton, J., Liu, S. B., & Hughes, A. (2007). *Crisis Informatics: Studying Crisis in a Networked World*. In Third International Conference on e-Social Science, Ann Arbor, MI.

Park, H. W., Park, S., & Chong, M. (2020). Conversations and Medical News Frames on Twitter: Infodemiological Study on COVID-19 in South Korea. *Journal of Medical Internet Research*, *22*(5), e18897. doi:10.2196/18897 PMID:32325426

Peng, L., Yang, W., Zhang, D., Zhuge, C., & Hong, L. (2020). *Epidemic analysis of COVID-19 in China by dynamical modeling.* arXiv preprint arXiv:2002.06563. doi:10.1101/2020.02.16.20023465

Pennycook, G., McPhetres, J., Zhang, Y., Lu, J. G., & Rand, D. G. (2020). Fighting COVID-19 misinformation on social media: Experimental evidence for a scalable accuracy-nudge intervention. *Psychological Science, 31*(7), 770–780. doi:10.1177/0956797620939054 PMID:32603243

Pesaresi, M., Ehrlich, D., Ferri, S., Florczyk, A., Freire, S., Haag, F., Halkia, M., Julea, A. M., Kemper, T., & Soille, P. (2015). Global human settlement analysis for disaster risk reduction. *The International Archives of the Photogrammetry, Remote Sensing and Spatial Information Sciences, 40*(W3), 837–843. doi:10.5194/isprsarchives-XL-7-W3-837-2015

Petrone. (n.d.). *The Skills Companies Need Most in 2019 – And How to Learn Them.* LinkedIn. com. https://learning.linkedin.com/blog/ top-skills/the-skills-companies-need-most-in-2019--and-how-to-learn-them

Phillips-Wren, G., & Ichalkaranje, N. (Eds.). (2008). *Intelligent decision making: An AI-based approach* (Vol. 97). Springer Science & Business Media. doi:10.1007/978-3-540-76829-6

Phneah, E. (2020). *China telcos, Internet firms restore services after Sichuan quake | ZDNet.* ZDNet. Retrieved 1 October 2020, from https://www.zdnet.com/article/china-telcos-internet-firms-restore-services-after-sichuan-quake/

Pinghui, Z. (2020). Sichuan quake: Food supplies finally arrived, but still it wasn't enough. *South China Morning Post.* Retrieved 1 October 2020, from https://www.scmp.com/comment/blogs/article/1222212/sichuan-quake-food-supplies-finally-arrived-still-it-wasnt-enough

Pink, S. (2016). *Digital ethnography. Innovative methods in media and communication research.* Academic Press.

Potash, S. (2017). *Focus: Big data for infectious disease surveillance, modelling.* NIH Fogarty International Center. Available from https://www.fic.nih.gov/News/GlobalHealthMatters/january-february-2017/Pages/big-data-infectious-disease-surveillance-modeling.aspx

Pournarakis, D. E., Sotiropoulos, D. N., & Giaglis, G. M. (2017). A computational model for mining consumer perceptions in social media. *Decision Support Systems, 93*(2016), 98–110. doi:10.1016/j.dss.2016.09.018

Pradhan, B., Tehrany, M. S., & Jebur, M. N. (2016). A new semiautomated detection mapping of flood extent from TerraSAR-X satellite image using rule-based classification and taguchi optimization techniques. *IEEE Transactions on Geoscience and Remote Sensing, 54*(7), 4331–4342. doi:10.1109/TGRS.2016.2539957

Projects – Google Open Source. Angular. (2020). Retrieved 13 September 2020, from https://opensource.google/projects/angular

Puente, L. (2016). *Mapping Twitter Followers in R | Lucas Puente.* http://lucaspuente.github.io/notes/2016/04/05/Mapping-Twitter-Followers

Qadir, J., & Anwaar, A. (2016). Crisis analytics: Big data-driven crisis response. *Journal of International Humanitarian Action*, *1*(1), 12. doi:10.118641018-016-0013-9

Qazi, U., Imran, M., & Ofli, F. (2020). Geocov19: A dataset of hundreds of millions of multilingual covid-19 tweets with location information. *SIGSPATIAL Special*, *12*(1), 6–15. doi:10.1145/3404820.3404823

Qian, H., Li, J., Zhang, Y., & Han, J. (2015). Privacy-preserving personal health record using multi-authority attribute-based encryption with revocation. *International Journal of Information Security*, 487–497.

Qin, L., Sun, Q., Wang, Y., Wu, K.-F., Chen, M., Shia, B.-C., & Wu, S.-Y. (2020). Prediction of Number of Cases of 2019 Novel Coronavirus (COVID-19) Using Social Media Search Index. *International Journal of Environmental Research and Public Health*, *17*(7), 2365. doi:10.3390/ijerph17072365 PMID:32244425

Qiu, W., Rutherford, S., Mao, A., & Chu, C. (2017). The pandemic and its impacts. *Health, Culture and Society (Pittsburgh, Pa.)*, *9*, 1–11. doi:10.5195/HCS.2017.221

Radford, A., Wu, J., Child, R., Luan, D., Amodei, D., & Sutskever, I. (2019). Language models are unsupervised multitask learners. *OpenAI Blog*, *1*(8), 9.

Ragini, J. R., Anand, P. M. R., & Bhaskar, V. (2018). Big data analytics for disaster response and recovery through sentiment analysis. *International Journal of Information Management*, *42*, 13–24. doi:10.1016/j.ijinfomgt.2018.05.004

Ramteke, J., Shah, S., Godhia, D., & Shaikh, A. (2016). Election result prediction using Twitter sentiment analysis. *2016 International Conference on Inventive Computation Technologies (ICICT)*, *1*, 1–5. 10.1109/INVENTIVE.2016.7823280

Ranjan, J. (2009). Data mining in pharma sector: Benefits. *International Journal of Health Care Quality Assurance*, *22*(1), 82–92. doi:10.1108/09526860910927970 PMID:19284173

RapidMiner Inc. (2019). *Sentiment Analysis using the new Extract Sentiment operator — RapidMiner Community*. https://community.rapidminer.com/discussion/55251/sentiment-analysis-using-the-new-extract-sentiment-operator

RapidMiner Inc. (2020a). *Introducing RapidMiner Auto Model | RapidMiner*. https://rapidminer.com/resource/automated-machine-learning/

RapidMiner Inc. (2020b). *RapidMiner | Best Data Science & Machine Learning Platform*. https://rapidminer.com/

RapidMiner Inc. (2020c). *Rapidminer Educational License | RapidMiner*. https://rapidminer.com/get-started-educational/

RapidMiner Inc. (2020d). *Text and Web Mining with RapidMiner*. https://academy.rapidminer.com/courses/text-and-web-mining-with-rapidminer

Raspini, F., Bardi, F., Bianchini, S., Ciampalini, A., Del Ventisette, C., Farina, P., Ferrigno, F., Solari, L., & Casagli, N. (2017). The contribution of satellite SAR-derived displacement measurements in landslide risk management practices. *Natural Hazards*, *86*(1), 327–351. doi:10.100711069-016-2691-4

Ravi, K., & Ravi, V. (2015). A survey on opinion mining and sentiment analysis: Tasks, approaches and applications. *Knowledge-Based Systems*, *89*, 14–46. doi:10.1016/j.knosys.2015.06.015

Ray, P.P., Mukherjee, M., & Shu, L. (n.d.). Internet of things for disaster management: State-of-the-art and prospects. *IEEE Access, 5*, 18818–18835.

Raza, M., Singh, N., Khalid, M., Khan, S., Awais, M., Hadi, M.U., Imran, M., Islam, S., & Rodrigues, J.J.P.C. (2021). Challenges and limitations of Internet of Things enabled Healthcare in COVID-19. *IEEE Internet of Things Magazine*.

Raza, M., Aslam, N., Le-Minh, H., Hussain, S., Cao, Y., & Khan, N. M. (2017a). A critical analysis of research potential, challenges, and future directives in industrial wireless sensor networks. *IEEE Communications Surveys and Tutorials*, *20*(1), 39–95. doi:10.1109/COMST.2017.2759725

Raza, M., Awais, M., Ellahi, W., Aslam, N., Nguyen, H. X., & Le-Minh, H. (2019). Diagnosis and monitoring of Alzheimer's patients using classical and deep learning techniques. *Expert Systems with Applications*, *136*, 353–364. doi:10.1016/j.eswa.2019.06.038

Raza, M., Awais, M., Singh, N., Imran, M., & Hussain, S. (2020). Intelligent IoT framework for indoor healthcare monitoring of Parkinson's disease patient. *IEEE Journal on Selected Areas in Communications*.

Raza, M., Le, M. H., Aslam, N., Le, C. H., Le, N. T., & Le, T. L. (2017b). Telehealth technology: Potentials, challenges and research directions for developing countries. In *International Conference on the Development of Biomedical Engineering in Vietnam* (pp. 523-528). Springer.

Revoredo-Giha, C., & Costa-Front, M. (2020). The UK's fresh produce supply under COVID-19 and a no-deal Brexit. *LSE Business Review*. Retrieved 4 July 2020, from https://blogs.lse.ac.uk/businessreview/2020/06/22/the-uks-fresh-produce-supply-under-covid-19-and-a-no-deal-brexit/

Rexiline Ragini, J., Rubesh Anand, P. M., & Bhaskar, V. (2018). Mining crisis information: A strategic approach for detection of people at risk through social media analysis. *International Journal of Disaster Risk Reduction*, *27*, 556–566. doi:10.1016/j.ijdrr.2017.12.002

Riche, N. H., Hurter, C., Diakopoulos, N., & Carpendale, S. (Eds.). (2018). *Data-driven storytelling*. CRC Press. doi:10.1201/9781315281575

Rick. (2020). *Over 24,000 papers on Coronavirus Research published on 16-March-2020, are now available at one place.* https:/tinyurl.com/MITTECHREV24000papers

Robertson, Johnson, Murthy, Smith, & Stephens. (2019). Using a combination of human insights and 'deep learning' for real-time disaster communication. *Progress in Disaster Science, 2*.

Roche, S., Propeck-Zimmermann, E., & Mericskay, B. (2013). GeoWeb and crisis management: Issues and perspectives of volunteered geographic information. *GeoJournal*, *78*(1), 21–40. doi:10.100710708-011-9423-9 PMID:32214617

Rosenberg. (1992). *Charles E Rosenberg Explaining Epidemics and other studies in the history of medicine.* Cambridge University Press.

RStudio PBC. (2020a). *R Packages - RStudio.* https://rstudio.com/products/rpackages/

RStudio PBC. (2020b). *RStudio - RStudio.* https://rstudio.com/products/rstudio/

Russell, S. J., & Norvig, P. (2016). *Learning from examples. Artificial intelligence: a modern approach* (3rd ed.). Pearson.

Sabuncu, İ., & Atmis, M. (2020). Social Media Analytics for Brand Image Tracking: A Case Study Application for Turkish Airlines. *Yönetim Bilişim Sistemleri Dergisi*, *6*(1), 26–41. https://dergipark.org.tr/tr/download/article-file/1104512

Saeed, N., Bader, A., Al-Naffouri, T. Y., & Alouini, M. S. (2020). When Wireless Communication Responds to COVID-19: Combating the Pandemic and Saving the Economy. *Frontiers in Communications and Networks*, *1*, 3. doi:10.3389/frcmn.2020.566853

Saif, H., He, Y., Fernandez, M., & Alani, H. (2016). Contextual semantics for sentiment analysis of Twitter. *Information Processing & Management*, *52*(1), 5–19. doi:10.1016/j.ipm.2015.01.005

Sakhardande, P., Hanagal, S., & Kulkarni, S. (2016). Design of disaster management system using IoT based interconnected network with smart city monitoring. In *Proceedings of the International Conference on Internet of Things and Applications (IOTA).* IEEE. 10.1109/IOTA.2016.7562719

Salathé, M., Bengtsson, L., Bodnar, T. J., Brewer, D. D., Brownstein, J. J., Buckee, C., Campbell, E. M., Cattuto, C., Khandelwal, S., Mabry, P. L., & Vespignani, A. (2012, July). Digital Epidemiology. *PLoS Computational Biology*, *8*(7), e1002616. doi:10.1371/journal.pcbi.1002616 PMID:22844241

Saleh, S. N., Lehmann, C. U., McDonald, S. A., Basit, M. A., & Medford, R. J. (2020). Understanding public perception of COVID-19 social distancing on twitter. *Infection Control and Hospital Epidemiology*, *2019*, 1–8. doi:10.1017/ice.2020.406 PMID:32758315

Sandler, M. (2018). *Mobilenetv2: Inverted residuals and linear bottlenecks.* Academic Press.

Sarker, A., Lakamana, S., Hogg-bremer, W., Xie, A., Al-garadi, M. A., & Yang, Y. (2020). Self-reported COVID-19 symptoms on Twitter: An analysis and a research resource. *Journal of the American Medical Informatics Association: JAMIA*, *27*(July), 1310–1315. doi:10.1093/jamia/ocaa116 PMID:32620975

Schmarzo, B. (2018). *Importance of Metadata in a Big Data World.* Data Science Central. Available from https://www.datasciencecentral.com/profiles/blogs/importance-of-metadata-in-a-big-data-world

Schreck, T., & Keim, D. (2012). Visual analysis of social media data. *Computer, 46*(5), 68–75. doi:10.1109/MC.2012.430

Schurink, C. A. M., Lucas, P. J. F., Hoepelman, I. M., & Bonten, M. J. M. (2005). Computer-assisted decision support for the diagnosis and treatment of infectious diseases in intensive care units. *The Lancet. Infectious Diseases, 5*(5), 305–312. doi:10.1016/S1473-3099(05)70115-8 PMID:15854886

Sear, R. F., Velasquez, N., Leahy, R., Restrepo, N. J., El Oud, S., Gabriel, N., Lupu, Y., & Johnson, N. F. (2020). Quantifying COVID-19 Content in the Online Health Opinion War Using Machine Learning. *IEEE Access: Practical Innovations, Open Solutions, 8*, 91886–91893. doi:10.1109/ACCESS.2020.2993967

Sedlmeir, J., Buhl, H., Fridgen, G., & Keller, R. (2020). The Energy Consumption of Blockchain Technology: Beyond Myth. *Business & Information Systems Engineering, 62*(6), 599–608. doi:10.100712599-020-00656-x

Sha, H., Al Hasan, M., Mohler, G., & Brantingham, P. J. (2020). Dynamic topic modeling of the COVID-19 Twitter narrative among U.S. governors and cabinet executives. *ArXiv Preprint ArXiv:2004.11692, 2*, 2–7. https://arxiv.org/abs/2004.11692

Shahi, G. K., & Nandini, D. (2020). *FakeCovid—A Multilingual Cross-domain Fact Check News Dataset for COVID-19*. ArXiv preprint arXiv:2006.11343.

Sharareh, N., Sabounchi, N. S., Sayama, H., & MacDonald, R. (2016). The ebola crisis and the corresponding public behavior: A system dynamics approach. *PLoS Currents, 8*. PMID:27974995

Sharma, A., & Muttoo, S. K. (2018). Spatial image steganalysis based on resnext. In *2018 IEEE 18th International Conference on Communication Technology (ICCT)*. IEEE.

Sheehan, D. (2020). *COVID-19 the biggest threat to the hotel industry*. Hospitalityandcateringnews.com. Retrieved 8 July 2020, from https://www.hospitalityandcateringnews.com/2020/03/covid-19-unwanted-solution-hospitalitys-people-skills-shortages/

Shen, C., Chen, A., Luo, C., Zhang, J., Feng, B., & Liao, W. (2020). Using Reports of Symptoms and Diagnoses on Social Media to Predict COVID-19 Case Counts in Mainland China: Observational Infoveillance Study. *Journal of Medical Internet Research, 22*(5), e19421. doi:10.2196/19421 PMID:32452804

Shmueli, G., Bruce, P. C., Yahav, I., Patel, N. R., & Lichtendahl, K. C. Jr. (2017). *Data Mining for Business Analytics: Concepts, Techniques, and Applications in R*. John Wiley & Sons.

Sichuan earthquake of 2008 | Overview, Damage, & Facts. Encyclopedia Britannica. (2020). Retrieved 1 October 2020, from https://www.britannica.com/event/Sichuan-earthquake-of-2008

Silge, J., & Robinson, D. (2017). *Text Mining with R: A Tidy Approach*. O'Reilly Media. https://books.google.com.tr/books?id=qNcnDwAAQBAJ

Silge, J., & Robinson, D. (2020). *2 Sentiment analysis with tidy data | Text Mining with R.* https://www.tidytextmining.com/sentiment.html

Singh, P., Dwivedi, Y. K., Kahlon, K. S., Pathania, A., & Sawhney, R. S. (2020). Can twitter analytics predict election outcome? An insight from 2017 Punjab assembly elections. *Government Information Quarterly, 37*(2), 101444. doi:10.1016/j.giq.2019.101444

Singh, R. P., Javaid, M., Haleem, A., & Suman, R. (2020). Internet of things (IoT) applications to fight against COVID-19 pandemic. *Diabetes & Metabolic Syndrome, 14*(4), 521–524. doi:10.1016/j.dsx.2020.04.041 PMID:32388333

Sitta, D., Faulkner, M., & Stern, P. (2018). What can the brand manager expect from Facebook? *Australasian Marketing Journal, 26*(1), 1–6. doi:10.1016/j.ausmj.2018.01.001

Skakun, S., Kussul, N., Shelestov, A., & Kussul, O. (2014). Flood hazard and flood risk assessment using a time series of satellite images: A case study in Namibia. *Risk Analysis, 34*(8), 1521–1537. doi:10.1111/risa.12156 PMID:24372226

Slatterly, L. (2020). Eat Out to Help Out: Diners claim 100 million meals. *BBC News.* Retrieved 4 October 2020, from https://www.bbc.co.uk/news/business-54015221

Soussan, T., & Trovati, M. (2020). Sentiment urgency emotion conversion over time for business intelligence. *International Journal of Web Information Systems.*

Southey, F. (2020). *Panic buying amid coronavirus fears: How much are we spending… and why is it a problem?* foodnavigator.com. Retrieved 4 September 2020, from https://www.foodnavigator.com/Article/2020/03/27/Panic-buying-amid-coronavirus-fears-How-much-are-we-spending-and-why-is-it-a-problem

Squicciarini, A., Tapia, A., & Stehle, S. (2017). Sentiment analysis during Hurricane Sandy in emergency response. *International Journal of Disaster Risk Reduction, 21*(May), 213–222. doi:10.1016/j.ijdrr.2016.12.011

Stanford, N. L. P. Group. (2020). *Overview - CoreNLP.* https://stanfordnlp.github.io/CoreNLP/index.html

Stewart, D. (2013). *Big Content: The Unstructured Side of Big Data.* Gartner. Available from https://blogs.gartner.com/darin-stewart/2013/05/01/big-content-the-unstructured-side-of-big-data/

Steyvers, M., & Griffiths, T. (2007). *Latent semantic analysis: a road to meaning, chapter probabilistic topic models.* Laurence Erlbaum.

Sun, E., Rosenn, I., Marlow, C., & Lento, T. M. (2009, May). Gesundheit! modeling contagion through Facebook news feed. ICWSM.

Sun, W., Bocchini, P., & Davison, B. D. (2020). Applications of artificial intelligence for disaster management. *Natural Hazards, 103*(3), 2631–2689. doi:10.100711069-020-04124-3

Swayamsiddha, S., & Mohanty, C. (2020). Application of cognitive Internet of Medical Things for COVID-19 pandemic. *Diabetes & Metabolic Syndrome*, *14*(5), 911–915. doi:10.1016/j.dsx.2020.06.014 PMID:32570016

Tagliabue, F., Galassi, L., & Mariani, P. (2020). The "Pandemic" of Disinformation in COVID-19. *SN Comprehensive Clinical Medicine*, *1–3*(9), 1287–1289. Advance online publication. doi:10.100742399-020-00439-1 PMID:32838179

Tang, C. (2021). The Intersection of Big Data and Epidemiology for Epidemiologic Research. *The AMIA 2021 Virtual Clinical Informatics Conference*.

Tang, Y., Salakhutdinov, R., & Hinton, G. E. (2012). *Deep lambertian networks*. arXiv:1206.6445.

Tang, B., Wang, X., Li, Q., Bragazzi, N. L., Tang, S., Xiao, Y., & Wu, J. (2020). Estimation of the transmission risk of the 2019-nCoV and its implication for public health interventions. *Journal of Clinical Medicine*, *9*(2), 462. doi:10.3390/jcm9020462 PMID:32046137

Tang, M., Mao, X., Yang, S., & Zhou, H. (2014). A dynamic microblog network and information dissemination in "@" mode. *Mathematical Problems in Engineering*, *2014*, 2014. doi:10.1155/2014/492753

The R Foundation. (2020). *R: The R Project for Statistical Computing*. https://www.r-project.org/

Thompson, S., Altay, N., Green, W. G. III, & Lapetina, J. (2006). Improving disaster response efforts with decision support systems. *International Journal of Emergency Management*, *3*(4), 250. doi:10.1504/IJEM.2006.011295

Tian, H. (2019). Privacy-preserving public auditing for secure data storage in fog-to-cloud computing. *Journal of Network and Computer Applications*, *127*, 59–69.

Tiernan, F. (2020). Australia's 2019-20 bushfire season. *The Canberra Times*. Retrieved 6 September 2020, from https://www.canberratimes.com.au/story/6574563/australias-2019-20-bushfire-season/

Ting, D. S. W., Carin, L., Dzau, V., & Wong, T. Y. (2020). Digital technology and COVID-19. *Nature Medicine*, *26*(4), 459–461. doi:10.103841591-020-0824-5 PMID:32284618

To Good To Go. (2020). Retrieved 10 July 2020, from https://toogoodtogo.co.uk/en-gb

Tomas, P. (2020). *Coronavirus: Why You Must Act Now*. https://medium.com/@tomaspueyo/coronavirus-act-today-or-people-will-die-f4d3d9cd99ca

Trovati, Asimakopoulou, & Bessis. (2018). An investigation on human dynamics in enclosed spaces. *Computers & Electrical Engineering*, *67*, 195–209. doi:10.1016/j.compeleceng.2018.03.031

Turnnidge, S., & Chao-Fong, L. (2020). *People Shielding From Coronavirus Question 'Confusing And Contradictory' Government Message*. Huffingtonpost.co.uk. Retrieved 4 August 2020, from https://www.huffingtonpost.co.uk/entry/shielding-coronavirus-lockdown-vulnerable_uk_5ed3c182c5b61691ddb5d11c

UKGOV. (2020). *Prime Minister's statement on coronavirus (COVID-19).* Retrieved 10 February 2021 https://www.gov.uk/government/speeches/pm-address-to-the-nation-on-coronavirus-23-march-2020

University of Oxford. (2020). *Coronavirus Government Response Tracker | Blavatnik School of Government.* https://www.bsg.ox.ac.uk/research/research-projects/coronavirus-government-response-tracker

Uribe-Sánchez, A., Savachkin, A., Santana, A., Prieto-Santa, D., & Das, T. K. (2011). A predictive decision-aid methodology for dynamic mitigation of influenza pandemics. *OR-Spektrum*, *33*(3), 751–786. doi:10.100700291-011-0249-0 PMID:32214571

Vaishya, R., Javaid, M., Khan, I. H., & Haleem, A. (2020). Artificial Intelligence (AI) applications for COVID-19 pandemic. *Diabetes & Metabolic Syndrome*, *14*(4), 337–339. doi:10.1016/j.dsx.2020.04.012 PMID:32305024

Valdivia, A., Luzón, M. V., Cambria, E., & Herrera, F. (2018). Consensus vote models for detecting and filtering neutrality in sentiment analysis. *Information Fusion*, *44*, 126–135. Advance online publication. doi:10.1016/j.inffus.2018.03.007

Valle, Sacco, Gallotti, Castaldo, & De Domenico. (2020). *Covid19 infodemics observatory.* Doi:10.17605/OSF.IO/N6UPX

Vanhoof, M., Reis, F., Smoreda, Z., & Plötz, T. (2012). Detecting Home Locations from CDR Data: Introducing Spatial Uncertainty to the State-of-the-Art. *Journal of Map & Geography Libraries: Advances in Geospatial Information. Collections & Archives*, *8*(2), 101–117.

Vardhanabhuti, V. (2020). CT scan AI-aided triage for patients with COVID-19 in China. *The Lancet. Digital Health*, *2*(10), e494–e495. doi:10.1016/S2589-7500(20)30222-3 PMID:32984793

Vatandoost, M., & Litkouhi, S. (2019). The Future of Healthcare Facilities: How Technology and Medical Advances May Shape Hospitals of the Future. *Hospital Practices and Research*, *4*(1), 1–11. doi:10.15171/hpr.2019.01

Wang, Y., Hao, H., & Platt, L. S. (2021). Examining risk and crisis communications of government agencies and stakeholders during early-stages of COVID-19 on Twitter. *Computers in Human Behavior*, *114*(June), 106568. doi:10.1016/j.chb.2020.106568

Wang, G., Mohanlal, M., Wilson, C., Wang, X., Metzger, M., Zheng, H., & Zhao, B. Y. (2013). Social Turing Tests: Crowdsourcing Sybil Detection. In *NDSS Symposium 2013.* Internet Society.

Wang, K., Lu, Z., Wang, X., Li, H., Li, H., Lin, D., & Ji, W. (2020). Current trends and future prediction of novel coronavirus disease (COVID-19) epidemic in China: A dynamical modeling analysis. *Mathematical Biosciences and Engineering*, *17*(4), 3052–3061. doi:10.3934/mbe.2020173 PMID:32987516

Wang, L. L., Lo, K., Chandrasekhar, Y., Reas, R., Yang, J., Eide, D., & Kohlmeier, S. (2020). *Cord-19: The covid-19 open research dataset.* ArXiv.

Wang, L., Lin, Z. Q., & Wong, A. (2020). Covid-net: A tailored deep convolutional neural network design for detection of covid-19 cases from chest x-ray images. *Scientific Reports*, *10*, 1–12.

Wang, Q., Lin, Z., Jin, Y., Cheng, S., & Yang, T. (2015). ESIS: Emotion-based spreader–ignorant–stifler model for information diffusion. *Knowledge-Based Systems*, *81*, 46–55. doi:10.1016/j.knosys.2015.02.006

Wang, W. Y., Pauleen, D. J., & Zhang, T. (2016). How social media applications affect {B2B} communication and improve business performance in {SMEs}. *Industrial Marketing Management*, *54*, 4–14. doi:10.1016/j.indmarman.2015.12.004

Wang, Y., McKee, M., Torbica, A., & Stuckler, D. (2019). Systematic literature review on the spread of health-related misinformation on social media. *Social Science & Medicine*, 240.

Wells, C. R., Sah, P., Moghadas, S. M., Pandey, A., Shoukat, A., Wang, Y., & Galvani, A. P. (2020). Impact of international travel and border control measures on the global spread of the novel 2019 coronavirus outbreak. *Proceedings of the National Academy of Sciences of the United States of America*, *117*(13), 7504–7509. doi:10.1073/pnas.2002616117 PMID:32170017

WHO. (2020). *Listings of WHO's response to COVID-19*. Retrieved 3 February 2021 https://www.who.int/news/item/29-06-2020-covidtimeline

Wicaksono, Suyoto, & Pranowo. (2017). A proposed method for predicting US presidential election by analyzing sentiment in social media. *Proceeding - 2016 2nd International Conference on Science in Information Technology, ICSITech 2016: Information Science for Green Society and Environment*. 10.1109/ICSITech.2016.7852647

Wicke, P., & Bolognesi, M. M. (2020). *Framing COVID-19: How we conceptualize and discuss the pandemic on Twitter*. ArXiv Preprint ArXiv:2004.06986. https://arxiv.org/abs/2004.06986

Wida, E. (2020). *Australian government airdrops more than 4K pounds of food to hungry animals*. TODAY.com. Retrieved 6 September 2020, from https://www.today.com/food/australian-government-airdrops-food-animals-amid-fires-t171683

Wittbold, K., Carroll, C., Iansiti, M., Zhang, H. M., & Landman, A. B. (2020). How Hospitals Are Using AI to Battle Covid-19. *Harvard Business Review*, 3.

Wood, Z. (2020). *Morrisons becomes first large supermarket to reinstate Covid rationing*. Retrieved 3 October 2020, from https://www.theguardian.com/business/2020/sep/24/morrisons-becomes-first-large-supermarket-to-reinstate-covid-rationing-purchase-limit-toilet-roll-empty-shelves

Woo, J., & Chen, H. (2012, June). An event-driven SIR model for topic diffusion in web forums. In *2012 IEEE International Conference on Intelligence and Security Informatics* (pp. 108-113). IEEE. 10.1109/ISI.2012.6284101

Woo, J., & Chen, H. (2016). Epidemic model for information diffusion in web forums: Experiments in marketing exchange and political dialog. *SpringerPlus*, *5*(1), 66. doi:10.118640064-016-1675-x PMID:26839759

World Health Organization. (2020). *World Coronavirus Disease (COVID-19) Dashboard*. https://covid19.who.int/

Wu, Leung, & Leung. (2020). Potential for domestic and foreign spreading the epidemic of 2019-ncov originating in Wuhan, China: a modelling analysis. The Lancet, 395(10225), 689-697.

Wukich, C. (2016). Government social media messages across disaster phases. *Journal of Contingencies and Crisis Management, 24*(4), 230–243. doi:10.1111/1468-5973.12119

Wu, Z., & McGoogan, J. M. (2020). Characteristics of and important lessons from the coronavirus disease 2019 (COVID-19) outbreak in China: Summary of a report of 72 314 cases from the Chinese Center for Disease Control and Prevention. *Journal of the American Medical Association, 323*(13), 1239–1242. doi:10.1001/jama.2020.2648 PMID:32091533

Xie, X., Zhong, Z., Zhao, W., Zheng, C., Wang, F., & Liu, J. (2020). Chest CT for typical coronavirus disease 2019 (COVID-19) pneumonia: Relationship to negative RT-PCR testing. *Radiology, 296*(2), E41–E45. doi:10.1148/radiol.2020200343 PMID:32049601

Yan, X. (2018). *GitHub BTM*. https://github.com/xiaohuiyan/BTM

Yang, F., Dong, H., Wang, Z., Ren, W., & Alsaadi, F. E. (2016). A new approach to non-fragile state estimation for continuous neural networks with time-delays. *Neurocomputing, 197*, 205–211. doi:10.1016/j.neucom.2016.02.062

Yan, X., Guo, J., Lan, Y., & Cheng, X. (2013). A biterm topic model for short texts. *Proceedings of the 22nd International Conference on World Wide Web*, 1445–1456. 10.1145/2488388.2488514

Yin, F., Lv, J., Zhang, X., Xia, X., & Wu, J. (2020). COVID-19 information propagation dynamics in the Chinese Sina-microblog. *Mathematical Biosciences and Engineering, 17*(3), 2676–2692. doi:10.3934/mbe.2020146 PMID:32233560

Yom-Tov, E., Lampos, V., Cox, I. J., & Edelstein, M. (2020). *Providing early indication of regional anomalies in COVID19 case counts in England using search engine queries*. arXiv preprint arXiv:2007.11821.

Youssef, M., & Scoglio, C. (2011). An individual-based approach to SIR epidemics in contact networks. *Journal of Theoretical Biology, 283*(1), 136–144. doi:10.1016/j.jtbi.2011.05.029 PMID:21663750

Yuan, Y., & Sun, F. (2014). Delay-dependent stability criteria for time-varying delay neural networks in the delta domain. *Neurocomputing, 125*, 17–21. doi:10.1016/j.neucom.2012.09.040

Yu, G. (2020). Enabling Attribute Revocation for Fine-Grained Access Control in Blockchain-IoT Systems. *IEEE Transactions on Engineering Management*.

Yu, J., Lu, Y., & Muñoz-Justicia, J. (2020). Analyzing Spanish News Frames on Twitter during COVID-19—A Network Study of El País and El Mundo. *International Journal of Environmental Research and Public Health, 17*(15), 5414. doi:10.3390/ijerph17155414 PMID:32731359

Yu, M., Yang, C., & Li, Y. (2018). Big Data in Natural Disaster Management: A Review. *Geosciences*, *8*(5), 165. doi:10.3390/geosciences8050165

Yu, Y., Dong, H., Wang, Z., Ren, W., & Alsaadi, F. E. (2016). Design of non-fragile state estimators for discrete time-delayed neural networks with parameter uncertain- ties. *Neurocomputing*, *182*, 18–24. doi:10.1016/j.neucom.2015.11.079

Zarei, K., Farahbakhsh, R., Crespi, N., & Tyson, G. (2020). *A first Instagram dataset on COVID-19*. arXiv preprint arXiv:2004.12226.

Zeng, L., Hall, H., & Pitts, M. J. (2012). Cultivating a community of learners: the potential challenges of social media in higher education. In *Social Media: Usage and Impact* (pp. 111–126). Lexington Books.

Zhang, F., Luo, J., Li, C., Wang, X., & Zhao, Z. (2014). Detecting and analyzing influenza epidemics with social media in China. In V. S. Tseng, T. B. Ho, Z.-H. Zhou, A. L. P. Chen, & H.-Y. Kao (Eds.), *Pacific-Asia Conference on Knowledge Discovery and Data Mining* (pp. 90–101). Springer. 10.1007/978-3-319-06608-0_8

Zhang, X., Fuehres, H., & Gloor, P. A. (2011). Predicting Stock Market Indicators Through Twitter "I hope it is not as bad as I fear". *Procedia - Social and Behavioral Sciences, 26*, 55–62. doi:10.1016/j.sbspro.2011.10.562

Zhang, J., Xue, N., & Huang, X. (2016). A secure system for pervasive social network-based healthcare. *IEEE Access : Practical Innovations, Open Solutions*, *4*, 9239–9250.

Zhang, Z. K., Liu, C., Zhan, X. X., Lu, X., Zhang, C. X., & Zhang, Y. C. (2016). Dynamics of information diffusion and its applications on complex networks. *Physics Reports*, *651*, 1–34. doi:10.1016/j.physrep.2016.07.002

Zhao, Y., Cheng, S., Yu, X., & Xu, H. (2020). Chinese public's attention to the COVID-19 epidemic on social media: Observational descriptive study. *Journal of Medical Internet Research*, *22*(5), 1–13. doi:10.2196/18825 PMID:32314976

Zhou, Y., Wang, F., Tang, J., Nussinov, R., & Cheng, F. (2020). Artificial intelligence in COVID-19 drug repurposing. *The Lancet. Digital Health*, *2*(12), e667–e676. doi:10.1016/S2589-7500(20)30192-8 PMID:32984792

Zhu, N., Zhang, D., Wang, W., Li, X., Yang, B., Sing, J., Zhao, X., Huang, B., Shi, W., Lu, R., & ... . (2020). *A novel coronavirus from pneumonia patients in China, 2019*. New England Medicine Journal. doi:10.1056/NEJMoa2001017

Ziemke, J. (2012). Crisis Mapping: The Construction of a New Interdisciplinary Field? International Network of Crisis Mappers, John Carroll University & the Harvard Humanitarian Initiative, University Heights, OH, USA. *Journal of Map & Geography Libraries: Advances in Geospatial Information. Collections & Archives*, *8*(2), 101–117.

About the Contributors

Eleana Asimakopoulou received the MA and PhD degrees in the area of Disaster Management from the University Westminster and Loughborough University, UK, in 2009 and 2008 respectively. She is been a lecturer and a visiting researcher in various institutions including the Hellenic National Defence College, Athens, Greece and an expert evaluator in national and European proposals for funding. Her research is in the area of utilizing disruptive technologies (IoT, grid and cloud computing) for disaster management. She has been involved in a number of projects and has published over 60 works. Dr Asimakopoulou is an editor of a book and an associate editor of a refereed international journal.

Nik Bessis is a full Professor of Computer Science and the Acting Head of the Department of Engineering at Edge Hill University, UK. Prior to that, Nik was a full Professor of Computer Science and the Director of Distributed and Intelligent Systems (DISYS) research centre at the University of Derby, UK. He holds a PhD and a MA from De Montfort University, UK and a BA from TEI of Athens, Greece. Professor Bessis is a Fellow of HEA, BCS and a Senior Member of IEEE. His research is on social graphs for network and big data analytics as well as on developing data push and resource provisioning services in IoT, FI and clouds. He has led several projects worth over £7m. He has published over 270 works and won 4 best paper awards. He has chaired over 40 international events, delivered 4 keynote speeches, edited 4 SIs, 8 books and 9 conference proceedings. His latest 2 edited books on IoTs & big data have been ranked as top 25 & top 40 on Amazon AI book lists. He is also the founding editor-in-chief of IJDST. Professor Bessis has served as an expert evaluator for the Hellenic QAA and, as an assessor for more than 10 Professorships conferment worldwide.

* * *

Umadevi A. is Assistant Professor in Department of Management Studies at SRM Valliammai Engineering College, Chennai. She is pursuing Ph.D in stream of Finance at Anna University. Has a 14 years of experience in handling Finance and Operations Management classes. Cleared National Eligibility Test (NET). Also have 2 years of corporate experience as Process executive. Has wide contributions to profession through many research journals and hold patents on Supply Chain area and Information system field. She is currently exploring research on Artificial Intelligence in Management field.

Chloë Allen-Ede is a final year Physics student at the University of Wolverhampton specialising in Quantum Technologies. She completed an additional year of her degree working for an acoustic based company on their computer modelling and programme team. Chloë is an IOP campus ambassador and actively works in outreach events to encourage more young people into STEM fields.

Muhammad Awais is Senior Lecturer at Edge Hill University, UK. Previously, he worked as a Research Fellow: in Data Analytics and AI at University of Hull, UK and in Signal Processing and Machine Learning at University of Leeds, UK. His research interests are in signal processing, applied machine learning and deep learning to develop ICT based systems for Internet of things, Industry 4.0, biomedical and health care domain.

Mehmet Aydin is Senior Lecturer in Computer Science in University of the West of England (UWE) started in January 2015. His research interests include machine learning, multi-agent systems, parallel and distributed metaheuristics, wired/wireless network planning and optimisation, evolutionary computation. He has conducted guest editorial of special issues for internationally peer-reviewed journal. In addition to the membership of advisory committee of many international conferences, he is a member of editorial board of a number of internationally peer-reviewed highly recognised journal. He is currently fellow of Higher Education Academy, member of EPSRC Review College, senior member of ACM and IEEE. He has published more than 100 journal and conference papers.

Herbert Daly is a Senior Lecturer in the School of Mathematics and Computer Science at the University of Wolverhampton. Organising the Guide SHARE Europe (GSE) UK "Mainframe Skills and Learning" group he works closely with industry and university students, advocating a practical role for technology in society and commerce. His research focuses on Software Engineering, Enterprise Systems, and the effective management of information ecosystems. He holds a Bachelors Degree in Computer Science, a Masters Degree in Software Engineering and a Doctoral

Degree in Systems modelling. He is a former Chair of the Computer Measurement Group UK.

Imran Haider Syed received his B.S. degree in Electronic Engineering from Capital University of Sciences and Technology (formerly known as Mohammad Ali Jinnah University, Islamabad, Pakistan) in 2008. He joined C.U.S.T. as Lab Engineer in 2008. There, he conducted laboratory demonstrations of signals and systems, communications systems and microcontroller interfacing. He was the founding member and also Vice-Chair of IEEE student chapter in C.U.S.T., Islamabad, Pakistan in 2008–2011. He managed all the branch activities including technical seminars, workshops, and grand open-house of final year projects of engineering and computer science departments in 2008–2011. He completed his M.S. degree in Electronic Engineering in 2013. His research interests include Electromagnetics, Microwave Devices, Radiated / Conducted EMI Analysis, EMC, Multiple Antennas (MIMO) Systems, OFDM, Vehicle to Vehicle (V2V) Communication, IoT Devices in 4G / 5G Networks, etc.

Iman Hussain received his MS in Computer Science from the University of Wolverhampton in 2020. In 2021 he joined the University of Lancaster as a researcher and currently holds the place of senior research assistant at the Centre for Global Eco-Innovation, an EU initiative based in the North West of England. He has won the Richardson's award for outstanding contributions to local businesses in his field of Computer Science, came third in CapGemini's international TechChallenge 2020 hackathon, and came second with his team in IBM's CallForCode 2020 international hackathon. His areas of expertise centres around distributed systems and data handling.

Lukas Jaks is a second year Computer Science student studying at the University of Wolverhampton. With a specialism in Mainframe technology, Lukas is an IBM zAmbassador and regularly contributes to various outreach events focusing on educating students on the Z platform. He is also part of the Broadcom mentorship program and is currently developing opensource applications with them.

Ehtasham Javed is a postdoctoral researcher in Neuroscience center at University of Helsinki, Finland. In general, his interests are in methods, models, and instrumentation for biomedical applications. Specifically, his work focuses on quantifying underlying trends and behaviors objectively from large datasets using temporal, spectral and spatial measures. The aim is to translate his research expertise to address real-life problems.

Guru K. is Assistant Professor in Department of Management Studies at SRM Valliammai Engineering College, Chennai. He is a dynamic professional with 7 years of experience in handling HR, Marketing, Operations and Information Management classes. Cleared State Eligible Test (SET) on Sep'2017. Also have 4 years of experience as Manager Marketing in the field of Health care service. Achieved Excellence in Teaching award and Best leader award with wide contributions to profession through more than twenty research journals, patent and as a guide for government funded projects. Published patent on title, "BLOCK CHAIN-BASED SHOPPING CART" (Application number 202041020687) and it was the first invention processed for grant in the year 2020 from IPI. Currently exploring research on MOOC and Online Learning platform in the educational field.

Bill Karakostas (PhD) has a 30+ year track record in IT in the Academia and industry. He served among other, as the R&D Director of VLTN, a Belgian SME specialising in IT Cloud services for the logistics sector, as senior lecturer with School of Informatics, City University, London, and as lecturer with the Department of Computation, UMIST, Manchester, UK. He is the author/co-author of three academic books and of over 250 scientific publications. He has led as technical manager 5 European Union funded R&D Projects, and participated as a researcher in over 20 other, in the period between 1988 and 2019. He is an acclaimed expert in business information systems, ERP systems, Big Data and metadata management and IoT platforms.

Georgios Kolostoumpis holds a Bachelor of Science (BSc), of the Department of Computer Science as Software Engineer from the University of Manchester. He has also received a Master Degree (MSc), in Business Systems Analysis & Design from the City University. He has completed his PhD from University of City, focused in the area of Medical Informatics to assist physicians with modern sophisticate systems, tools, to improve prognosis, diagnosis, therapeutic response prediction and health care. Most of my specialized experience is in investigating the underlying regulatory disturbance of cancer and prevention and hopefully the effective treatments in late stage recognized cancer. Also, the use of intelligent tools, statistical methods and computer programs to collect, organize and analyze data for improving and innovating reports to fully exploit data rich clinical systems and providing interpretive analytics and commentary. His research interests include Bioinformatics, Clinical Decision Support Systems, Artificial Intelligence in cancer diseases and systematic reviews in a health technology assessment, research quality of improvement the health services. Since 2007 until today, he joined as a Scientific Expert for Research & Innovation Projects of EU Programme under EUREKA, ERC, ECDC, and other EU organizations, providing and supporting frontier research, proposals and pioneering ideas which manage unconventional and innovative approaches. Involved and encourage the highest quality research across Europe, USA, Canada, Africa, through competitive funding and support investigator – driven frontier research across the field of Medical Informatics, based on scientific excellence.

Mohsin Raza is a senior lecturer at Department of Computer Science, Edge Hill University, UK. He completed his PhD at Math, Physics and Electrical Engineering Department, Northumbria University (NU), UK and BS (Hons) and MS degrees in Electronic Engineering from Mohammad Ali Jinnah University (MAJU), Pakistan. Prior to his work at Edge Hill University, he worked as a Lecturer (2019-20) at Northumbria University, UK, as a post-doctoral fellow (2018-19) at Middlesex University, UK, as a Demonstrator/Associate-Lecturer and Doctoral Fellow (2015-17) at Northumbria University UK, Junior lecturer (2010-12) and later as Lecturer (2012-15) in Engineering department at Mohammad Ali Jinnah University, Pakistan, and Hardware Support Engineer (2009-10) at Unified Secure Services, Pakistan. He served as a technical committee member for ICET 2012, SKIMA 2015, SKIMA 2017, WSGT 2017, CSNDSP 2018, SKIMA 2018, ICT 2019 and CSoNet 2019. He has also been a guest editor in several special issues in wireless communications, Industry 4.0 (Industrial IoT), and smart healthcare (Internet of Medical Things, AI) and severed as reviewer of several journals. His research interests include IoT, 5G and wireless networks, autonomous transportation systems, machine learning, Industry 4.0 and digital twins.

İbrahim Sabuncu was born in Istanbul and graduated from Çukurova University, Department of Industrial Engineering in 2002. In 2005, he completed his master's degree in Gaziantep University Industrial Engineering Department. Between 2003 and 2004, he worked as a research assistant in the same department. Between 2006-2014, he worked as a lecturer in the Department of Computer Engineering, Faculty of Engineering, Harran University. He completed his PhD in International Trade and Finance at Yalova University, Institute of Social Sciences. He had worked as research assistant at the Industrial Engineering Department of Yalova University from 2014 to 2017. Now he has been working as a Assistant Professor at same department. He has studies and publications within the scope of business analytics. He teaches analytical methods in marketing, customer relationship management, e-commerce, process management, marketing management and system simulation.

Tariq Soussan is a PhD student in the Department of Computer Science, Edge Hill University. He obtained his bachelor's degree in Computer Science in 2010 at the Lebanese American University. He received a graduate assistantship as a teaching and research assistant to pursue and obtain his master's degree in Computer Science at the Lebanese American University in 2012. In 2016, he obtained his second master's degree in Information Technology at the University of Derby at which he did research on text mining, web mining, and sentiment analysis. He worked at one of the biggest SAP partners in the world during which he received a consulting excellence award in 2018 in recognition of his outstanding contribution to SAP Business One Projects. Tariq has taught courses at many universities around the world, such as Lebanese American University, Nottingham Trent University, and the American University in the Emirates. Tariq's main interests include: Data and Text Mining, Web Mining, Opinion Mining, Sentiment Analysis.

Hugo Tianfield has been a Professor of Computing with Glasgow Caledonian University, Scotland, United Kingdom since early 2001. Prof Tianfield is extensively involved in professional activities. He is member of EPSRC Peer College, Chair of Technical Committee on Cyber-Physical Cloud Systems of IEEE Systems, Man, and Cybernetics Society, Editor-in-Chief of Multiagent and Grid Systems - An International Journal of Data Science and Engineering, and Associate Editor of IEEE Transactions on Systems, Man, and Cybernetics: Systems. Prof Tianfield is Director of AI+IoT Research Lab. His research areas include Edge AI, Data Science, and Health Data Science. He is (co-)author to over 200 research articles published in refereed journals and conferences, and is a frequent invited speaker at conferences and institutions all over the world. Hugo Tianfield earned his Bachelor Eng (Hons), Master Eng and Doctorate Eng degrees all in Electronic Engineering (Industrial Automation).

Marcello Trovati is a Professor in Computer Science in the Department of Computer Science, Edge Hill University. After having obtained his Ph.D. in Mathematics at the University of Exeter in 2007, specializing in theoretical dynamical systems with singularities, he accepted a position as algorithm tester and research specialist at a medium sized software development company. His main responsibility was to create, test and documents state-of-the-art statistical algorithms to analyse big datasets. He then moved to the newly created Dublin IBM Research Lab to carry out research mainly in the field of knowledge discovery, text mining, and mathematical modelling, where he gained valuable business and research experience through collaboration with several scientists both at IBM, and at academic institutions. He was involved in a number of research projects in collaboration with other IBM Research Centres and academic institutions. He then joined Coventry University to take up a position as Teaching Fellow, and subsequently the University of Derby as a lecturer, during which he was involved various multi-disciplinary projects focussing on mathematical modelling, algorithm design, and big data analytics. In 2016 Marcello joined the Computer Science Department at Edge Hill University as a senior lecturer and he was recently awarded a Readership in Computer Science. He is involved in several research themes and projects. He is co-leading the STEM Data Research centre and is actively involved in the Productivity and Innovation Lab, aiming to collaborate and support SMEs in Lancashire. Marcello's main interests include: Mathematical Modelling, Data Science, Big Data Analytics, Network Theory, Machine Learning, Data and Text Mining.

Thu Yein Win is a Senior Lecturer in Cyber Computing in the School of Computing & Engineering at the University of Gloucestershire, United Kingdom. He specializes in virtualization security and big data-based security analytics using different privacy-preserving approaches. His work examines the security issues in virtualization, with the aim of developing a security system which protects the virtualization environment against security attacks. He obtained his Master degrees from the University of Bedfordshire and Asian Institute of Technology. His research interests encompass a wide range of topics in security including virtualization security, privacy-preserving big data security analytics, cloud computing and information security as well as operating systems security. He is a professional member of the British Computing Society (BCS) as well as a member of the IEEE.

Index

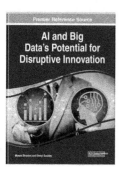
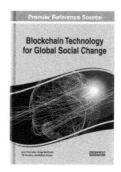
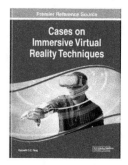
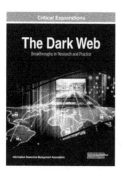
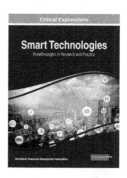
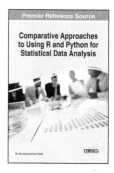
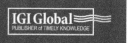

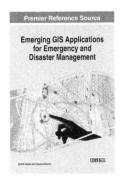
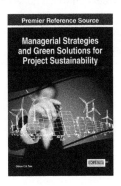
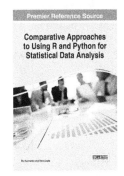
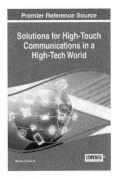

IGI Global Author Services

Providing a high-quality, affordable, and expeditious service, IGI Global's Author Services enable authors to streamline their publishing process, increase chance of acceptance, and adhere to IGI Global's publication standards.

Benefits of Author Services:

- **Professional Service:** All our editors, designers, and translators are experts in their field with years of experience and professional certifications.

- **Quality Guarantee & Certificate:** Each order is returned with a quality guarantee and certificate of professional completion.

- **Timeliness:** All editorial orders have a guaranteed return timeframe of 3-5 business days and translation orders are guaranteed in 7-10 business days.

- **Affordable Pricing:** IGI Global Author Services are competitively priced compared to other industry service providers.

- **APC Reimbursement:** IGI Global authors publishing Open Access (OA) will be able to deduct the cost of editing and other IGI Global author services from their OA APC publishing fee.

Author Services Offered:

 English Language Copy Editing
Professional, native English language copy editors improve your manuscript's grammar, spelling, punctuation, terminology, semantics, consistency, flow, formatting, and more.

 Scientific & Scholarly Editing
A Ph.D. level review for qualities such as originality and significance, interest to researchers, level of methodology and analysis, coverage of literature, organization, quality of writing, and strengths and weaknesses.

 Figure, Table, Chart & Equation Conversions
Work with IGI Global's graphic designers before submission to enhance and design all figures and charts to IGI Global's specific standards for clarity.

 Translation
Providing 70 language options, including Simplified and Traditional Chinese, Spanish, Arabic, German, French, and more.

Hear What the Experts Are Saying About IGI Global's Author Services

 "Publishing with IGI Global has been *an amazing experience* for me for sharing my research. The *strong academic production* support ensures quality and timely completion." – **Prof. Margaret Niess, Oregon State University, USA**

"The service was *very fast, very thorough, and very helpful* in ensuring our chapter meets the criteria and requirements of the book's editors. I was *quite impressed and happy* with your service." – **Prof. Tom Brinthaupt, Middle Tennessee State University, USA**

Learn More or Get Started Here: For Questions, Contact IGI Global's Customer Service Team at cust@igi-global.com or 717-533-8845

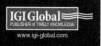

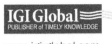

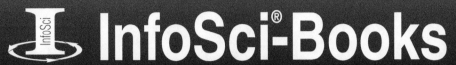
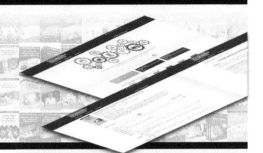

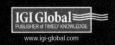

CPSIA information can be obtained
at www.ICGtesting.com
Printed in the USA
BVHW010029310321
603752BV00003B/24

9 781799 867364